• About the author •

Denise Winn is a journalist who has
specialised in medicine and psychology for
more than 20 years. She has written regularly
for numerous national newspapers and
magzines, and is author of ten previous
books on health and psychological topics.

WELL WOMAN HANDBOOK

Your Complete Guide to Healthy Living

Denise Winn

In association with SHE magazine

VERMILION

LONDON

First published 1995

1 3 5 7 9 10 8 6 4 2

First published in the United Kingdom in 1995 by Vermilion
an imprint of Ebury Press
Random House, 20 Vauxhall Bridge Road, London SW1V 2SA

Random House Australia (Pty) Limited
20 Alfred Street, Milsons Point, Sydney,
New South Wales, 2061, Australia

Random House New Zealand Limited
18 Poland Road, Glenfield,
Auckland 10, New Zealand

Random House South Africa (Pty) Limited
PO Box 337, Bergvlei, South Africa

Random House UK Limited Reg. No. 954009

A catalogue record for this book is available from the British Library

ISBN: 0 09 178457 3

Editor: Margot Richardson
Designer: Bob Vickers
Illustrations: Vana Haggerty

Printed and bound in Great Britain by Mackays of Chatham plc, Kent

Papers used by Ebury Press are natural recyclable products made from wood
grown in sustainable forests.

CONTENTS

INTRODUCTION

PART III: OUR SEXUAL SELVES

PART IV: A–Z OF WOMEN'S HEALTH PROBLEMS

INTRODUCTION

· How to use this book ·

There are many guides to women's health. This one is different because it aims to be as accessible and relevant to the reader as *SHE* magazine succeeds in being.

It aims to provide a wealth of information clearly and simply, without being clinical and remote, and yet also to be a good 'read', in the style of articles on health in women's magazines. As well as being a source of health information as and when you need it, I hope that you find you can dip into it anywhere and find something that intrigues you and makes you want to read on.

As a guide to women's health, the contents concentrate on those areas that are of especial interest or concern to women although of course the information in some of these areas may be equally applicable to men.

Part I: Everyday Health looks in detail at all you can do to keep yourself in tip-top working order, both physically and emotionally. It tells you all you need to know about healthy living (and that doesn't mean no fun; you'll find a few refreshing surprises), how to handle bad habits, look after your body, and prevent or deal with problems.

Part II: Emotional and Mental Health Although emotional health receives a lot of attention throughout the book, this section specifically provides very practical guidance for dealing with a whole range of common emotional or mental health problems, as well as self-help ideas for improving how we handle our lives.

Part III: Our Sexual Selves treats in detail the different concerns women may have at different stages of their lives. It covers gynaecological matters, breasts, sexual problems, contraception, wanted and unwanted pregnancy, infertility and aspects of the menopause, looking not only at what happens when there are problems but at the great range of normal situations when everything is working well

There is one very large area, however, that is intentionally omitted: pregnancy and childbirth. This is because it is a large and important subject in itself and there are many good guides to pregnancy available. You will, however, find many references in this book to pregnancy, in terms of conditions which are more common in pregnancy or which may occur mainly after childbirth.

Part IV: A–Z of Women's Health Problems   covers physical conditions and complaints not treated elsewhere in the book, which specifically, or more commonly, affect women; and what to do about them.

Even a book as big as this one can't cover everything in the detail it warrants. So there are plenty of pointers towards acquiring more information – from specific organisations or good books – about particular areas that may interest you.

Useful Contacts and Further Reading contains full, easy-reference lists of all the helpful organisations and books mentioned in the text.

The book acknowledges both orthodox and complementary health care methods. However, as the range of complementary therapies is vast and treatment approaches are highly diverse, these are included for specific conditions only where they are very well known, commonly tried or have a proven high success rate.

I do hope you enjoy this book, as well as finding it a useful reference work. It doesn't tub-thump, but it does take the view that women's physical and emotional health is important and that we are all entitled to the best care, both from and for ourselves. The more knowledge we have, the better equipped we are to attain it.

Denise Winn

Part I

EVERYDAY HEALTH

WHEN we are young we often assume that all the bits of our bodies take care of themselves. As we grow a little older, we realise that they need a little help. How we eat, how active we are, how we sleep, relax and enjoy ourselves, how we behave in our home and work lives and how we take care of our bodies, all either take their toll on us physically and mentally or help to keep us healthy.

Unfortunately, with the physically and emotionally demanding lives that women tend to lead, it isn't always easy to take the best care of our health. All too often it is children and families needs that we put before our own.

But caring enough for our own health needn't be too dauntingly difficult either. This section of the book takes a look at what we can all do within the limits of our lifestyles to make the most of what we've got. It also helps you look with fresh eyes at how you could, if you wanted to, make small or major changes – such as adding more exercise, allowing yourself a few luxuries or stopping smoking – that could have an enormously beneficial impact on your life.

· LIFESTYLE ·

1
....
HEALTHY EATING

FOOD means different things to different women. For some, it is a pleasure to buy, to cook and to eat; for others it is a chore, or must be grabbed on the run, or is hedged around with fears of overweight, whether real or imagined. Unhappiness or anxiety may be channelled into comfort eating in an effort to find relief from painful feelings. For some, compulsive eating or compulsive dieting becomes a habit and food is seen as the enemy.

Whatever our attitude to food, we cannot avoid it, nor can we avoid the consequences of not taking care over what we eat. Bad diet, whether through eating too many of the wrong things or not enough of the right things or too much or too little of everything, is strongly associated with physical and mental ill health. Our attitudes to eating have an impact upon our children's attitudes towards food, too. We can best serve both ourselves and our families by trying to come to healthy terms with food and eating nutritiously, whatever sort of lifestyles we lead.

· What do we need to eat? ·

For our bodies to work properly and for us to feel healthy and energetic we need to eat enough of the right substances (called nutrients) in food. We need a combination of carbohydrates, fats, protein, vitamins and minerals and we also need fibre, the part of food which aids the digestion and absorption of other nutrients.

All these types of foods can be found in the four main food groups: that is starchy foods; dairy foods; meat, poultry, fish and nuts; and vegetables and fruit. Foods from each of these groups should be contained in our normal daily diet.

OUR DAILY NEEDS

Starchy foods eg, potatoes, bread, pasta, rice, breakfast cereals, maize, millet, chapattis, plantain and bananas
Dairy foods eg, milk, cheese, yoghurt, fromage frais
Meat, poultry, fish and nuts
Vegetables and fruits

• Carbohydrates •

Carbohydrates are starches and sugars. They are broken down, converted into glucose by the liver and used by the body as its main source of energy. Any glucose that isn't needed for energy is stored as fat. However, it is wrong to think that carbohydrates are themselves particularly fattening. Eaten in normal portions, and not in foods where fats are also present (such as fried foods, or cakes and biscuits), they are far less likely than fats to cause you to put on weight.

A starch-rich diet is thought to help protect against colon cancer. World-wide studies have shown that ordinary starch is even more protective against this type of cancer than fibre (see page 453). Good sources of starch are potatoes, bread, pasta, rice, breakfast cereals, maize, millet, chapattis, plantain and bananas. Ideally, starches should make up just over half our food intake.

Sugars are simple carbohydrates. They are absorbed more quickly than starch, giving a quick 'high' to blood glucose but just as quickly falling again. They occur naturally in foods such as fruit and milk, but we don't need refined sugar in our diet as it is all 'empty' calories and has no nutrients. Refined sugar is heavily present in cakes, biscuits, ice-cream and chocolate, but also in many savoury tinned foods. It may show on a food label as sugar – or as glucose, dextrose, sucrose, fructose or maltose.

• Proteins •

Protein is important for the growth and repair of all our body cells. When protein foods are eaten, amino acids are released and it is these which help to make new cells. Animal proteins, which come from meat, poultry, fish, dairy foods and eggs, contain all the amino acids the body needs. Plant proteins, found in whole-grain cereals, wholemeal bread, pasta, peas, beans, soya-bean curd (tofu) and nuts, do not have all the necessary amino acids. However, by combining different types of plant protein, it is perfectly possible to get all the types of amino acids we need. In the West, we don't need to worry about getting enough protein – we are almost all likely to be eating double the amount we need.

Excessive intake of protein needs to be avoided by anyone with liver or kidney problems.

• Fats •

Fatty acids are released from digested fat. The body needs them to help form and repair body cells, and also to form chemical messengers, responsible for activating many of the body's functions. Fats can also provide energy. Any excess is stored in the body as fat. There are two types of fat: saturated and unsaturated.

• Saturated fats •

These fats are found in animal and dairy foods and are hard at room temperature. They are found in beef, pork, lamb, meat products such as pies and sausage rolls, eggs and whole milk. Even some vegetable oils are high in saturated fats, notably palm and coconut oil. And, of course, there is plenty in sweet foods such as cakes, biscuits, chocolate and puddings.

The more saturated fats you eat, the higher your levels of blood cholesterol are likely to be. Cholesterol is not all bad. (See heart disease, page 463, for explanation of 'good' and 'bad' cholesterol.) It is a substance vital to the body and is used for many essential aspects of body functioning, including the formation of hormones needed for reproduction. The liver manufactures it from many foods but mainly from saturated fats. However, enough is enough. Cholesterol is carried around the body by the blood, and any that isn't taken up by cells remains in the bloodstream.

If too much cholesterol builds up, it gradually clogs the arteries and blocks blood flow, leading to heart attack or stroke. Some foods, such as eggs, liver, kidneys and some shellfish, are naturally rich in cholesterol. However, cholesterol from these foods does not usually translate into cholesterol in the blood.

• Unsaturated fats •

These come in two types: polyunsaturated fats and monounsaturated fats. The difference is in their chemical make-up. They are both liquid at room temperature. Polyunsaturated fats include the fat in fish and chicken, soft margarines labelled high in polyunsaturates, or very low-fat spreads made with unsaturated oils (which cannot make claims because overall fat content is too low, so read the label) and vegetable oils such as corn oil, sunflower oil, safflower oil and soya-bean oil. Monunsaturated fats are found particularly in olives, olive oil, rapeseed oil, peanuts, peanut oil and avocado.

Polyunsaturated fats used to be seen as the good guys, essential to our bodies and not damaging in the way that saturated fats are. However the pendulum has started to swing again and it is now thought that oxygen attack (making oils go rancid quickly and fish quick to rot), to which polyunsaturates are more vulnerable than saturated fats, could also be to blame for some furring of the arteries. (See Free Radicals, page 20). So it is important not to have too many polyunsaturates in the diet either.

Monounsaturated fats are now thought to be especially linked with healthy hearts. Take care, however, with spreads made from either monounsaturated or polyunsaturated oils. Hydrogenated oil, used to harden them into spreads, creates what are called trans fatty acids, which act much like saturated fats once in the blood. So watch out for the words 'hydrogenated vegetable fat/oil' in ingredients lists on these spreads and on other food labels. Hydrogenated vegetable fats and oils may be found in crisps, biscuits, cakes and cereals, etc.

Whole Earth SuperSpread and Vitaquell spreads, available from health food shops, are almost trans-free. Other manufacturers are now working hard to lower their levels of trans fats. Flora was the first of these to claim that its sunflower spread is low in trans fats. Look out for other manufacturers following suit.

• Some good news about fish and meat •

Polyunsaturates that are still strongly in nutritional favour are fish oils. Oily fish, such as mackerel, salmon, tuna, herring, kippers, sardines and pilchards, contain polyunsaturated fatty acids known as omega-3 (whereas vegetable oils contain omega-6). Eating them appears to be very good for the heart and possibly for relieving symptoms of conditions such as arthritis and diabetes.

Fish oils also appear to have a role in brain development, in helping pregnancy run to term and may even have some part to play in shrinking cancer tumours. Once it was thought that you had to eat rather a lot to get the benefits. However it has now been shown that eating the equivalent of just 30g (approx 1oz) a day is sufficient to give the benefit to your heart, and that eating more is not necessarily better, at least for your heart. Most experts recommend eating oily fish at least twice a week.

Meat is in with the bad guys because it accounts for nearly a quarter of the saturated fats taken in the British diet, but it also provides 17.4 per cent of our polyunsaturated intake, as it contains both types of fats. As well, a review of dietary factors in heart disease found no connection between red meat consumption and heart disease in EC countries. The Greeks eat the most red meat and have the least heart disease, whereas Britain is second lowest on meat but second highest in heart disease rates. However, always eat lean red meat and cut off the visible fat.

• Too much fat? •

Our diets should not contain more than 30 per cent fat. Of this, only a third should be saturated fats and the rest slightly more monounsaturated than polyunsaturated, if possible. The polyunsaturated component should contain plenty of fish oils. There is a good reason why women, particularly, should make sure they keep all fats down to the recommended levels. Triglycerides are a type of blood fat created from digested fats and used for energy. Norwegian research has shown that raised triglyceride levels are an independent predictor of increased risk of death from heart disease and other causes in women, but not in men. The more fat of any type is taken in the diet, the more triglyceride levels rise.

• Keeping down the fat •

1 Use any spreads, whether butter, margarine or vegetable oils thinly. Avoid using any whenever possible.
2 Use semi-skimmed or skimmed milk. If you don't like the taste, you can always thicken it with dried milk powder: about 20ml per 200ml (two dessertspoons per 7fl oz) significantly increases your calcium intake too.
3 Remember that cottage cheese has less than a quarter of the fat of hard cheeses.
4 Grill, steam and bake rather than fry.
5 Take the skin off chicken and cut off all visible fat from meat.
6 Avoid too many biscuits, cakes, crisps, chips, etc.

• Vitamins and minerals •

Vitamins and minerals help our bodies function and are required in small amounts, so they are also known as micronutrients. They are essential to our health and are mostly found, in plenty, in fresh fruits and vegetables.

Some vitamins (A, D and E) are fat-soluble, which means they dissolve in fat and can be stored in our bodies: others (B and C) are water-soluble, dissolving in water and not able to be stored. We have to make sure we take in sufficient water-soluble vitamins each day to meet our needs.

Most vitamins are found in our food. Vitamin K, however, is provided by bacteria in the bowel and some vitamin D comes from sunlight.

Minerals are found in the soil in which our food grows. Those of which we need a very tiny amount are known as trace elements.

• Recommended amounts •

For a number of vitamins and minerals the government used to give guidelines on how much we need to eat each day to avoid deficiency symptoms. This appeared on food labels as the RDA, or recommended daily amount. However, this system has now changed because different people have different requirements and so one blanket recommendation was felt to be insufficient. Now, although RDA is still commonly used on food labels in the UK, you may come across any of the following terms:

Reference nutrient intake (RNI)   This is closest to the old RDA and meets the needs of almost all the population. In fact, it is higher than most people need.

Estimated average requirement (EAR)   The average requirement for a nutrient, but many people will need more and many will need less.

Lower reference nutrient intake (LRNI)   The amount deemed adequate for people with low needs. However, most of us will need more to avoid deficiency.

Safe intake   A term used to indicate the intake which is judged safe for a nutrient about which there isn't much information, thus preventing a clear recommendation about our requirements for it.

Dietary reference values (DRVs)   The overall term for all the above types of recommendation.

• How much is enough? •

There are EC guidelines for twelve vitamins and six minerals, which were drawn up in 1993. These are the amounts the EC advises consuming every day and are roughly equivalent to our reference nutrient intake (RNI).

Vitamin or mineral	Daily requirement	Vitamin or mineral	Daily requirement
Vitamin A	800mcg	Vitamin D	5mcg
Thiamin (B_1)	1.4mg	Vitamin E	10mg
Riboflavin (B_2)	1.6mg	Calcium	800mg
Niacin	18mg	Phosphorus	800mg
Vitamin B_6	2mg	Iron	14mg
Folic acid	200mcg	Magnesium	300mg
Vitamin B_{12}	1mcg	Zinc	15mg
Biotin	0.15mg	Iodine	150mcg
Pantothenic acid	6mg		

Although these amounts aren't likely to mean very much here, they can be a useful guide when looking at labels of foods that are fortified with vitamins and minerals, or at the contents of vitamin and mineral supplements.

It is important to remember, however, that these are levels at which deficiency is avoided. There is now a strong school of thought that we may need much more of some vitamins and minerals, because in greater amounts they may have important protective effects on our health. (See Antioxidants, page 20.)

• Measurement of vitamins and minerals •

Measurement is usually in milligrams (mg) or, if the amount needed is very tiny, micrograms (mcg). There are 1000 milligrams in 1 gram and 1,000,000 micrograms in 1 gram. There is also an old fashioned measurement called international units (iu) that is still sometimes used for vitamins A, D and E and which measures biological activity.

● 0.3mcg of vitamin A is equivalent to 1iu of vitamin A
● 1mcg of vitamin D is equivalent to 40iu of vitamin D
● 1mg of natural vitamin E is equivalent to 1.49iu of vitamin E.

• Quick guide to vitamins and minerals •

Below is a brief summary of useful facts about the main vitamins and minerals we need. Their actual functions in the body are various and often complicated, so these have mostly been left out. Also, deficiency symptoms are only included where there is a real possibility that deficiency could occur. A balanced and varied diet, including the foods mentioned below, is likely to give us all the necessary vitamins and minerals, unless stated.

Vitamin A   comes in two forms: retinol from animal foods such as meat, fish, eggs and dairy foods; and beta carotene, found in orange and yellow fruit and vegetables and green leafy vegetables, particularly carrots, broccoli, spinach, sweet potatoes, peppers, apricots and cantaloupe melon. Vitamin A is fat soluble and so any not used is stored by the liver.

Too much retinol can be toxic: long-term daily doses of about eight times the RNI can cause problems, with symptoms such as joint and bone pain, blurred vision, dry skin, and hair and weight loss. However beta carotene can be stored by the body safely. Half a raw carrot, an ounce of boiled broccoli or one small slice of lamb's liver would provide the RNI per day. Both vitamin A and beta carotene have a valuable function as antioxidants. (See Antioxidants, page 20.)

Vitamin B₁ (thiamin) The B vitamins work as a group but all have their own specific functions too. Yeast extract is a rich source of B_1. Other good ones are wholemeal bread, brown rice, pasta, whole-grain cereals, fortified breakfast cereals, liver, kidney, peas, beans, nuts and eggs. B_1 cannot be stored in the body.

Vitamin B₂ (riboflavin) The best source is yeast extract but B_2 is also found in milk, cheese, yoghurt, eggs, green leafy vegetables, liver and fortified breakfast cereals. Women on the contraceptive pill need more B_2. So does anyone who smokes or drinks a lot.

Niacin (sometimes known as B₃) Can best be obtained from yeast extract, brewers' yeast, liver, meat, poultry, fish, nuts, dried beans, milk, cheese and fortified breakfast cereals. It cannot be stored. People who drink a lot of alcohol need more.

Vitamin B₆ (pyridoxine) Good sources are yeast extract, brewers' yeast, wholemeal bread, whole-grain cereals, fortified breakfast cereals, fish, liver, bananas and potatoes. There is a little B_6 in most fruit and vegetables. Cannot be stored. Women taking the contraceptive pill or before a period may need more.

Vitamin B₁₂ (cobalamin) B_{12} is only found naturally in foods of animal origin: meat, poultry, liver and kidneys, fish, eggs, milk and cheese. However, fortified breakfast cereals contain it in useful amounts. Unlike most B vitamins, B_{12} can be stored in the liver so regular daily intake is not quite so important. Vegans may need a B_{12} supplement.

Folic acid (folate) Works alongside vitamin B_{12} and can also be stored by the body. It is very important for pregnant women and is thought to reduce risk of spina bifida. Good sources are leafy green vegetables, liver, nuts, wheatgerm, peas and dried beans. Women wishing to become pregnant should start taking daily 400mcg folic-acid supplements and keep taking them until 12 weeks pregnant. Women on the contraceptive pill may need to ensure a good intake from diet.

Biotin Another B vitamin, but without a number. Richest sources are yeast extract, brewers' yeast, wheatgerm, wholemeal bread, milk, cheese and yoghurt. Cannot be stored.

Pantothenic acid Another B vitamin without a number. Yeast extract and brewers' yeast, liver, kidney, nuts and soya flour provide plenty. Also you'll find some in egg, wholemeal flour and dried fruit. It cannot be stored.

Vitamin C Best sources are blackcurrants, citrus fruits and kiwi fruit. Bananas also provide a reasonable amount. Green leafy vegetables, green

KEEP UP THE KIWI

Eating kiwi is a pleasant way to get many health benefits. It contains nearly one milligram of vitamin C for every gram of fruit (98mg in a l00g (4oz) serving), is higher in vitamin E than other fruits, contains soluble fibre which helps reduce cholesterol levels, insoluble fibre which helps prevent constipation, potassium to offset salt intake and folic acid, important when pregnant or if on the pill.

peppers and potatoes contain it too. For best amounts of vitamin C, foods should be eaten raw as this vitamin is very easily lost in cooking, and the least interference with it beforehand (eg cutting or chopping), the better.

Vitamin C cannot be stored in the body. When you are under stress, you may benefit from an increased intake. Also, smokers need two or three times the recommended amounts because they derive less benefit from the vitamin C they consume. Vitamin C is an important antioxidant (See Antioxidants, page 20.)

Vitamin D Without sufficient vitamin D, the body cannot make proper use of the calcium and phosphorus it receives. Our bodies make vitamin D when we are out in the sunshine but we also need some from food. Oily fish, cod, liver, milk, dried milks and fortified breakfast cereals contain it. It is stored by the liver and excess must be avoided. An upper limit of 15mcg daily should not be exceeded. Excess is toxic and can interfere with heart muscle activity.

Vitamin E (tocopherol) Another antioxidant (see page 20). It is found in wheatgerm, peanuts and other nuts, green leafy vegetables, fish and meat. Vitamin E is fat soluble and can be stored in the body.

Calcium This is a very important mineral for keeping bones and teeth healthy. The National Osteoporosis Society recommends that women aged 20 to 40 should consume 1000mg a day and women over 45 should have 1500mg a day (or 1000mg if on hormone replacement therapy). That is considerably more than the RNI but may help prevent osteoporosis. Women who are breast feeding should take in 1250mg of calcium daily, according to government guidelines. However, government health advisers no longer think increased intake during pregnancy is necessary because a woman's body absorbs calcium more efficiently when pregnant.

Calcium can be found in milk, cheese, yoghurt, sardines, bread (all bread other than wholemeal has calcium added), green leafy vegetables and hard water. Skimmed milk contains slightly more than ordinary milk. A third of a pint of skimmed milk will provide 250mg. So will a 150g (5oz) pot of yoghurt or 50g (2oz) of tinned sardines. Cheddar cheese weighing 50g (2oz) gives 200mg, 100g (4oz) of broccoli 85mg, two slices of white bread 60mg and 100g (4oz) of baked beans or 50g (2oz) of dried apricots 50mg. Dried milk added to skimmed or whole milk will increase calcium content too. However, tea, coffee and raw bran can reduce the absorption of calcium.

Phosphorus This mineral is also important for healthy teeth and bones. It is found in the same foods as calcium, and also in meat and poultry.

Iron Iron helps in the formation of red blood cells, amongst other things. Women are quite commonly deficient because of blood loss at menstruation, during which iron is lost as well. About a third of women under 50 are estimated to be low in iron.

Best sources of iron are from liver, kidneys and red meats, eggs and dried apricots. It is also found in wholemeal bread, beans and green leafy vegetables, but uptake isn't so good from these sources. Fortified breakfast cereals contain it. There is even quite a lot in liquorice allsorts!

Eating a food containing vitamin C or drinking a fruit juice containing it at the same time as eating iron significantly increases the body's ability to absorb the iron. Conversely, heavy tea drinking and a diet extremely high in fibre can reduce iron absorption.

The main symptom of iron deficiency is tiredness. Severe deficiency can cause anaemia (see page 451). However too much iron is harmful too so don't take an iron supplement without consulting your doctor.

Magnesium This mineral is another which helps form teeth and bones, amongst other functions. It is found in nuts, soya beans, brewers' yeast, fish, wholemeal bread, milk, seafood, dried fruits and hard water. Adequate intake appears to play a part in reducing premenstrual syndrome.

Zinc Among its many roles in the body, zinc is thought to be connected with fertility. Women wishing to become pregnant (and their partners) should ensure a good intake of zinc. Best sources are meat, chicken, pork, seafood (a meal-time portion of one of these would give you the RNI) but also wholemeal bread, whole-grain cereals, nuts, eggs and some green vegetables. Eating too much calcium may lead to reduction in zinc absorption.

Iodine This is important for proper functioning of the thyroid gland. Best sources are seafood and sea salt.

Sodium This is salt. We need it in our diets but we get more than enough from the foods we eat because almost all contain it. We certainly don't need to add it.

Potassium Potassium works with sodium to keep our water balance right. You find it in very many foods but not always in high amounts. Best sources are fruits such as bananas, apples and oranges, vegetables such as carrots, broccoli and tomatoes, meat, poultry, fish, bread and beans.

Selenium This is a trace mineral, meaning very little of it is needed to prevent deficiency. However it is an antioxidant and may have, at greater intake, a valuable role to play in helping protect health. (See Antioxidants, page 20.) It works alongside vitamin E and is found in whole grains, meat, fish, shellfish and dairy foods.

• Making the most of your vitamins •

1 Eat fruits and vegetables as soon as possible after buying.

2 Fruits and vegetables containing vitamins A and C are sensitive to light, heat and air, so over-exposure to any of these results in a heavy loss of vitamins. Keep them in a cool, dark place. Cover vegetables and any thin-skinned or soft fruit, as oxygen can penetrate.

3 Don't handle more than you have to before eating.

4 Don't soak. You will lose more than half the C and B vitamins.

5 Avoid peeling or chopping fruit.

6 Cooking will destroy over half of the vitamin C in green leafy vegetables and some of their vitamin A, too. Eat raw where possible.

7 Eating carrots lightly cooked gives you more beta carotene than eating them raw. Mature carrots also have more beta carotene than young pale ones. Eat your carrots with a little fat, to aid absorption.

8 Don't be dismissive of frozen fruits and vegetables. They often have more of their vitamins intact than the fresh variety.

9 Don't shake cartons or bottles of fruit juice as this will increase the rate at which vitamin C is lost once opened.

10 Avoid frying meat. It destroys almost a third of the vitamin A, which is fat soluble.

11 Don't leave milk on the doorstep in sunlight. It will lose its vitamin B_2.

• Antioxidants and free radicals •

Vitamins A, C and E and the trace mineral selenium are all antioxidants. Folic acid and constituents of garlic and onion also have antioxidant properties. All antioxidants can mop up free radicals. These are molecules which are natural by-products of the body's metabolism but which are also produced after exposure to sunlight, X-rays, environmental pollutants, ozone and cigarette smoke. Our bodies can cope with small amounts – in fact we need them – but it is thought that we can't cope with such an overload. The excess are believed to play a part in triggering degeneration and disease. Heart disease, cancers and even cataracts and rheumatoid arthritis have all been linked with them, although as yet there is not sufficient proof to satisfy everybody.

Consuming antioxidants is an important way to reduce free-radical damage. Most nutrition experts now recommend that we should all eat five good servings of fruit and vegetables a day and some suggest that supplements may be helpful too as, they claim, it is hardly practical to eat the large amounts of antioxidants which we need for full benefit.

However, is it possible to eat too much this way? There is no known harm in taking much larger amounts of vitamin E than the RNI, but sceptics would say that optimal blood levels of vitamin E simply haven't been established, and high E levels could affect the action of anticoagulant drugs. Vitamin C at high levels is excreted if not used but can, in the long term, cause kidney stones, and when stopped it may even cause rebound scurvy, a symptom of vitamin C deficiency caused by the sudden drop in high levels. Vitamin A must not be taken in high doses, although beta carotene is safe (but might turn your skin orange). Stick to manufacturers' recommendations if you do take these supplements.

Regardless of the outcome of the free-radical disease theory, plenty of research now shows that a good daily intake of fresh fruit and vegetables seems to play a valuable part in reducing risk of a number of cancers. Supplements, if taken, are no substitute as fruit and vegetables may contain other natural substances which work with the antioxidants to give them their good effects and also have a positive impact of their own. (See The importance of Freshness, page 22.)

• Supplements •

Are supplements a good thing in general? Certainly more and more people are taking them, with multivitamins, iron and vitamin C the favourites. There are differing views, of course. While some nutrition experts now think that taking daily supplements is essential for health, others are more sceptical, and certainly there are risks which should be avoided.

The biggest problem in this complex area is that increasing intake of one particular vitamin or mineral in a supplement may interfere with absorption of another which may then affect another, and so on. For instance, one expert has claimed that high doses of vitamin C may decrease absorption of the trace mineral copper which is important in the metabolism of iron. When iron is not metabolised properly, toxic levels may accumulate in body tissues.

Taking too much of one thing – and not only too much of those vitamins known to be toxic in excess, such as A and D – may be bad for the body. There have been reports of problems with taking 30 times the RNI for niacin (vitamin B_3) and vitamin B_6. Some multi-vitamin and mineral supplements contain far more than the RNI for very many of their micronutrients – sometimes up to 1000 times more – which is thought unnecessary; 50mcg of vitamin D may be found in some, which may actually be dangerous. Look at the amounts and the percentages of RNI (or RDA) on the labels.

There is another thing to be aware of. The Food Commission, an independent body concerned with the quality of food, found from experiments that many vitamin pills tested didn't break down in the stomach and were therefore completely ineffective.

People who may benefit from judicious supplementation include those who don't eat a wide range of good foods, such as children who are faddy eaters, people on diets, and people recovering from illnesses or whose immune systems are suppressed by treatments for illnesses. Pregnant and breast-feeding women particularly need to ensure a good intake of vitamins and minerals one way or another.

Make sure, with a water-soluble vitamin supplement, to take it with food and early in the day, otherwise it will just be excreted in the urine.

Regardless of their views on supplements, one that many experts do particularly recommend is vitamin E because it is difficult to obtain from the diet at the levels needed to help protect against heart disease. If buying a vitamin E supplement, it is important to choose a natural-source vitamin E, not a synthetic one. Natural vitamin E is officially recognised as at least 36 per cent more powerful than synthetic versions and recent studies even claim that natural is twice as effective. Natural vitamin E is listed on a label as d-alpha tocopherol. Synthetic vitamin E is listed as di-alpha tocopherol.

A folic-acid supplement is definitely recommended when trying to get pregnant and during the first three months of pregnancy, to reduce risk of a spina bifida baby. (See Folic Acid, page 17).

• The importance of freshness •

Even if you do take a supplement, still try to ensure you eat at least five portions of fruit and vegetables a day. Scientists are discovering that chemicals which give plants their colour and protect them from sunlight (known as protective factors) work together, and with vitamins in food, to stimulate the immune system to fight many kinds of disease.

A family of chemicals found in cabbage, broccoli, Brussels sprouts, cauliflower and turnips are exciting particular interest, but protective factors can be found in plenty in a very wide range of fruits and vegetables. Tomatoes, onions, green peppers, pineapples, strawberries and carrots have all been found to contain thousands and thousands of different protective chemicals. Even if these could ever find their way into pill form, their relationship with the vitamins naturally occurring in foods is extremely complex and unlikely to be reproducible in a capsule.

• Fibre •

Fibre is the undigestible part of unrefined grains, vegetables and fruits. There are two types: soluble fibre, found in fruits, vegetables, oats and beans, which affects the absorption of fat and lowers blood cholesterol levels; and insoluble fibre, found in wholemeal bread, whole-grain pasta and brown rice, which softens and bulks out faeces, aiding their passage through the intestines and helping to prevent constipation. It is thought that quicker transit time of faeces may be linked with healthier colons and that fibre in the diet helps protect against cancer of the colon.

We should aim for about 25g (1oz) of fibre in our diet every day. Portions of 100g (4oz) of baked beans, spinach, raisins and peas all give 7g, the same amount of prunes contains 14g, a slice of wholemeal bread 4g and apples and bananas 2g. Unprocessed bran gives very high amounts – 44g per 100g (1¾oz per 4oz) – but has no other food value and interferes with calcium absorption, so it is is better to get fibre in other ways.

• Sugar •

We don't need sugar in the form of snacks, chocolates, cakes and biscuits, etc. Although we are led to believe by some advertisers that sugar is a good energy food, all the energy we need can be derived from other, more nutritious, foods.

If you like sugary foods, try to keep overall consumption down and, for the sake of your teeth, eat any sugary treats in one go rather than repeatedly over the day (eg, sucking a sweet every hour or so) as this does less damage. Remember that honey is all sugar, whatever medicinal value it may be vaunted to have, and fruit juices are full of natural sugar, even when no extra is added. Look at the labels of manufactured foods for unexpected sugar, eg in tins of sweetcorn.

• Salt •

Lowering salt intake may help people who have high blood pressure but is unlikely to affect people with normal blood pressure. However, as there are very often no symptoms to high blood pressure and as we all get as much salt as we need naturally from our food, it is best either not to add it or to keep consumption low. Look at the labels on manufactured foods to see if salt is added.

• Coffee •

The story about coffee seems to change all the time. It used to be thought that caffeine over-stimulated the heart and might be implicated in heart disease but American research found no effect on heart disease from drinking coffee. These findings were confirmed by research at Ninewells Hospital in Dundee which actually found a protective effect from drinking more than five cups of coffee a day. Another plus is that coffee may protect against depression, according to American reseachers. Coffee appears to be linked with low suicide rates and with less likelihood of dying of cirrhosis of the liver.

However, caffeine definitely over-stimulates many people, causing symptoms of agitation, and is not advised when pregnant. It can also be addictive, even when drunk moderately. A study of people who averaged two and a half cups a day were asked to stop for a while. Half reported moderate or severe headaches and one in ten suffered symptoms of anxiety or depression. Stopping abruptly, if you want to cut your caffeine intake down, is obviously not a wise course. Some women crave extra-strong coffee just before their period starts; if so, it may be better to drink it weak or not at all, to avoid increased anxiety, irritability and mood swings.

• Alcohol •

The recommended upper limit for alcohol intake is 14 units a week for women: a unit is a small glass of wine, a pub measure of spirits or half a pint of normal strength beer or lager. Half a pint of extra-strength beers, lagers or cider may count for up to three units. Keeping within these limits is thought to be low risk.

A moderate amount of alcohol consumption may be protective against heart disease and two drinks a day may even improve memory and learning. However, the negative side of excessive drinking is considerable. (See Drinking, page 57.)

• Health foods •

Health-food shops contain lots of healthy foods and supplements but they also carry many that aren't altogether healthy. For example, there is plenty of fruit sugar in pure fruit spreads which will rot teeth almost as effectively as cane sugar. Raw sugar, muscovado sugar, honey and molasses are all still sugar. Wholemeal pastry still contains the normal amount of fat found in any other pastry. Some vegetarian sausages actually have higher amounts of fat than meat sausages. Carob bars are caffeine-free chocolate substitutes, but may contain more fat and only slightly less sugar than chocolate. So choose carefully in the health-food shop, or you may be paying more for no real benefit.

• Being a vegetarian •

More and more women are choosing to become vegetarian: one in 14 no longer eats meat compared with one in 24 men. True vegetarians eat no meat, poultry or fish but many people who still eat fish consider themselves vegetarian. Vegans exclude not only meat, poultry and fish but dairy foods and eggs as well.

A vegetarian diet that is varied can be a very healthy one. Research has shown that vegetarians tend to have lower blood cholesterol, lower blood pressure and less incidence of colon cancer than meat eaters. Other benefits include lowered risk of diabetes, appendicitis, piles, hiatus hernia, varicose veins, gallstones and osteoporosis (except vegans, who have more osteoporosis). However, not all these benefits can necessarily be attributed to the diet. Vegetarians as a group tend to be less obese, for instance, which could account for lower incidence of gallstones and lower blood pressure. Also, vegetarians tend to be interested in their health and therefore may lead generally more healthy lifestyles. One study found that cutting down on fat and refined food and eating more fruit and vegetables is more associated with health than whether we eat meat and fish.

If you are vegetarian, you should eat plenty of vegetables, fruits, grains and pulses and not too many dairy foods. Plant protein is not complete for our needs but combining different plant proteins makes up perfectly adequately for the loss, eg by eating beans on toast, cereals with added nuts or macaroni cheese.

Contrary to belief, vegetarians aren't prone to anaemia. The biggest problem may be a deficiency of vitamin B_{12} if you eat little or no dairy food. Fortified breakfast cereals and yeast extract spreads, such as Marmite, have useful amounts for vegetarian needs. If you don't eat those, take a suitable supplement.

• Food safety at home •

Taking care when buying, storing and cooking food can help prevent food poisoning. Here are some tips.

1 Always check that products you buy are not beyond their sell-by date.
2 Avoid any cans that have dents: the can's seal which prevents metallic corrosion may have been damaged and particles from the tin could dissolve into the food inside. Also avoid cans that look swollen at the ends as this could mean there are bacteria within which may cause food poisoning. To check how long ago the can was filled, look at the top row of numbers stamped on the end of the tin. The first three figures indicate on which day (out of 365) the can was filled and the final number refers to the last number of the year that it was filled. So 0055 would mean a can was filled on January 5, 1995.
3 Pack your shopping carefully, so that raw chicken and meat in easily damaged cellophane wrappings and polystyrene trays are not next to ready-to-eat foods such as cheese. Take shopping home as soon as possible. Leaving it sitting in the boot of a car or in a warm office for an hour is sufficient for the temperature of the food to rise and give bacteria a chance to grow.
4 Pack your fridge carefully. Raw meats and chicken should be kept at the bottom of the fridge so that they cannot drip on to cooked foods. Make sure they don't drip into the salad or vegetable box either. Keep raw and cooked foods away from each other.
5 Check your fridge is never at a temperature higher than 5 °C or 41 °F (a fridge thermometer is the easiest way to be sure). Avoid leaving the door open or improperly closed, or putting hot foods into the fridge, as all these things raise the temperature of the fridge.
6 Freezers should be kept at minus118 °C or 0 °F.
7 Wash your hands after handling raw meats and chicken. Wash your hands after touching pets if you are about to prepare food.
8 Keep chopping boards clean (wooden boards are now thought to be more hygienic than plastic ones) by washing them in hot soapy water, and drying them with disposable paper towels if possible. Disposable all-purpose cloths are rarely disposed of after one use and can harbour germs if kept moist.
9 Don't use the same chopping board or knife for chopping raw food, cooked food and fruit or vegetables without thoroughly washing the board and knife in between.

10 Defrost foods thoroughly, preferably in the fridge or microwave oven.

11 Put cooked food into the fridge within an hour of being cooked. Eat it within a couple of days and do not reheat more than once. Reheat until the food is piping hot to ensure that all bacteria have been killed.

12 Avoid eating homemade mayonnaise, mousses, and anything that contains uncooked egg. Pregnant women and others especially vulnerable to infection should avoid eating unpasteurised soft cheeses such as brie, camembert and blue-vein cheeses as these can be contaminated with dangerous bacteria called listeria.

• Food allergy •

True food allergy means allergic symptoms such as vomiting, swelling and severe rashes which occur almost immediately after eating the culprit food. The most severe form of allergic response is anaphylaxis when, in addition to the above, there may be breathing difficulties, a swelling in the throat which can itself be fatal, a drop in blood pressure and unconsciousness. The foods most commonly associated with anaphylaxis are nuts and shellfish.

More commonly, people may suffer from food sensitivity but this is still a contentious area in the medical world. However, there is evidence that problems such as migraine, headaches, respiratory difficulties, hay-fever symptoms, joint and muscles aches, tension, depression, irritability, stomach upsets, cramps and indigestion may, for some people, be caused by eating regularly one or more foods that their bodies cannot tolerate. Intolerance to the food can develop quite suddenly, after a lifetime of eating it without problems. It is as if the body, which has previously struggled successfully to cope with the problem food, suddenly can't cope any more, perhaps because of other simultaneous strong stresses and strains placed on the immune system.

Although dairy foods and wheat are a particularly common source of problems, sensitivity of this kind can be experienced with any food, fresh or processed. Some food additives have a similar effect for some people.

The problem is that it is difficult to pin down the culprit. There are a number of ways to test for food allergies, some of which are controversial, and you may come out seemingly allergic to virtually everything you like to eat but with no real respite to your problems. If you do suspect that some foods may be your problem, try keeping a diary of all the food you eat (including brands for packaged foods) and all your symptoms, so that you can see if the two match up.

Often the problem is referred to as masked allergy because if the food is one eaten every day, you just constantly feel below par in one way or another. To detect a masked allergy, you need to eliminate a common food from your diet for five days and then reintroduce it. If the eliminated food is indeed the culprit, you may experience some withdrawal symptoms while you are not eating it but when you reintroduce it, symptoms should be particularly marked, as your body will be reacting to the food as if presented with it for the first time.

If you get no joy by this method and wish to try allergy-testing, see your GP for advice. If you decide to approach a private allergy-testing clinic, check that the person running it is medically qualified. You can look up his or her name in the Medical Register which you should be able to consult at your local library.

• Food additives •

Food additives are often thought of as E numbers, because these are the numbers allotted to additives approved by the European Community. Many people fear them but they are far from all bad. Some additives are necessary for food safety or for the convenience we have come to expect when buying and using food. For example, we could not keep certain foods any length of time if they did not contain preservatives.

The main functions of food additives are to prevent the growth of bacteria which could cause food poisoning, to improve texture of processed foods and to add colour and flavour. Clearly only a small minority are actually essential for food safety. Because of scares about toxic effects found in animals, links with cancers and worries about the cumulative effects of additives – none as yet proven a significant hazard in humans – manufacturers now often try to cut out as many additives as they can. There is, therefore, more consumer choice.

If additives concern you, read the labels. As a rough guide, colourings are numbered from E100 to E199, preservatives from E200 to E299, antioxidants from E300 to E399 and emulsifiers, stabilisers, thickeners and gelling agents from E400 to E499. There may also be additives with numbers not preceded by an E, meaning that the additive has been approved in the UK but not yet by the EC.

For two helpful guides on additives, see Further Reading.

• Obesity •

Being obese means being 20 per cent above your ideal maximum weight. About 5 per cent of the population in the UK falls into this category.

If you are surprised to find yourself seriously overweight, consider first whether there may be any reasons for the gain other than overeating. Some drugs prescribed by your doctor, particularly steroids, may cause a gradual increase. A hormonal disorder such as an underactive thyroid can also cause weight gain, along with other symptoms, such as weakness, dry skin, lethargy and feeling cold. Stopping smoking may lead temporarily to extra weight, but usually not more than half a stone if you don't eat to compensate for not smoking.

Most often, however, obesity is caused by eating too much. You may come from a family who all have weight problems and there certainly is a genetic component to weight gain, but even in these circumstances you can still lose weight if you really want to, though you may have to work harder at it.

Obesity is an unpleasant word. It also carries unpleasant health risks such as high blood pressure, high blood cholesterol, higher risk of heart disease and stroke, higher risk of breast and endometrial cancer, backache, joint strain, osteoarthritis, gallstones, hernias, varicose veins, diabetes, breathlessness and skin problems. It can also be connected with infertility.

The highest risk of illness is in those who have what is termed central obesity: they have a high waist to hip ratio (WHR) and are often called 'apple shape'. You find your WHR by dividing your waist measurement by your hip measurement. Very overweight women with a WHR higher than 0.75 are at greater risk. The good news is that 'apples', with their mainly abdominal fat, can lose weight more easily than pear-shaped women with more subcutaneous fat. Also, giving up smoking can help because overweight smokers are more likely to become apples than pears.

If you are suffering any problems or fear for your health, for your own sake you ought to try to lose weight. Although some people resort to appetite suppressants or seek drastic cures such as stomach stapling, the best way to lose weight is to eat fewer but more healthy foods and to exercise more. Gradual reduction programmes which re-educate the appetite are far more successful and more healthy than crash or fad diets.

• Being underweight •

Being underweight is less of a health hazard than being overweight, although serious underweight can of course be fatal (see Anorexia Nervosa, page 182). However, any woman planning to get pregnant would do well not to be underweight at conception if possible. Low weight at conception increases the likelihood of having an underweight baby.

• Compulsive eating •

If you are a compulsive eater you may unconsciously use food to avoid expressing difficult emotions. Or, you may overeat for other complicated and not necessarily conscious reasons, such as to make a jealous partner feel more secure because they think your severe overweight may prevent rivals from being attracted to you.

If you want change, you will need to identify and tackle such underlying causes and find new healthier solutions before you can successfully lose weight and keep it off. You will also probably be happier with yourself and your life, not just because you may be experiencing constant guilt, self-disgust and physical discomfort while eating compulsively, but because you will be able to acknowledge openly your important emotional needs and try to find more satisfying and fulfilling ways to have them met.

See pages 182 and 185 for information about the eating disorders anorexia and bulimia; and page 62 in the chapter on Indulgences and Addictions for general advice on trying to break habits.

A helpful book to read is *The Food Trap*: see Further Reading.

2

EXERCISE

REGULAR exercise is good for many aspects of physical and mental health, as well as helping to improve our appearance, keep off excess weight and ward off illnesses. Even so, if you find you baulk at the thought of regular exercise, take heart. A variety of normal, everyday activities can give you the benefits you need, and accumulated short periods of activity in a day can be broadly equivalent in benefit to a sustained and sweaty workout.

• Ten good reasons to exercise •

1 Exercise can help your heart. The muscle fibres in the walls around the heart become stronger and thicker when you exercise regularly, allowing the heart to pump out more blood with less effort. Your risk of heart attack or angina (pain in the heart) is reduced, especially as exercise is also thought to help keep cholesterol from building up in the arteries.

2 Vigorous exercise in early adulthood has been found to be protective against stroke in later life but exercise, particularly walking, not taken up until later in life still has a beneficial effect.

3 Exercise keeps a good supply of blood coming to the skin, improving the skin's appearance. It also can help you sleep better, which in turn has effects that show in healthier skin. Lungs work better, allowing you to take in more oxygen. Muscles can work longer and harder and joints keep mobile, reducing the risks of backache and of pain and stiffness as you age.

4 Exercise can help protect against several cancers. A sedentary lifestyle is especially linked with increased risk of cancer of the colon, breast, cervix and ovary, for instance. One recent study found that the risk of endometrial cancer is considerably increased in older inactive women.

5 Bones benefit from regular physical activity. Just three hours of walking a week, for instance, helps build bone density in people under 30 and slows down loss of bone in those who are older.

6 Exercise is a good way, coupled with healthy eating, to deal with or prevent obesity and the health problems that often come with it, such as diabetes, high blood pressure, heart disease and gallstones.

7 Exercise can lessen premenstrual tension or period pain for some women.

8 Exercise can improve the mood, making you feel good about yourself and happier about your body. It can also markedly increase energy, a brisk 10-minute walk being enough to boost it for up to two hours afterwards as well as decrease fatigue and tension. Some studies show increased intellectual functioning and better memory powers.

9 Both depression and anxiety can be reduced. Exercise can also be a healthy way to express negative pent-up feelings such as anxiety or anger.

10 Finally, regular exercise can even give your sex life a boost. A survey of 8000 women in Los Angeles found that nearly a third claimed more frequent sex after starting to exercise regularly; 40 per cent noticed an increase in arousal; and a quarter were more able to reach orgasm.

• Who should exercise? •

Everyone should get exercise in some form that suits them, including the young, the old, the disabled and the chronically ill.

Children are more likely to avoid many later illnesses if they get into the habit of enjoying physical activity every day.

Suitable exercise during pregnancy can help you stay more fit and comfortable, reduce your risk of varicose veins and backache, ease labour and childbirth and help you to lose your weight gain more quickly afterwards. Take advice about what sort of exercise and how much: ligaments soften to prepare the body for labour, which can increase the risk of an injury.

Regular exercise when elderly helps slow down some of the physical effects of ageing, such as stiffness. It is never too late to start, as long as the type of exercise is chosen with care and only increased gradually. Walking, for instance, is excellent value and easy to incorporate into any lifestyle. In a study at a Massachusetts hospital, ten 86 to 96 year olds were encouraged to lift weights three times a week for 10 to 20 minutes. They started with just 2.25kg (5lb) weights. After eight weeks, they had all doubled their strength and two no longer needed canes for walking.

If you have a disability or chronic illness, you may need to choose your form of exercise with care (see below). At certain times it is unwise for anyone to exercise: for example, when feeling feverish and flu-ish.

If you have any special medical condition, are overweight or are a heavy smoker, it is advisable to consult your doctor about any form of exercise which would be especially beneficial to you, and any that you should avoid.

• Short bursts rather than the burn •

The experts now say that the old advised regime of at least 20 minutes vigorous exercise at least three times a week is not the minimum required for good health after all: in fact just half an hour's moderate physical activity a day – not even taken all at once but added up together – is sufficient to have significant health benefits.

This was decided after numerous studies which have shown the benefits of less exercise, and it was announced in 1993 by a number of America's leading authorities on health and exercise, including the US Centers for Disease Control and Prevention, the American College of Sports Medicine and the President's Council on Physical Fitness and Sports. Authorities in Britain have now followed suit. 'We are keen to encourage more people to be more active more often,' is the official line from the Health Education Authority.

While it is good to carry on doing more than this – if that is what you are already doing and enjoy it – the evidence is very clear that moderate exercise is a lot better than none. One study carried out at the University of Minnesota School of Public Health found that men who were at high risk of coronary heart disease, who undertook moderate amounts of light or medium physical activity, had lower rates of heart disease and death than men whose lives were more sedentary. Particularly interesting was the finding that 30 minutes-worth of moderate leisure-time physical activity had as much benefit in terms of protection from fatal heart attacks as did exercising three times as much.

Sometimes, it seems, less can be better than more. For example, moderate activity can lessen chances of catching colds and infections because it strengthens the immune system whereas high-intensity and long-duration activity can weaken the immune system and make us more likely to catch infections, particularly upper respiratory ones.

Low-impact aerobic exercise has been shown to help reduce pain, fatigue, swelling and depression in people who suffer from rheumatoid arthritis, but they are usually advised to avoid vigorous exercise as it may be harmful instead.

In another study, for eight clinically depressed people the effects of just 30 to 45 minutes of walking three times a week compared well with those of psychotherapy. Six people were virtually recovered within three weeks. However, overdoing exercise or training can increase depression instead of reducing it.

If you still like the idea of giving it all you've got, research findings show that three 10-minute bouts of exertion at least four hours apart are comparable in health benefit with one sustained, longer workout. It may be easier for some women to incorporate shorter workouts into a busy day, and it may also be easier to sustain them.

• What kind of exercise do we need? •

To keep fit or become fully fit we need to improve our strength, stamina and suppleness. These are the three distinct elements of fitness and while some forms of exercise or activity may help improve one of them, they may not be so good for the others.

Strength This means muscle power. You need to exercise each muscle group separately in order to build up your muscle strength: that is, you must work the muscles in each arm and each leg. If you have good muscle strength you will more easily be able to lift heavy objects, carry heavy loads and carry out countless other daily activities that require muscle power. Very effective activities to increase strength include running, swimming, rowing, tennis, squash, digging, aerobics, weight-lifting and vigorous housework. Dancing and golf are also fairly good.

Stamina   This allows us to keep going. The better your heart, lungs and muscles can work, the longer you will be able to exercise without a break. Excellent activities to build up stamina include cycling, jogging, rowing, swimming, tennis, aerobics, running and heavy housework.

Suppleness   Suppleness is the ability to bend, stretch, twist and turn easily, for which we need flexible muscles and joints. Dancing, tennis, gymnastics, swimming, yoga and aerobics are all very good for this. Games like badminton, golf and basketball are reasonably good and so too is walking.

• Exercise options •

The important thing about exercise is to keep it up. Just as some good effects of exercise are instant (just one session can make muscle cells more sensitive to insulin, for example, and increase ability to break down blood clots), so too are the effects of stopping. So, if deciding to build regular exercise into your day, try to choose activities which you think you will enjoy or which need to be done, and you know you have a good chance of keeping up.

Instead of setting yourself the task of attending an aerobics class three times a week, for example, you might choose a variety of different activities throughout your week, such as dancing, golf, going for a hill walk, raking leaves, and even having a session of vigorous sex. You might also decide that ball games, bicycle trails, visits to the zoo or bonfire-building in the garden with the children or grandchildren are a good way to get you both moving and enjoying each other's company.

Another way to accumulate your half hour of exercise a day is to count in necessary physical chores: the type we might usually want to put off, such as spring cleaning, decorating, digging in the garden, mowing the lawn and building shelves. The chores themselves may even appear more appealing if we know they are doing us good.

A third option is to adapt your usual day to include a little more exercise. For example, you might choose to climb all stairs instead of taking lifts (or get out of the lift at a floor two below or above the one you really want); walk to work or walk part of the way (by getting off the bus or train at an earlier stop or parking the car at a distance). Walking is particularly good because it is so easy to fit into a normal routine. It may not offer much in terms of increasing strength and suppleness but it can help burn up almost as many calories as running, if you do it briskly, and it can increase levels of high density lipoproteins ('good' cholesterol) even if you do it slowly.

Whatever you choose to do, start off slowly if you haven't been doing much exercise before. You don't need to worry about taking your pulse to check your heart rate and see how much good you are doing; just judge by your own body. Allow yourself to get a little breathless and to feel your heart beating faster than normal but do not go to the point of exhaustion. You should feel tired but good afterwards – not good for nothing!

AEROBIC EXERCISE

Although the term aerobics is popularly used for dance-type exercises performed to music, aerobic exercise actually refers to any form of exercise which is carried out without stopping for at least 12 to 15 minutes at a time. The muscles are not pushed harder than they can function and the blood can supply enough oxygen to keep the muscles going. Aerobic exercise is what increases fitness. Anaerobic exercise means exercise that is carried out in brief bursts, such as sprinting or squash, where the blood can't supply enough oxygen to the muscles quickly enough and they tire quickly. Because by its nature anaerobic exercise can't be carried out for long, it doesn't improve heart and lung function, essential for fitness.

• Avoid exercise if. . . •

You are anaemic   Before or while you are being treated you could put a serious strain on your heart if you exercise at all vigorously.

You are feeling feverish or fluey   While you are fighting an infection, exercise can cause it to persist and make you feel far worse and for longer. Certain types of virus, for example those which cause gastric flu, chicken pox and glandular fever, can take a very firm hold instead of being eliminated from the body if you put the body under stress while suffering – or incubating – them. Myalgic Encephalomyelitis (ME) characterised by intense physical and mental fatigue after any trivial exertion, and neurological disturbances such as loss of short-term memory and concentration, is thought mainly to be caused in this way (see page 473).

• Dos and don'ts •

Always warm up before and cool down after   This is essential before and after any kind of sustained vigorous exercise, otherwise you are at risk of tearing a ligament or pulling a muscle. Warm up by doing a series of gentle bends and stretches. Make circling movements with your arms, hands and ankles. Do a little running on the spot or walking to increase the blood flow to your muscles and help them function more freely. Do the same sorts of movements to cool down after your exercise is over because, if you just stop abruptly, you may get cramp and sore muscles. If you just collapse in a heap the minute your vigorous exercise is over, the blood won't flow fast enough through your muscles to bring in fresh oxygen and eliminate waste products that build up during exercise.

Eat sensibly before you take exercise   Don't do any vigorous physical activity after eating a heavy meal because your body will not be able to digest it properly while blood flow is diverted from the stomach to the muscles you are using. You may also feel sick if you have eaten too heavily too recently.

Carbohydrates, such as pasta, potatoes or bread, are good to eat, preferably a couple of hours prior to exercising, as they supply the energy you need most quickly. Drink adequate fluid.

Wear suitable clothes   These must allow you to move freely and shouldn't make you excessively hot and sweaty. Cotton is good because it absorbs a considerable amount of sweat. If you need sports shoes for your exercise, ensure that they fit well and are suitable for the exact sport you have in mind.

Don't overdo it   Stop if you feel really uncomfortable at any time. If you exercise for ten minutes but are gasping for breath for five of them, you might as well not have done those five because it means you are lacking the oxygen to work your muscles. As a rough guide to what to expect of yourself, you should be able to talk at the same time as carrying out your chosen physical activity. Do not over-train. If you find that you want to keep up a punishing exercise schedule despite feeling stiff, sore and exhausted, you are becoming unhealthily obsessed with exercise and also not doing your body much good. For your body to strengthen, your muscles must be allowed sufficient rest. (Professional athletes never exercise at full pelt every day.)

Avoid getting over-competitive   You may enjoy the competitive element of games such as tennis and that may be what attracts you to them in the first place. But becoming over-competitive or too obsessed with playing every stroke well can soon remove the pleasure of the game and all the psychological benefits of exercise. Try to keep your mind on the game, not on whether you missed a good backhand, whether you think you are looking an idiot or you fear you look too fat.

Keep your motivation up   If you are not someone who naturally enjoys physical activity, try to find ways to keep yourself going. Remind yourself of the rewards: physical, mental and appearance-wise. Or give yourself a responsibility, such as arranging to play a particular sport with a particular friend at regular times, arranging to take an elderly neighbour's dog for a walk, or getting one of your own. Incorporate physical activity into something you do like doing, such as taking a brisk walk to a lovely country pub for Sunday lunch.

• Beware of sports injuries •

The most common injuries are:

- Ankle sprain, when the foot turns over, particularly in tennis, badminton and squash.
- Pulled hamstring: tearing some fibres at the back of the thigh through over-stretching when sprinting or kicking a ball.
- Inflammation of the Achilles tendon at the back of the heel, usually from running long distances, running on unsuitable surfaces or running in unsuitable shoes. Doing step aerobics without proper warming up can also cause it.

- Torn knee cartilage, from twisting with the body's full weight on the bent knee; common in skiers.
- Back pain, caused by injury to the ligament or muscle during sports such as rowing, weight-lifting or gymnastics.

After any injury, rest the damaged part, raising it higher than the heart to reduce bleeding and swelling. Put on a firm bandage and apply ice; both will help to reduce swelling further. If you are no better and still in considerable pain after two days, see your doctor. Don't exercise again until you can move the part freely and without pain. Get back into stride slowly.

DEALING WITH EXCUSES

I don't want to do an exercise class because I'll look fat Check the class out first. There may be others there of your build who aren't embarrassed at all, and from whose presence you'll draw confidence. Wear something loose in which you feel more comfortable. Or don't do a class; do some physical activity for which you can wear your usual clothes and where the emphasis will be on enjoyment rather than on feeling inadequate or inferior to young, svelte things.

Exercise is boring If you feel this way, you may do best to go for the 'adapting your normal day' option: that is climbing stairs instead of using lifts or escalators, or doing necessary physical chores. You could make a point of varying your activities every day or making the same activity different, such as by walking to different places or listening to favourite music on a personal stereo while you run.

I haven't got time The accumulated 30 minutes of exercise a day is obviously for you. A brisk 10 minute walk twice a day to somewhere you need to go, a bit of stair-climbing, a few necessary daily chores and you are there. It isn't necessary to go somewhere special to exercise. Many people have a lot of fun and derive considerable benefit from dancing in the front room at home.

I feel guilty taking the time from the family for myself If you think that, you probably deserve some time to yourself more than most. Taking a bit of space to be yourself, to do something you enjoy and that makes you feel good is probably the best thing you can do for your family life. If you feel you don't have enough time to do things with your family, let alone by yourself, try involving them in some form of activity that everyone can enjoy together.

3

SLEEPING WELL

A REGULAR good night's sleep is essential for our health and well-being. It is the only time that the brain can shut down and 'relax', whereas the body and muscles can relax at any time. During sleep, our bodies undergo repairs and, according to an increasing number of research findings, our immune systems are given a boost. Yet countless people have difficulty getting enough sleep – and most of them are women.

While one night's loss of sleep is insignificant, the effect of chronic sleep loss is considerable, including difficulty in concentration, poor memory powers, irritability, slow thinking, unhappiness, unpredictable behaviour and a general feeling of being unwell. Not surprisingly, insomniacs have more car accidents and more accidents at work because they are constantly tired. When we have gone without a good night's sleep for a while, for whatever reason, we are likely to be more susceptible to illnesses such as colds and flu.

Concern about sleep is very widespread. A third of those who visit their GPs for health problems say they are dissatisfied with their sleep; and twice as many women as men go to their GPs specifically because of worry about not being able to sleep. Fortunately, some of these concerns may be groundless. According to experts, we often underestimate how much sleep we have had, and we may also have misconceptions about how much we actually need.

• What is sleep? •

Sleep is divided into two different types, called either paradoxical and orthodox sleep or REM (rapid eye movement) and non-REM sleep. During a normal night, 20 per cent of our sleep is REM sleep, when our eyes move around rapidly under our lids and our brain waves are irregular. It is during REM sleep that we dream most vividly, and we are most likely to remember these dreams if we are woken during them. The other 80 per cent of our sleep is non-REM. It is divided into four stages from light to deepest sleep, and our brain waves are long and slow.

Although experts are still not totally clear about the full functions of each type of sleep, it is believed that REM sleep is beneficial and restorative for the brain, while non-REM sleep is the time when body repair takes place: for example, fresh protein is manufactured to replace tissue worn out during the day.

• How much sleep do we need? •

The mythical eight hours   Professor Jim Horne of Loughborough University, a renowned expert on sleep, is adamant that six hours sleep a night is sufficient for most needs. After six hours' sleep, he says, we are unlikely to feel sleepy in the day, which is the key symptom of poor or insufficient sleep. (Feeling drained and heavy in the day, rather than feeling sleepy, is more likely to be a symptom of stress rather than insomnia.) We may enjoy our eight hours' sleep and miss the extra two if denied them, but this is just habit. The last two hours are not essential for the brain or body.

Some people may manage quite happily on even less sleep. As we grow older, we tend to need less sleep although, contrary to belief, the elderly don't need significantly less than the middle-aged. If you have a short sleep cycle but feel adequately refreshed by it, you have no need for worry. However, if your sleep cycle is short and you don't feel well you may have a problem that needs attention. (See below.)

Cat-napping   Many people who claim to manage on very little sleep take cat-naps during the day. (Winston Churchill was a famous cat-napper.) These naps, together with a shorter night-time sleep, can add up to a normal sleep cycle.

Many elderly people may not be able to sleep very long at night because of increased inability to remain awake for long periods during the day. This, exacerbated by illness, loneliness or boredom, may lead them to take naps, particularly after lunch, in the late afternoon and in the middle of the evening. As a result, they may be fully awake after only a few hours of night-time sleep. If they go to bed early because of cold or boredom, or because they feel tired and it doesn't seem appropriate just to nap, they may be wide awake at 1am; not a happy hour to start the next day. The best solution may be to make the mid-evening sleep a nap and then go to bed correspondingly later for the night-time sleep.

One night without sleep doesn't hurt   One night's loss of sleep doesn't do us any harm, irritating though it is the next day. If you have the occasional night when you just can't stop tossing and turning, try to accept that it isn't very important, and perhaps get up and read or, if it is too cold and uncomfortable to stir out of bed, lie and think about something pleasant without subconsciously willing yourself to sleep. It can be helpful to remember that when we stay up late and miss sleep by choice, because of a late party or overnight travel for example, our mood the next day is much better than when we have tossed and turned, even though the sleep loss is the same. One night's bad sleep is unlikely to affect our performance much next day and the following night we quickly make up on all our lost deep sleep, making do with less of the lighter, less essential sleep.

We may get more than we think   Sometimes we believe we have been awake when in fact we have been asleep. What can happen is this. In the early stages of sleep we often return briefly to consciousness. If this flicker of wakefulness lasts longer than 15 seconds we remember it, but how we remember it varies according to how long we have been asleep. If we have been sleeping for more than 10 minutes, we probably realise we have been asleep, whereas if we have been sleeping for any less than 10 minutes we are more likely to claim that we have been awake all the time. If several such awakenings occur each time we drop back to sleep, we may think we have had no sleep at all, whereas in reality we have already had an hour. If you are seriously deprived of sleep, however, you need to find the cause.

• Common causes of sleep problems •

Worry   Once medical problems which can cause insomnia have been discounted, the biggest cause of loss of sleep is stress and worry, according to consumer surveys. One found that worries about personal life, family, work or being unable to 'switch off' accounted for more than half of all sleep difficulties. Once we perceive ourselves as having a sleep problem, we start to worry about that too, which in itself then helps to perpetuate the problem.

If people are under extreme stress or are very anxious or depressed, they may start suffering regular nightmares in which they are persecuted or threatened in some frightening way. This is really a signal to identify and deal with the underlying problem.

Change   All manner of changes can affect sleep patterns. For example, a change in diet, weight, alcohol intake or sexual activity; large lifestyle changes such as marriage, bereavement, changing job, moving house; or environmental changes such as a different bed, a different bedroom, different temperature or lighting can all take their toll on sleep.

Bad beds   Your mattress may be too soft, too hard or too old. Although we often don't think about it, a mattress bought new only lasts about ten years before it becomes lumpy and uncomfortable. Sleep will suffer too if a bed isn't long or wide enough for its occupant(s).

Noise   This is a very common cause of sleep disturbance, particularly the unwelcome sound of a partner's heavy snoring, noise from the road or noise from neighbouring houses. Some people, however, need noise to sleep and can't drop off if all is quiet.

Untimely exercise   While exercise in general helps create good sleep patterns, the timing of it is crucial. A late-night jog or indeed any vigorous exercise within two or three hours of bedtime may be stimulating rather than calming, and may keep you awake.

Disturbed body clock   Our inner body clock, which usually tells us when to wake and when to sleep, can be thrown out by crossing time zones when flying or by having to work odd hours when normally we would be asleep.

Physical causes   Poor sleep may be associated with all sorts of illnesses and conditions as various as angina, stomach ulcers, chronic pain, arthritis, asthma, Parkinsonism and depression. Many women suffer a day or two of disturbed sleep before a period. The discomfort of late pregnancy also prevents easy sleep, and so too may hot flushes when they are a symptom of the menopause.

• Tips to help you sleep •

1 Don't have a heavy meal shortly before you plan to go to bed, but don't go to bed hungry either. A light carbohydrate snack, half an hour before bedtime, may help you sleep because carbohydrates increase the brain levels of a chemical called serotonin which helps to get us off to sleep.

2 Avoid stimulants such as coffee, tea, alcohol and cigarettes before bedtime. Be wary of hidden caffeine. A strong cup of tea contains two thirds as much caffeine as a cup of coffee; cocoa contains one third as much. You will find caffeine in chocolate and in many soft drinks, pain killers, anti-allergy drugs and diuretics. If you have to take any medication before bed and suspect this could be the problem, check with your pharmacist. However, some people are actually helped by a cup of coffee before bed, particularly, it has been found, those who need noisy environments in which to sleep. Sometimes a cup of coffee may be a way of winding down after the day and the calming effects of the ritual may be more powerful for them than the stimulant.

Some people swear by alcohol as a means of dropping off to sleep. It may make you sleepy but the downside is that it can also cause frequent night awakenings. Don't drink too much of anything non-alcoholic before bedtime either, otherwise a full bladder will wake you, even if nothing else will.

3 Make sure your bedroom is as you need it to be. We sleep best when we are neither too warm nor too cold: a room temperature of 17 to 21 °C (65 to 70 °F) is ideal. If too much light comes into your bedroom, try a sleep mask.

4 Make sure your bed is as comfortable as possible. Don't have too many layers of bed clothes. Stick to natural materials such as cotton and wool for bed coverings and feathers for pillows unless you have an allergy to them. If your mattress is too soft and you aren't yet ready to replace it, put a wooden board underneath it.

5 Take exercise during the day. Morning exercise, though fine in itself, won't have much impact on your sleep. To help get yourself comfortably tired at the right time, do something physical in the late afternoon or early evening.

6 If noise bothers you, try ear plugs. If it is noise that is not of your choosing which is the problem – for example, the neighbours' TV – you may find music of your own choice soothing. Find a radio station with music you like and preferably have the kind of radio which can turn itself off after a pre-set time.

7 If anything is on your mind before bedtime, such as tasks to be carried out the following day, write them all down in a list so that you can forget them. If anything is worrying you, try writing that down too and getting it off your chest, instead of taking it to bed with you.

8 Sex at bedtime may not be such a good idea. Whereas sex tends to put men to sleep afterwards, it more often keeps women awake.

9 If your sleep patterns are suffering from jet-lag or from doing shift work, readjust by extending your day and going to sleep when everyone else does, rather than going to sleep when you are tired, which is likely to be the wrong time of day.

10 Consider sleeping pills an absolute last resort. Benzodiazepines, the most common kind prescribed, can quickly become addictive and don't improve sleep for more than a few nights anyway. There are, however, other sleeping pills available now which are claimed not to be addictive. Sleeping pills may be helpful for some people in the very short term: for breaking a cycle of insomnia, for example, if anxiety about not being able to sleep is creating much of the problem.

11 Natural remedies which may help include herbal teas such as camomile and vervain; taking a bath before bedtime to which you add three aromatherapy oils: five drops of camomile, three of vetifer and two of melissa or lime; the homoeopathic remedy *nux vomica* for insomnia caused by overwork, and the remedies *aconite* or *coffea cruda* for insomnia caused by anxiety.

• If you really can't sleep. . . . •

1 Don't take a nap in the day, even if you are really tired.

2 Do not read, watch television, eat, talk on the telephone or have arguments in your bedroom. Associate bed just with sleep (and sex).

3 Don't go to bed until you are really sleepy.

4 If you are still awake after 10 minutes of trying to fall asleep, get up, go into another room and do something to occupy your mind pleasurably, such as reading or doing a jigsaw. Think of yourself as relaxing.

5 Go back to bed only when you feel really ready to sleep.

6 Get up the next morning at exactly the same time as usual, setting your alarm clock if necessary. Don't stay in bed even if you have the opportunity. You will feel tired during the day but you should sleep better the following night.

7 If you are in a chronically bad sleeping pattern, such as only being able to fall asleep at 4am and then having to rise at 8am, you may need to re-programme your body clock. The best way to do this is to push on your sleep times until you have gone around the clock and arrived at a reasonable hour. So, if you normally fall asleep at 4am, next day go to bed three hours later at 7am, then the next day at 10am, then 1pm and so on until – sleeping a maximum eight hours at a time – you work round to a suitable bedtime. This is, however, only likely to be possible if you can take a week off from work or your usual commitments.

Free advice on sleep problems is available from the Insomnia Helpline, run by a charity called the Medical Advisory Service. See Useful Contacts.

4

RELAXATION

RELAXATION isn't a luxury, a nice little reward for hard work if we get a moment; nor is it an indulgence. Sufficient relaxation to offset the demands of our lives is actually essential for health. It is a means of undoing damaging physical and emotional tension caused by stress (see page 141).

Stress is inevitable in daily life. Sitting immobile in a traffic jam watching the moments tick by before the plane you were racing to catch takes off, getting a dressing down from the boss, worrying about getting a dressing down from the boss, trying to look after a sick parent as well as a young family, facing a failing marriage or redundancy, dealing with the death of someone close: all these are stresses that can take a toll on our bodies, even though the stress may be more mental than physical.

There are only two ways to deal with the damaging effects of stress: to deal with the causes, if possible; and to learn to relax, so that the body ceases to be in a permanent tense state of readiness for something to happen. Renowned physiotherapist, Laura Mitchell, who has developed her own effective and down-to-earth method of relaxation, makes the important and telling point that rest is one of the in-built rules of the human body. The heart, after every heartbeat, and the uterus, after every contraction during labour, actually rest for longer than they work.

Learning to relax is very valuable for helping overcome phobic anxieties, sleep problems, stomach complaints, headaches, high blood pressure and much else.

• Different types of relaxation •

Relaxation doesn't have to mean sitting in a darkened room, concentrating on tense muscles. Some people are good at switching off and really can relax fully by reading, watching television or enjoying hobbies and sports. If you are able to balance your everyday activities so that you have sufficient relaxation, you do not need to worry about doing anything special. However, you may find that certain types of tension respond best to certain types of activity.

For example, if you are experiencing tension in terms of physical symptoms such as a racing heart, sinking stomach and aches and pain, something designed to relax your body may be particularly beneficial: a soothing bath, a massage, a walk or deep breathing. If your symptoms of stress are more mental, for example inability to concentrate, constant worrying, racing thoughts or intrusive frightening thoughts, something that occupies your mind may be more helpful, such as playing a game, doing a jigsaw, watching television, trying a visualisation technique.

Some methods of relaxation make certain people more tense rather than relaxed. For example, highly anxious people often feel more anxious and even fearful if trying to meditate or carry out muscle relaxation. This may be because tension can be a means of holding in frightening emotions; trying to let go of the tension may leave the person feeling defenceless.

Particular relaxation methods don't always work all the time, even if you find they do work sometimes. It may be better to experiment with your mood and be open to changing tack. You may even find that a body relaxation method works for an overactive mind and vice versa.

If you are carrying areas of tension around which stay tense even when you think you are relaxed, you might benefit from trying something more structured to help you relax. Here are some suggestions.

• Deep breaths •

Take some slow deep breaths whenever you find yourself getting over-stressed or panicky, particularly at times when you can't control your situation, such as when stuck in a car in traffic or in a slow-moving supermarket queue. Make sure that you are breathing the right way round: when you breathe in through your nose your diaphragm should rise, so you look as if your stomach is filling out. When you breathe out, your stomach gets sucked in.

• Physical techniques •

A very commonly used technique is to tense each muscle group before you relax it, so that you can feel the difference between tension and relaxation. Lie or sit somewhere comfortable, wearing loose clothing. Working from the toes up to the head, tense and relax each part of your body in turn. Screw up your toes, feel the sensation of tension and then let go. Move to your calf muscles, your knees, your thighs, your buttocks and your back. Tense and relax your fingers, hands and arms, then your shoulders, neck, jaw, eyes and forehead.

Laura Mitchell's method differs from the above because it doesn't advocate any deliberate tension. She recommends sitting with the head and body comfortably supported and then giving specific orders to each part of the body which you are trying to relax, to enable it to find its position of relaxation naturally and without strain. For example, pull your shoulders gently down towards your feet to relax them and then simply stop. Lengthen your fingers as far as possible to relax them and then stop. Push your body into the support at your back to relax it and then stop. The method is described more fully in her useful book *Simple Relaxation*: see Further Reading.

For further specific information about relaxation techniques or if you would like to find a trained relaxation teacher, send a large stamped address envelope to Relaxation for Living; see Useful Contacts.

• Meditation •

Meditation as practised and taught by spiritual leaders is a means of quietening the mind so that, undistracted by the thoughts and feelings of the day, you can just 'be', achieving along the way peace and contentment and, eventually, clarity of vision and understanding. It just so happens that it is a very valuable means of achieving relaxation as well and it is a good way to help learn to turn off a racing mind.

There are many different methods of meditation, for example concentrating on the breath, a mantra (a special word that is chanted), or an object (see below). No religious or spiritual element is required.

1 Sit in a quiet place in a comfortable position. Shut your eyes and try to relax your muscles. Breathe calmly, counting each breath as you exhale. When you reach ten, start at one again.
2 In a quiet place in your comfortable position, concentrate your attention on your stomach rising and falling with each breath.
3 In a quiet place in your comfortable position, become gently aware of your breathing. Every time you breathe out silently say to yourself the word 'one', (or any other word that appeals).
4 Place a simple object in front of you; a lighted candle, a flower or a stone are good choices. As you sit comfortably and quietly, focus on the object as you breathe. The aim eventually is to be able to see the object so clearly in your mind's eye that you can do without it altogether.

If distracting thoughts come into your mind – which they will – during any of these methods, try to let them come and go without concentrating any attention on them. Don't stay with them but don't push them away too hard either. Gently draw yourself back if your attention wanders. Keep going for about 20 minutes. If you find that you can't stop your mind taking over even after several attempts at meditation, try progressive muscle relaxation first.

• Imagery •

Choose a scene for yourself which you think you might find calming and peaceful. For example, you might choose to imagine yourself on a deserted beach, by a mountain stream or a babbling brook. Create the scene for yourself or choose a real place that gives you pleasure, or has done in the past. Try to conjure it up in every detail and use all your senses to make it come alive. For example, if you choose a beach, feel the warm sun on every part of your body, feel the gentle breeze caressing you, feel the sand between your toes. See the colours of the sea, the soft movement of the waves, hear the seagulls and the soft splash of water against rock, smell and taste the sea salt in the air. Imagine yourself strolling along the shore, drinking in all these sensations, then stretching out on a towel on the sand and drifting deeper and deeper into peaceful relaxation as you lie with eyes closed, the sounds and smells now a calming muted background.

Make sure you pick your own scene rather than adapting one from a book. You know what specific sights, sounds, colours and activities are appealing and peaceful for you. If you are a person who doesn't like beaches, no amount of imagination is going to make it work for you as a relaxation tool.

• Self-hypnosis •

Learning and using the skill of self-hypnosis can help make relaxation easier. Sit or lie comfortably in a relaxed position. Fix your gaze on a particular object in front of you, such as a vase of flowers or a picture, and take a few deep breaths. Then, as you gaze at your object, say to yourself something like 'my eyelids are starting to feel heavier and heavier, so heavy that they want to shut'. Say this a few times and then allow your eyes to shut and say to yourself, 'I am going to relax and count slowly from one to ten. As I say each number, I shall feel more and more deeply relaxed.' Start counting and after each number, add one phrase such as, 'yes, I am feeling more relaxed,' 'I am feeling even more and more relaxed,' 'I am getting so relaxed and feeling so peaceful,' etc.

When you have reached ten and have spent as long as you want in your relaxed state, say 'now I am going to count from ten to one. As I say each number I shall become more and more alert, and when I reach number one, I shall open my eyes feeling fully alert and refreshed.'

• Yoga •

Yoga is an Eastern discipline which uses special movements, positions and controlled gentle breathing to achieve a peaceful state of mind. It is both excellent exercise and good for relaxation, as you work only within the natural limits of the body, never pushing it further than it is ready to go. The physical postures in yoga are called *asanas* and the breathing exercises are called *pranayama*. It is best to start yoga in a class taught by a qualified teacher rather than on your own from a book, as a teacher can better tell whether you are achieving the right positions or trying too hard. Many local authorities offer day or evening classes in yoga. Look also at health-food shop notice boards or ask at your local library.

• T'ai Chi •

This is a Chinese exercise based on long slow sequences of flowing rhythmic movements which look rather like gentle dance movements. They help to concentrate the mind and relax the body. The aim is to achieve inner peace through co-ordination, balance and breathing. T'ai Chi is one of the martial arts but, if practised for relaxation purposes its softer aspects are emphasised. The movements are very simple to master and satisfying to perform. In China it is very popular with the elderly while here it appeals to all ages. Look at notice boards in health-food shops or ask at the local library for classes.

• Massage •

Massage is a very pleasant means of relaxation and you don't have to master any complicated strokes to derive the benefit. It is a proven method for releasing tension and lessening stress-related problems such as migraine, insomnia and chronic back or neck pain.

Either treat yourself to a professional massage or arrange with a friend or partner to give and receive a massage. When giving a massage, ask the person to lie on their stomach first, on a firm surface softened with blankets, and then use different movements to achieve different effects. Stroke the body slowly to soothe, briskly to stimulate. Achieve variety by changing speed and pressure. Knead shoulders and fleshy areas such as hips and thighs to stretch muscles and relax them. Try pummelling: bouncing the side of your relaxed fists one after the other against your partner's skin. Experiment with what feels good, always keeping your hands in contact with your partner's skin. Continuous relaxed touch feels pleasant and safe whereas sudden removal and then replacing of hands on another part of the body is unsettling and uncomfortable. Make sure the person is warm and try using oils, if the idea appeals to you both.

Giving a massage can be almost as good as receiving one because the act of offering massage is soothing too. If you haven't much time, opt for just a partial massage, such as head, feet or hands. As long as you listen to your own and the other person's responses, you shouldn't go wrong. However, never carry out massage on someone who has a fever, a skin infection or an inflammatory condition such as thrombosis or phlebitis. If pain shoots down their arms and legs as you massage their back, stop at once.

For further information, see Further Reading.

5

FEELING GOOD

MANY people have to face considerable adversity and difficulties in their lives, perhaps caring for a severely handicapped child or looking after a chronically sick parent at the same time as raising a family of young children, and yet they still manage to laugh and smile and be active and energetic. They are also quite likely to stay healthy, despite the emotional and physical demands made upon them. A great deal of exciting research now shows that if you are optimistic and can enjoy the small pleasures of life, you are likely to stay healthier or handle ill health better, whatever else may happen to you.

When we are feeling depressed, miserable or bad about ourselves we are more vulnerable to infections and specific diseases. In one interesting experiment carried out at the University of Vienna, a few people who tended to suffer cold sores were hypnotised and asked to remember something very painful from their past, such as the loss of someone they loved dearly. All proceeded to develop cold sores immediately afterwards, seeming to show that we are more susceptible to infection (in this case the herpes virus) when our emotions are very negative.

• Illnesses linked with feelings •

Allergies, epilepsy, asthma, arthritis, skin, hair, scalp, teeth and gum problems, back pain, pelvic pain, irritable bowel syndrome, ulcers, insomnia and headaches are common conditions which all seem to be linked with feelings. Attacks or flare-ups are far more common when we are feeling bad or are under stress that we cannot handle confidently or comfortably. In one study of patients carried out by a Boston dermatologist, life stresses were clearly linked with outbreaks of psoriasis, eczema and hives: with warts, acne and severe itching the stress link at the onset of the outbreak or problem was at least 94 per cent.

A link between stress and dental decay seems to be indicated by work carried out at a dental school in Philadelphia. Researchers took saliva samples from students before asking them to meditate and took samples again when the meditation session was over. Analysis showed that bacteria levels in saliva dropped after meditation (which reduces stress), indicating less risk of dental decay. Elsewhere, in a different experiment, researchers measured substances in saliva which help the body fight off infections such as colds. They found immunity stronger when people were in a positive mood than when they were feeling low.

As far as the big killer diseases go, heart disease is more common in people who are overly ambitious, impatient and easily made angry. Cancer is more common in those who are deeply depressed or especially fearful and anxious.

• Accidents and stress •

Accidents happen more often when we are under stress. In one rather impressive study researchers were able to predict, from studying the stresses nurses were facing and how they were handling them, which of the nurses would suffer accidents such as dropping things or scraping their cars – and when it might happen.

• The feel-good factor •

If all this seems rather disturbing, it needn't be. It isn't how much stress or unhappiness you have to face which lowers body defences so much as how you handle it. The way we think about our lives affects the way important brain chemicals act on our immune systems. It has been found from blood samples that those who are usually optimistic have more of the white blood cells which are important in fighting illness than people who tend to have a more pessimistic outlook on life.

The more things we can make happen for ourselves, in order to feel good about life, the better our health is likely to be. Research clearly shows that taking pleasure, in many little ways, is far from a luxury: it is positively essential for wellbeing. In fact, indulging all of our senses can help us to health.

• The positive power of touch •

Touch, in the form of stroking or massage, can help premature babies' chances of survival. When a hand reaches out to touch and comfort us, the racing heartbeat can slow down. This was seen in one study, when researchers lightly touched subjects on the wrist, but heartbeats were unchanged when the researchers just stood nearby or when the subjects touched their own wrists. Massage, another study showed, can help reduce tension in extremely anxious patients when drugs and relaxation techniques have failed, and can also free people to open up more about their worries.

• Seeing is believing •

What we choose to look at can be beneficially calming. Gazing into a fish tank, for example, lowers blood pressure and having a hospital room with a view of trees and grass can speed recovery after an operation, reduce the amount of post-operative pain killers needed and reduce the length of time you need to stay in hospital. Even recalling the image of a particularly pleasant and peaceful scene can have a relaxing effect.

• Hearing helps •

Listening to music appears to be linked with the release of endorphins, body chemicals which are powerful natural pain killers and which can also induce heady feelings of euphoria. Music can lower blood pressure, slow breathing and reduce the level of circulating stress hormones in the body. It can also excite and arouse. When music is played before, during and after operations, it has been found that patients are less anxious, have less need for post-operative pain relief and are ready to leave hospital more quickly after recovery. However, it is music that you like which will have good effects on you, not music that others feel you ought to like, and which in fact may leave you cold.

• Aah. . . the aroma •

Smells can affect our mood for better or worse. A whiff of spiced apple, for example, can lower stress and blood pressure, slowing breathing and relaxing the body. Smells may make us relax because of pleasant associations or just because of the act of breathing more deeply to savour them. There is much research going on to find out which odours help what conditions. For example, in one study, inhaling the smell of peach helped people with chronic pain to relax. Probably, however, rather than any one smell having the same effect, different smells will have different connotations for each of us.

Not all odours that affect us have a conscious effect on us. Aromatic chemicals secreted in a man's body odour appear to have a subliminal effect on women: those who have sex at least once a week with a man are more likely to have regular menstrual cycles, and a non-troublesome menopause, than women who have sex less often or not at all.

• The taste test •

Different foods can affect the production of brain chemicals which in turn affect our mood; conversely, the prevalence of certain brain chemicals can affect our appetite for particular foods. To stay alert and energetic we need more protein (which stimulates production of the 'alertness' chemicals dopamine and noradrenalin) and less carbohydrate. An evening meal high in carbohydrate (which stimulates production of calming serotonin) and low in protein is likely to ease us into sleep when bedtime comes, especially for anyone who has difficulty turning off mentally and sleeping.

• Positive feelings and good health •

Here are some suggestions for incorporating positive attitudes, feelings and pleasures into our daily lives and making them work for our health.

• Be optimistic •

If you worry about your health without any real reason, you are far more likely to fall prey to illness than those who are optimistic about their own wellbeing. One study showed that those who don't think they are very well, even when examination shows them to be in perfect health, tend to end up suffering more illnesses than those who think they are healthy, despite doctors' reports that they are not.

Being optimistic simply means hoping for the best, not putting a black view on things and not assuming that, because something has gone wrong, everything else will go wrong too. Being optimistic does not mean being unrealistic, however. You can't just hope that you'll get a better job without applying for one, or plan your future on the basis of winning a big money prize.

• Laugh, smile and be merry •

Laughing is like having an inner-body workout. A good laugh exercises almost all of your muscles, including those of the face, arms, legs and stomach. It stimulates your circulation and your metabolism and then, when you stop, you feel wonderfully relaxed. One leading medical expert on laughter claims that having a laugh at least 100 times a day is equivalent to 10 minutes' hard rowing. Laughter can reduce the sensation of pain and stimulate the immune system: when we laugh we produce higher levels of a chemical that helps us fight off infection, but the effect doesn't last long so we need to laugh often. Laughter also has good mental effects, distracting us from anxieties and helping us relieve the tension of any unexpressed anger, hostility or frustration.

If you can't manage a laugh, or even if you can, smile a lot instead or as well. You can help your mood if you smile even when you don't feel happy because the physical expression of smiling increases blood flow to the brain and stimulates the release of endorphins, the chemicals that block pain and increase wellbeing. Then suddenly you do feel happier. Smiling makes the blood pressure and heart rate drop and also helps relax the body.

• Read the good news •

What you read can affect your mood quite powerfully. Doctors often recommend that depressed people shouldn't read newspapers or watch television news because all the bad news depresses them more. Fortunately, the opposite is true too. A researcher gave some people positive and negatives statements to read. The positive ones made them demonstrably happier, even if they hadn't felt happy to start with, and when they read the negative ones, they felt sad.

So, if you are feeling down, look for things that will lighten your mood, even if you don't feel like it at all. Write down some positive statements about yourself, read from a book that always makes you feel cheerful, think some positive thoughts, watch a funny film or flick through some cartoons.

• Explain failures positively •

If something goes wrong, you can either blame yourself or blame the circumstances. It is far more healthy to see the problem as something that can be rectified or which need not happen next time, than to see one's own shortcomings as the cause of disaster.

It is an important distinction to make because the explanation you give to yourself can powerfully affect your mood as well as your attitude towards yourself and life. In one study, for example, students were deliberately failed on a test. Half were given to understand that the failure was due to their own incompetence while the other half were told they were not to blame. The students who thought themselves incompetent became depressed while those who didn't think they were to blame were unconcerned by their own failure.

Unfortunately, women have more of a tendency towards what psychologists term 'an internal locus of control' (meaning they see themselves as responsible for whatever happens to them), whereas men have more of an external locus of control (they think circumstances are to blame). If a woman loses a tennis game, she will more likely think it is because she is no good, can't concentrate, is too fat, etc. The man who loses more likely blames indigestion, poor weather, a stone in his shoe. Neither extreme is good. If we don't take responsibility where relevant, we can't make changes for the better; but if we take responsibility where there is none to be taken, we do ourselves significant disservice.

• See success •

If you have some daunting or challenging task to perform, be it giving a speech at your child's school or returning faulty goods to a shop, imagine yourself doing it successfully. The more you rehearse success, the more successful you are likely to be. Spend as much time as you can with people who encourage you or who are naturally optimistic themselves and can be an inspiring example.

• Feel your power •

The more we can feel in control in our life, the healthier and happier we are. That doesn't mean trying to control other people or even trying to control everything that happens to ourselves: that could mean too much safety and sameness and no stimulating challenges or risks. Feeling our power and feeling in control means recognising that we can always have an impact on a situation, however little or however limited, at times. For example, when about to have an operation, using breathing exercises to lessen anxiety or choosing to listen to a music tape before and during the operation are simple actions which can have an enormously beneficial effect on outcome, recovery and speed of discharge.

In one interesting experiment, volunteers were asked to undertake a complicated arithmetic problem but were disturbed by some irritating and intrusive noise. Half were told that, if absolutely desperate, they could press a button to have the noise stopped (although in reality pressing the button would achieve nothing), while the others were not given any chance of controlling it. Those who thought they could control the noise suffered far fewer stress symptoms, such as speeding heart rate and sweaty palms (and therefore didn't even need to try to control the noise).

In similar vein, when people go to the dentist, many feel more relaxed about undergoing dental treatment if they know they can raise a hand to stop it at any time. Feeling helpless, on the other hand, can lead to depression.

Even if a situation is itself uncontrollable – a marriage where your partner is unfaithful, a job where you cannot get advancement – you can still alter your own situation, develop your own interests or move on.

• Aim for happiness now •

Don't set up expectations for your future that can detract from your chances of happiness today. If you don't feel satisfied because you have not yet achieved the job status or affluence or lifestyle that you imagine means happiness, it means you are concentrating on what you don't have rather than what you do have. If you take a look at what you have right now, you might see you have much of considerably higher value than you realised. So maybe you aren't boss of your own small company, don't have the salary you would like or don't have a really good relationship and two children. True happiness lies in narrowing the gap between where you see yourself and where you tell yourself you want to be.

• Be loving •

Having good lovers and/or good friends or loving family can do more to keep you healthy than taking the right amount of exercise, eating properly and not smoking or drinking, an important American study once found. It is not just our bodies that need touching but our hearts. A large study of Israeli men who had had heart attacks found that they were more likely than those who stayed healthy to claim that their wives did not show them affection. Feeling loved and showing love are good for all of us. So cuddle someone, pat a pet or tend a plant. It all counts.

• Do things for others •

No one quite knows why but doing things to help others, whether it is those we know or those we don't, seems to benefit us as well as them. One Michigan study in which the health and lifestyle of nearly 3000 inhabitants were monitored for ten years, found that those who did voluntary work had a death rate two and a half times lower than those who didn't. There does seem to be some effect on the immune system. A group of people were shown some videos, one of which was of Mother Teresa caring for the sick and the others of neutral subjects. People's immune function, as measured by levels of certain chemicals in the blood, rose only when watching Mother Teresa. It seems even just having one's compassion stirred does something positive to the body's defences.

• Take a lot of little pleasures •

Real happiness is about feeling happy a lot of the time rather than feeling ecstatically happy on a few occasions, says American psychologist Dr Robert Ornstein, an expert on attitude and health. Better to build in a lot of little pleasures – a ten-minute walk when it is sunny, playing a game with the children, sitting by an open window, drinking the perfect cup of coffee – than to put your energies into creating the wedding of the year or the holiday of a lifetime. Feeling good in little ways a lot of the time means a fairly permanent positive outlook that will be a plus whenever difficulties come along to be handled.

....

6

INDULGENCES AND ADDICTIONS

MOST pleasures that we indulge in can lead to dependence or addiction (two words for the same thing) if for some reason they get out of hand. Sometimes the cause of addiction may be physical: nicotine and hard drugs are pharmacologically addictive. Sometimes the reason may be primarily psychological: for example, a very frequent need to have sex and with numerous new partners.

When does a pleasure or indulgence become a dependence or an addiction? It happens when an activity is engaged in to excess, be it drinking, gambling, dieting, working, spending money, watching television or anything else that takes over too much of a life. If you feel 'compelled' to indulge, can't stop yourself, think about the activity a great deal whenever you are not doing it, deny to all and sundry that it is a problem and continually backtrack on plans or promises to give up or cut down, you probably have a dependence you would do well to face.

• Smoking •

Smoking is not a healthy habit, as we all know, but it isn't always addictive. Some people are able to have a cigarette or two every day and not crave for more, others can have 10, 15 or even 40 in a single evening and then none at all for a week. It may be relatively easy for those who smoke so little to stop if they decide they really want to. However, some people who are used to only one or two cigarettes a day, after meals, may find even this habit extraordinarily difficult to give up. Dependence on nicotine develops the more you smoke. For women, pharmacological dependence tends to occur at 20 cigarettes a day or over, and this then compounds the psychological dependence.

Whereas 40 years ago, women smoked only half as much as men, statistics show that today women tend to smoke in the same numbers as men. The number of men who smoke has dropped considerably over the years, but women are giving up much more slowly. About 33 per cent of men smoke and 30 per cent of women. A particularly worrying recent finding from the Institute of Cancer Research in Surrey is that women who smoke have a significantly greater chance of developing lung cancer than men who smoke the same number of cigarettes.

If you are smoking over 20 cigarettes a day, or even if you smoke fewer, it is likely that you worry about it, even if you find the thought of trying to stop daunting. The most important factor in giving up successfully is really wanting to give up. Facing the undeniable facts about smoking's effects on you may be a spur, or you may be more motivated by looking at the benefits of not smoking (see below).

• What smoking does to you •

1 Tobacco causes 90 per cent of UK lung cancers and kills over 12,000 women every year. Lung cancer has overtaken breast cancer as the leading cause of death in women in many parts of the UK and women smokers appear to be even more susceptible to it than male smokers.

2 Smoking can also cause cancer of the lip, mouth, pharynx, larynx, oesophagus, pancreas and bladder. It may have a link with cancers of the nose, stomach, kidneys and liver and with myeloid leukaemia.

3 Smoking is associated with cancer of the cervix, probably because it causes changes in the tissues of the cervix and also appears to lower immune function in the cervix.

4 Coronary artery and vascular disease account for a third of all deaths related to smoking. At least 80 per cent of heart attacks suffered by smokers in early middle age are caused by smoking. Ultrasound can now show that even teenage and young adult smokers have evidence of early thickening of the arteries.

5 Over 90 per cent of people who have peripheral vascular disease (PVD, obstructed circulation in the limbs) are smokers. Every year surgeons carry out over 2000 amputations, mainly as a result of PVD.

6 Bronchitis, emphysema and other respiratory diseases account for a fifth of deaths from smoking. Airways in the lung become gradually more and more obstructed and breathing becomes progressively more difficult for years before death.

7 Smoking significantly increases the likelihood of breast abscesses that are not connected with breast feeding.

8 One in three women smokers is at risk of developing urinary incontinence (see page 467).

9 Smoking is associated with backache. The more cigarettes smoked, the more severe the backache.

10 The menopause occurs two or three years earlier in women smokers.

11 Smokers have significantly fewer teeth than non-smokers. They also have more wrinkled and sallow skin.

12 Smoking kills one person in the UK every five minutes. Every cigarette smoked shortens your life by about five and a half minutes.

• What smoking can do to your children •

1 Smoking can reduce fertility. If a woman smokes when pregnant, she has twice the risk of miscarriage, a higher risk of complications and more likelihood of suffering a stillbirth than a woman who doesn't smoke.
2 If you smoke during pregnancy, a daughter has a 29 per cent higher risk of miscarriage and complications when she becomes pregnant and a son has a higher risk of minor reproductive abnormalities, particularly undescended testes.
3 Children of mothers who were smoking ten or more cigarettes a day after the fourth month of pregnancy tend to progress more poorly at school, at least up until the age of 16.
4 Children of smoking parents suffer more frequent and more severe respiratory illnesses, particularly asthma.
5 Children of smokers themselves inhale the equivalent of 80 to 150 cigarettes a year.
6 Passive smoking is now the biggest single factor in cot deaths, with one in three babies at risk.

• The health benefits of stopping •

1 Ex-smokers have fewer problems with ill-health and fewer days of illness than smokers.
2 One year after stopping smoking, you have only half the smoker's extra risk of heart disease. Within two or three years, your risk of heart attack may be no higher than that of women who have never smoked in their lives – however much you smoked before.
3 After 15 years of not smoking, you have almost no higher risk of death than anyone else from any of the smoking-related illnesses.
4 Your skin looks better, your teeth are healthier and you smell better.
5 Any weight gain is unlikely to be more than half a stone, if you do not eat significantly more to compensate for not smoking, and should be lost after a few months. If fear of any weight gain is what puts you off trying to stop smoking, you might consider chewing nicotine gum for a while once stopped, which seems to help keep weight stable.
6 The psychological benefits are endless, and individual. You may feel increased self-esteem, more attractive, relief not to be treated as a social outcast and a powerful sense of achievement.

• How to stop smoking •

Most people just make the decision and stop. If that seems too daunting, there are many methods which claim success in helping people stop smoking, but they can only help – if they do help – when you are absolutely determined that you want to stop. Nothing can make that decision for you.

Be very wary of high-success claims – often of 80 per cent or more – from some of the methods. According to QUIT, a UK charity which aims to help people stop smoking, a method can only be counted as a success if someone who has used it is still not smoking after a year. However, relatively few stop-smoking therapies do follow-up, let alone for a year, and often count as a success someone who leaves the session not smoking. Whichever way you try to give up smoking, don't get downhearted if you don't succeed first time. Evidence shows that, far from breeding failure, the more efforts people make to stop, the higher their chances of succeeding in the long run.

Hypnotherapy   In this type of treatment, you are put into a state of deep relaxation in which you may be more open than usual to suggestions, such as that you will never want to smoke again or that you will, from now on, think of smoking as a dirty, unattractive habit. The therapist may also try to boost your confidence and your belief in your ability to stop smoking. During hypnotherapy you are aware of everything that is going on and are at no time unconscious. Some therapists teach you self-hypnosis techniques so that you can carry on sessions at home, as needs be, or they may give you a tape to listen to at home. Costs vary enormously but the average is about £30 per session. To find a local properly trained hypnotherapist send a large sae to the Institute for Complementary Medicine: see Useful Contacts.

Acupuncture   Acupuncture is an ancient Chinese medicine which views disease as the result of blockages in the essential life energy that flows through our bodies. Inserting special needles in specific places on the body, according to where the blockage is, is believed to be able to free this important energy. The part of the body that is treated for smoking addiction is the ear. The acupuncturist inserts a tiny staple in the ear which is left in place for about a week. During this time, twiddling the staple every time you feel an urge to smoke is supposed to reduce or stop the craving. Costs vary but average at £30 per session. To find a reputable acupuncturist, send a large sae to the Institute for Complementary Medicine: see Useful Contacts.

Laser Therapy   This is the name of a company and its therapy. A cold laser beam is directed at acupuncture points in the ear, nose and hand, to stimulate the release of the body's own natural pain killers which reduce withdrawal symptoms. Counselling is also part of the process. Three sessions cost £85, but clinics are only available in a few parts of the UK and Northern Ireland. See Useful Contacts.

Immunology   This is a method only offered to 20-a-day-plus smokers who have failed with other methods. Clinics around the country are run by a research group called the National Health Association and the method involves taking tiny amounts of tobacco dissolved in sterile water to stop your craving. The actual amounts of tobacco required are decided according to the amount you smoke. You also pay according to the amount you smoke: the fee is whatever it costs you to smoke for six months. See Useful Contacts.

Nicotine gum   You should chew up to 15 pieces a day over a three-month period to reduce craving once you have stopped smoking, then gradually reduce the amount you chew until you aren't using any at all. If you are a heavy smoker, you may need the 4mg-strength gum which is only available on private prescription from your doctor. The 2mg, lower-strength gum can be bought direct from pharmacies. Using nine or more pieces of gum a day appears to lead to significantly less weight gain after stopping smoking than chewing five pieces or fewer per day. Some people complain that they don't like the taste, get indigestion, or suffer nausea from chewing the gum. Anyone with dentures may have difficulties and anyone with a peptic ulcer should not use it.

Nicotine patches At the time of writing, Nicabate, Nicorette Patch and Nicotinell TTS are the only patches which are licensed by the government. They are available direct from pharmacies or on private prescription. Only use a licensed patch, so buy from a pharmacy and not from any other outlet. The patches are used for a full course or set period. There are three strengths of patch, with the idea that you use the strongest at the beginning and then gradually reduce the strength through the course. The patches look a bit like plasters and are worn on your arm, chest or back, so that the nicotine is absorbed through the skin. They are replaced daily. Side-effects may include disturbed sleep, vivid dreams, nausea, skin rashes and itchiness around the patch.

Quitline A free information and advice service for help and support while giving up smoking, or for referral to stop-smoking groups. The line is open on weekdays from 9.30am to 5.30pm. See Useful Contacts.

Stop-smoking groups These are groups run usually by doctors, nurses or other health professionals for groups of up to 12 people who want to stop smoking. There are about five sessions, during which participants are helped to prepare themselves for stopping, set a date, stop and stay stopped. People often find the group support extremely helpful. Free or very cheap. Ring Quitline (see Useful Contacts) for details.

Allen Carr method Allen Carr encourages you to make a positive commitment never to smoke again, by showing that in giving up smoking one is giving up nothing of value. The positive attitude is necessary, he says, to prevent a sense of deprivation and a return to smoking. He believes that nicotine addiction and an unwillingness to face up to being addicted is what keeps people smoking. For further information, read his book, *The Easy Way to Stop Smoking*: see Further Reading.

Full Stop This is the name of a course that runs for two weekends with follow-up phone support. The method aims to help smokers overcome feelings of deprivation and irritability, and provide a practical technique to prevent returning to smoking. It encourages the would-be ex-smoker to accept that desires to smoke will continue at first but will fade in time, and that these are best coped with by the methods taught, rather than denied or your life lived so as to avoid them, such as not going into pubs, avoiding coffee or other smokers, etc. You can phone for details – see Useful Contacts – or read the self-help book, *How to Stop Smoking and Stay Stopped*: see Further Reading.

_____ **USEFUL TIP** _____

However you give up smoking, it might be wise to cut down on your caffeine intake. Smokers tend to drink more coffee than non-smokers because they metabolise caffeine faster; but caffeine metabolism slows down within days of stopping smoking which means that, if you keep drinking the same amount that you were drinking as a smoker, your blood levels of caffeine may rise by 250 per cent and significantly increase smoking withdrawal symptoms. This reduced rate of caffeine metabolism continues for at least six months after stopping smoking.

Adifax   If weight gain is an enormous problem after stopping smoking, it may be due to a lack of serotonin, a brain chemical which affects mood. The brains of smokers develop large numbers of nicotine receptors which release serotonin but this stops when smoking stops. Serotonin is supplied by carbohydrates, so a craving after stopping smoking for bread, cakes and chocolate, etc, could be the body's attempt to make up the shortfall. Adifax is the brand name for the serotonin-releasing agent dexfenfluramine which has been found, in at least one American study with overweight women smokers, to prevent weight gain after stopping smoking. It is only licensed in the UK as a treatment to be given for a maximum of three months for obesity although a doctor can prescribe it for another purpose if he or she personally sees fit.

Tips for breaking the habit   For general advice which applies to handling any kind of addiction, see Breaking the Habit, page 62.

• Drinking •

The standard advice given by health professionals is that women should drink no more than 14 units of alcohol a week with, preferably, two days in the week when no alcohol is consumed at all. A unit is half a pint of ordinary-strength beer or lager (strong beers, strong lagers and cider can be up to three times as strong), a pub-measure glass of wine or sherry or a single pub-measure of spirits.

We all react differently to alcohol, however. Our weight, frame, size and height have a major bearing on how alcohol affects us and we probably all know someone who just can't take any alcohol, or who appears unaffected by much larger amounts than seems wise.

• Effects on women •

As a rule, women cannot handle as much alcohol as men. Not only are women smaller and slighter in general than men, but our bodies have a greater proportion of fat whereas men's have more water, leaving us, compared with men, with a more concentrated amount of alcohol in our systems when we drink.

In the few days before a period and also when we ovulate, we are more susceptible than normal to the effects of alcohol. We absorb it more quickly and therefore may get drunk more quickly.

Whenever we drink, alcohol passes through the stomach into the bloodstream and on to the brain. We feel the effects within 20 minutes, or probably in less than ten when taken on an empty stomach. The liver has to burn up the alcohol and does this at the rate of one unit per hour.

• The positive side of alcohol •

1 Drinking in moderation seems to raise levels of high density lipoproteins, HDL or 'good' cholesterol which helps prevent blood clots and therefore may reduce risk of heart disease.
2 Alcohol can reduce anxiety and release inhibitions, which can be useful at times but dangerous at others. (More accidents happen in the home when women have been drinking.)
3 Consumed in moderate amounts, it also appears to stimulate compassion towards others. An American study found people more willing to offer to help others in need after they had had a few drinks.

• The negative effects of alcohol •

Unfortunately, this is a much longer list.

1 Drinking heavily can lead to inflammation of the liver (alcoholic hepatitis) or scarring of the liver (alcoholic cirrhosis). Women can develop liver problems after a shorter heavy-drinking period than men and the problems may also be more serious.
2 Alcohol can cause inflammation of the stomach lining and make a stomach ulcer worse. It can also damage the pancreas.
3 Drinking well above the recommended limits doubles the risk of cancer of the oesophagus. If you smoke as well as drink, the risk increases by 150 times. It trebles risk of cancer of the pharynx and quadruples risk of cancer of the larynx.
4 Heavy drinking can double the risk of stroke.
5 Drinking too much is commonly associated with high blood pressure.
6 Despite sometimes appearing to raise someone's spirits, alcohol is, in fact, a depressant.
7 One study has found a link between breast cancer and even moderate drinking but this is a matter of contention and not widely accepted. Much more research is needed before any certain link between alcohol and breast cancer can be proved.

• Drinking in pregnancy •

1 Women who drink over 35 units a week reduce their fertility.
2 Alcohol consumed while pregnant can cross the placenta and affect the foetus

in the womb, with the most serious effects likely in the early weeks of pregnancy when crucial body organs and the nervous system are developing. Doctors have tended to play it safe and recommend that women should drink no alcohol while pregnant. This is fine for the doctors but is a restriction on women which may not be wholly warranted. Researchers in Edinburgh have concluded, from studying over 1000 pregnancies, that one alcoholic drink a day or the equivalent a week (but not all at once) does no harm.

3 There may be a link between drinking more than 14 units a week and miscarriage.
4 Drinking more than ten units a week increases the risk of having an underweight baby.
5 Birth defects are much more likely to occur if pregnant women drink extremely heavily. Foetal alcohol syndrome, which includes growth deficiencies, facial malformations, central nervous system problems and lowered IQ, can affect the babies of women who regularly drink more than 56 units a week.

• Do you drink too much? •

You may not know how much you are drinking but be a little concerned in case it is too much. A good way to find out is to keep a drink diary for a few weeks: note down every drink you have each day and tot up your units of alcohol per week.

There are likely to be some obvious signs if alcohol is affecting you adversely. The organisation Alçohol Concern suggests you watch out for:

• Needing to have alcohol at hand.
• Getting into trouble (for example, at work, with money, with the police) because of your drinking.
• Being angry when people discuss your drinking.
• Making drink a top priority in your life.
• Having to increase the amount you drink to feel the effect.
• Feeling sick, irritable, having the shakes, sweating in the morning or in the middle of the night.
• Having accidents or injuries because of drinking.
• Other people telling you they are worried about your drinking.

If you are only drinking a little too much, you may be able to cut down just by deciding to and sticking to it. It may help to look at when you tend to drink most – such as when you are nervous, bored or lonely – and try to find ways to deal with the problem or circumstance differently. See also the section at the end of this chapter on breaking habits. If you cannot go it alone, don't be ashamed to seek help.

• Where to find help •

There are at least 100 independent and confidential advice centres in England and Wales, known variously as councils on alcohol, alcohol information centres, alcohol advice centres or alcohol counselling centres. By approaching one of these, you should be able to find out about all types of help available, including medical and counselling services, self-help and therapy groups, in your area. Going to the advice centre is free.

Women are often concerned that if they reveal they have a drinking problem their children will be taken away from them, so they resist seeking help. These fears can be discussed in confidence with a counsellor at an alcohol advice centre and usually be allayed. There are increasing numbers of women alcohol counsellors so, if seeing a woman is important to you, this can quite likely be arranged.

You can find the number of your local centre in the phone book under 'alcohol' or contact Alcohol Concern: see Useful Contacts.

If your GP is sympathetic, he or she may be able to help you withdraw from alcohol gently or may, if you like, refer you to a specialist alcohol-treatment unit at a hospital, as an out-patient or in-patient, as appropriate.

Alcoholics Anonymous has over 2000 self-help groups in Britain. Your local group is listed under alcohol in the phone book, or you can contact the head office in York: see Useful Contacts

• Tranquillisers •

Benzodiazepines (such as Valium, Ativan and Librium) are a class of minor tranquillisers which were seen as wonder treatments for anxiety, panic attacks or for insomnia until it became apparent in the 1980s that they could be addictive, even at a normal dose. Unfortunately, the problem is still far from over. Although fewer of these drugs are now prescribed – 20 million a year, compared to 30 million in the late 1970s – not all are repeat prescriptions for long-term users who cannot kick the addiction or don't dare try. Benzodiazepines are still the most commonly prescribed drug for anxiety, and many GPs still prescribe them to new patients as sleeping pills, with the risk that another pool of long-term users could be created.

• Important facts about benzodiazepines •

1 Benzodiazepine tranquillisers can indeed relieve anxiety or stress but there is no evidence that they continue working after four months, and they certainly don't in any way deal with the cause of the problem.
2 Benzodiazepine tranquillisers should be prescribed only in cases of extremely severe anxiety and should not be given for longer than a month, at least without a thorough review.
3 Benzodiazepine sleeping pills, such as Dalmane, Mogadon and Normison, are not essentially different from benzodazepine tranquillisers. They have the same action but just a slightly different purpose. They are not likely to be effective after 12 nights of use, and may be of little or no value even after three nights.

4 Dependence on benzodiazepines can occur after a few months of taking them according to the prescribed dosage.

5 Benzodiazepines are prescribed twice as often for women as for men.

Possible side-effects   Common side-effects as a result of taking these drugs can include lack of motivation, loss of energy, lack of co-ordination, inability to concentrate, poor memory, dizziness, weakness, difficulty forming sentences, weight loss, tiredness, a dry mouth, low blood pressure and high fevers.

• When not to take them •

If you can possibly manage without benzodiazepines, don't start taking them at all. Never use them for very short-term anxiety or as a way to avoid dealing with a problem. Sometimes, if you are in such a state that you cannot think straight, using these drugs to calm down for a few days may help you get into the frame of mind where you can tackle a demanding issue. However, they are not the solution themselves to short- or long-term problems, and they are positively harmful if used as a way to reduce anxiety before occasions such as giving a speech or taking an exam as they will reduce your alertness and adversely affect your concentration.

NAMES TO NOTE

If your GP prescribes you a drug for anxiety, depression or inability to sleep, check whether it is a benzodiazepine. Common types are listed below under the problem they are usually prescribed for, but some are prescribed for either anxiety or insomnia.

	generic name	brand name
for anxiety	chlordiazepoxide	Librium, Libritas, Tropium
	clobazam	Frisium
	clorazepate	Tranxene
	diazepam	Alupram, Atensine, Diazemuls Evacalm, Sedapum, Solis, Tensulm, Valium, Valrelease
	ketazolam	Anxon
	lorazepam	Ativan
	medazepam	Nobrium
	oxazepam	Serax, Serenid D, Serenid Forte
sleeping pills	flunitrazepam	Rohypnol
	flurazepam	Dalmane
	lormetazepam	Noctamid
	nitrazepam	Mogadon, Nitrados, Remnos omnite, Surem
	temazepam	Euhypnos, Normison
	triazolam	Halcion

Only ever use tranquillisers for a maximum of a month and sleeping pills for under a fortnight, preferably for only a few days. Sometimes people are prescribed sleeping pills after a bereavement. Pills may help if you really can't sleep in the first few days after the loss of someone very close, but you also need to give full rein to your grief, not let it be masked by tranquillising drugs, under whatever name they are prescribed.

Benzodiazepines should never be prescribed for depression. Antidepressants, if required, are an entirely different class of drugs and are not addictive.

Another drug which can be prescribed short-term for anxiety is buspirone. This is a completely different type of drug from the benzodiazepines. Trials show that, used short term at least, there appears to be no risk of dependence. Side-effects are far fewer. Although effective in relieving anxiety, buspirone does not work as quickly as the benzodiazepines. Unfortunately, anyone who has until now been a user of benzodiazepines is unlikely to find that buspirone works for them.

• Withdrawal •

According to surveys, over half of long-term users would like to stop taking benzodiazepines. Sadly, stopping may not be easy and must never be done suddenly, as the withdrawal symptoms are likely to be very severe. Gradual reduction of dosage, preferably under the supervision of a doctor, will reduce the severity of symptoms.

Withdrawal symptoms can include anxiety, palpitations, panic attacks, restlessness, extra sensitivity to noise and light, shaking, sweating, lack of concentration, feelings of being unreal, tension, nausea and headaches. Obviously these feelings can be very frightening, as well as debilitating and unnerving, and need to be minimised at all costs.

The best idea is to agree with your doctor a sensible amount by which to cut your dosage each week or each fortnight. Self-help and support organisations can also give useful advice. The Council for Involuntary Tranquilliser Addiction runs a telephone helpline (see Useful Contacts) and also publishes books and an audio tape to help sufferers cope with benzodiazepine addiction.

You should expect to suffer some withdrawal symptoms – although not all people do – and they may last up to six weeks. However, it has been argued that withdrawal symptoms last longer if you have used benzodiazepines for a long time, and a more realistic estimate would be 35 days of withdrawal symptoms per year of using the drugs.

If you fear giving up your tranquillisers or sleeping pills, or just don't want to, don't feel you must if your life is not adversely affected. As more than one psychiatrist has pointed out, despite all the bad press benzodiazepines are not lethal.

• Breaking the habit •

Whatever the sort of addiction you are wanting to deal with, some general guidelines may help.

Be sure   The motivation to stop needs to come from you. If you are still denying you have a problem, you are not ready to change. Reluctantly agreeing to try to stop, to keep your partner or children happy when you wouldn't bother for yourself, is not likely to lead to success either; just resentment towards loved ones.

Look at why   Why are you doing whatever you are doing to such excess? If the addiction is physical, you will have to kick it. But there may be a large pyschological component too. You may need to work out how you are going to deal with situations that normally lead you to indulge or what it is that is lacking in your life for which your addiction is a replacement. Maybe you need to let out your emotions more, take assertiveness training, go for marriage guidance, do some therapy, get help with financial or housing problems or something of this ilk.

Ensure you have support   Get support from family, friends, a counsellor or self-help organisation. Make sure it is the kind of support you will find helpful: anxious looks from a spouse who is wondering whether you are thinking of relapsing might be rather irritating and unhelpful. You may need someone who can listen uncritically to your worries and difficulties, and not berate you. Or you may just want people to treat you normally, not with kid gloves.

Recognise your cravings   Expect to feel a desire to do whatever it is you are trying to give up, and realise that feeding it will ensure you feel more and more cravings more and more frequently. Try to look at what you are feeling as if you are floating somewhere above yourself. Rather than saying to yourself, 'I'd kill for a cigarette/cream cake,' think, 'This is an urge to smoke/eat compulsively that I am experiencing now.' By removing the emotive, suffering element of the craving, you may be more able to let the urge pass.

Don't be deceived   You will hear a determined little inner voice telling you that life is boring without your addiction, your health isn't so bad anyway, you always were weak and can't change now, etc. The negative thoughts will be powerful but that is all they are, negative thoughts.

Don't triumph too soon   Once you have kept off your addictive substance/activity for a short while, don't decide to test yourself and see if you can have one/do it once without a problem. You probably can't.

A lapse needn't be lasting   If you do give in and have one/do it once, don't instantly think it is all over and return to full-blown addiction. Some experts like to say that you can turn a lapse not into a relapse but a prolapse, that is, a falling forward into renewed commitment. Stop doing whatever it is or take yourself out of the danger situation as soon as possible, then think about why you lapsed and what you can learn from it to prevent it happening again.

7

HEALTH AT WORK

PAID employment can take up a lot of our lives and much of our energy, so it is important that work should be as satisfying an experience as possible. Feeling good about work can boost confidence and self-esteem whereas unhappiness or anxiety about a job may lead to stress and serious physical and mental problems. Women, of course, commonly have the double responsibility of work and family and may have to struggle hard to find ways to juggle both.

• Are you satisfied with your job? •

There are a number of factors which have a special bearing on whether people are happy with their jobs. Look at the following points and see how they apply to you. Are you satisfied with:

- Your working environment: do you find your physical surroundings comfortable, pleasant, conducive to concentration, etc?
- Your working hours: does your starting and finishing time suit you and your family requirements? If you are expected to work all hours, is this acceptable (because of the reward in salary perhaps) or a problem?
- The people you work with: do you respect your boss, value and feel valued by your peers and enjoy the company of at least some people in your work place?
- Your job content: does your job interest you, challenge you, suit you for some reason, or bore you? Are all your skills required or do you feel that some of your talents are wasted? Is your job content varied or is it very repetitive?
- Your responsibilities: do you feel comfortable with the amount of responsibility you have, or is it too much or too little?
- The way you work: can you organise your time and your priorities yourself and decide on your own methods of achieving a goal, or do you have to do things as and when told by a superior?
- The way you are managed or manage: do you feel you are given credit for good work and good ideas? Do you feel that your department/team is run effectively? Are you kept in the know and are channels of communication open to your boss? If you are in charge, can you delegate comfortably, recognise others' good work, communicate well and be a good listener? Do you feel respected?

- Your future: do you feel you have the chance of advancement, and do you want it? Are you more interested in job security than in promotion to a higher position?
- Your salary: do you feel that what you earn is right for what you do? If you think you are underpaid, do you accept that for a particular reason, such as job satisfaction or because the hours fit in with family needs? Or do you resent it?

· Stress at work ·

Stress at work is a common complaint. It is easy to assume that the work element of our lives – hectic, demanding and full of responsibilities – is most stressful and most often linked with anxiety, depression, heart attacks or other stress-related disorders such as ulcers. However, a demanding and very responsible job may not be stressful to someone who thrives on those elements. On the contrary, a boring repetitive job may be more stressful if you yearn for some occupation in which you can demonstrate your talents or enjoy a bit of variety.

Bearing in mind that different things bother different people, common stressful elements of work can include all the following: having too much responsibility; having too little responsibility; having responsibility but no authority; experiencing too much rapid change; lack of strong direction from the boss; poor prospects; threat of redundancy; incompetent colleagues; poor relationships with colleagues or boss; dealing with hostile members of the public; poor communication in the workplace; sexual harassment; too much noise; too many interruptions; lack of consultation; poor office environment; malfunctioning equipment.

Most people attribute any mental-health problems to their jobs, whether this is actually the case or not. In fact, about 60 per cent of problems at work stem from outside stresses, according to work health expert Professor Cary Cooper. Marital problems, family problems and financial problems can all contribute to and exacerbate stresses at work.

· Symptoms of stress ·

Symptoms of stress are the same, whatever the cause. The tell-tale signs may be any number of the following problems: difficulty falling asleep at night; difficulty relaxing; feeling short-tempered; feeling constantly on edge; loss of energy; lack of motivation; experiencing palpitations and dizziness; indigestion; extreme tiredness; suffering lots of headaches, neck ache or backache; getting constipation or diarrhoea; smoking or drinking more than usual.

· What's the problem? ·

If you aren't satisfied with your job and believe it may be doing your health harm, you need to find out the problem. Dissatisfaction may not in itself be a cause of stress, however. Some people may deliberately choose a job which is less than perfectly fitted to their talents because, for example, the hours are flexible and give them the freedom to pursue other interests more important to them, or because they can take holidays that fit in with school holidays and choose to spend time with their children rather than having fulfilment at work. If, however, you haven't made any such choice, here are some areas to think about.

• Control •

Too much control and too little control can both be unhealthy. If you so firmly need to keep control over your work that you cannot or fear to delegate, it may be because of your own insecurity in your role or a dissatisfaction with the abilities of colleagues.

Not having control can mean that you are expected to act instantly when asked, regardless of your other commitments and your views on the matter; or having to cope with sweeping changes made by bosses without any prior warning. This is usually the result of poor management or an authoritarian management style. Managers who want to motivate and fulfil staff, whatever their level, can always find or encourage ways for individuals to have some role in devising their own work-styles, contributing suggestions and expressing concerns.

If you and your colleagues feel downtrodden by the work style of an unrealistic and authoritarian boss, you might try asking for a meeting in which you explain your difficulties with current practice and make some specific, constructive suggestions for doing some things differently – but without putting anyone's nose out of joint. If this idea is not well received or the process comes to nothing, you may have to accept the status quo or think seriously about moving on.

Supervisors can find themselves in a particularly invidious position. They have usually been promoted to manage others doing the job that they themselves used to do. They are now above their old colleagues, who may feel resentful, but are still below management level. They aren't on a par with anyone. It can be hard to have to stop being 'one of the girls', and they may dread having to give directions to or discipline a former co-worker. They are also frightened to make mistakes, because they haven't yet been able to prove their worth. It is control at a price. If you find yourself flung into this position, ask about the possibilities for training in supervisory skills.

• Overwork •

If you always have a pile of work waiting for you and feel overwhelmed; if you continually miss deadlines or are constantly anxious about getting behind; if you regularly have to break family or social arrangements to stay late or work at weekends, then you have more work than you can comfortably do. You may just have a greater workload than you can possibly manage and in this case you should tackle your boss. However, poor time management could possibly be contributing to the problem: see the box on the next page.

TEN STEPS TO BETTER TIME MANAGEMENT

1 First realise that, if you can't get everything done, you are not placing enough importance on your own time. Plan to make your time work for you instead of against you.

2 Write down a list of things you need to do each day and put them in order of priority. Be ruthlessly realistic. Some things just don't need doing. Cross them off the list altogether or put the papers in the bin.

3 Plan realistically how you are going to achieve what you have decided to do. Schedule how much time each activity needs, including all elements. For example, writing a report may include collecting together the necessary background material, three quick phone calls for updates from different departments, preparation time and writing time.

4 Tackle the big jobs first. Do not be tempted to put them off by tidying cabinets or doing unnecessary chores which are less daunting.

5 Don't be diverted. If you are able to, put a do not disturb sign up and tell the switchboard you won't take calls until a certain hour. Or find a place to do your work where no one who is looking for you will find you. If you have to stay visible and at your post, learn to say no, not possible now, when unrealistic demands are added to your existing burden, or ask your boss to decide which parts of your work you should give priority and delegate some of the rest.

6 Delegate, if you are in a position to. If you resist delegation, consider why. Are you frightened that subordinates will shine and soon displace you? If so, you need to tackle your insecurity and find ways to show your own abilities without blocking the chances of others. You may well find that, without so much work to do, you have more time to be creative and impressive in what you do do.

7 Expect some interruptions. Emergencies will happen. Certain events just have to be handled the instant they crop up. Don't plan your time so tightly that your entire timetable is thrown out by an unexpected problem or circumstance.

8 Take sufficient breaks and relax. Time spent at your tasks is irrelevant; it is the end result of that time that is important. So if you can do something in an hour if you take a half-hour coffee break first, that will be more effective than struggling unproductively for three hours. Make sure you switch off and relax in your life outside work as well.

9 Know yourself and your limitations. Know what stimulates you, what daunts you and find a working style that lets you make the most of yourself. For example, if you hate a certain task, make sure you plan one you really enjoy to follow it. If you think best when bouncing ideas around, arrange regular brainstorming sessions that will benefit all parties.

10 If possible, ask to be sent on a course on effective time management.

Having too much work can be a symptom of workaholism. But here the work is often self-instigated because the workaholic cannot bear to have no work. The workaholic will skip or hurry meals, be late home and bring work with him or her, be reluctant to arrange weekends away or holidays, and continually break family engagements to carry on working. When a holiday is finally taken, the workaholic is usually restless and anxious, because the workaholic needs work more than the work needs him or her. Usually, the cause is some underlying problem that is not being faced, such as an unhappy home life or a neurotic need to be highly admired or successful.

• Too little work •

Not enough work, with resultant boredom, can be just as stressful as having too much to do.

If you just don't have enough work, try to think of ways you could extend your job description. Look around and see what needs to be done that isn't being done or where someone could do with some help, and make a plan and a case for doing it. If your boss won't have it, either find ways to suit yourself to fill the time (such as study for a degree), or look out for another job.

• Personality mismatch •

If you feel comfortable plodding along, knowing exactly what you have to do and when, you may well become stressed in a job where there is a whirlwind of frenetic activity and unexpected demands that have to be met in an instant. Alternatively, if you thrive on variety and challenge, you won't want predictability and an organisation that is set in its ways. Perhaps you are obliged to work on your own too much when you really work best in a team or vice versa.

You may just have to accept that you are in the wrong type of job for you and look for another more suited to your style.

• Other people •

You need to be comfortable with colleagues, whether peers, superiors or subordinates. A very bad personal relationship with one person can make your life a misery. Similarly, feeling that your boss doesn't value or respect you, or that you don't know how to handle people in your charge so that they do what you ask but still like you, can be very destructive for self-esteem and achievement. Good communication skills and assertiveness skills are essential: both for dealing with co-workers or with awkward or rude customers. There are numerous books and courses available on both. (For more on Assertiveness, see page 194).

• The stress of change •

Any major changes in life are stressful, and major changes at work are no exception. These might be personal, in the form of changed responsibilities, or affect the whole organisation, such as the introduction of new technologies, or relocation. An open organisation will try to minimise the stress of major change by alerting staff to what is happening, involving them in discussions, helping them to make psychological as well as physical adjustments, and so on. If your company is not so forward-thinking, try to find at least one person with whom you can discuss your concerns, or get a group of staff together to seek information from management and voice collective worries to them.

If it is your own circumstances that have changed and not for the better, you need to work out how best you can cope and progress from here. Express your feelings about the change to someone you trust, try to see why it has come about and what it makes most sense to do or aim for next. Give yourself practical goals.

• Dual roles: the stress of being a working mother •

Women who are or want to be mothers are still expected to take career breaks, to work part-time to accommodate the children or to shoulder all the guilt of working full time. (Full-time fathers do not, as a rule, feel guilty.) Despite moves towards equality, every survey on the subject shows that working mothers do more of the household chores and carry more of the child care than working fathers. It is more often mothers who take the days off to care for sick children or attend school parent meetings. As most working mothers have to organise their work lives very precisely so that they can drop or collect their children at the requisite times, there is little opportunity for putting in extra hours and doing whatever might be necessary to compete with male colleagues for advancement.

What can be done? Try to make child-care arrangements in which you know your children are happy; then don't waste valuable energy feeling guilty that you are not with them. Assert yourself in your relationship and insist on equal shares of the chores and child rearing, as appropriate. Think creatively and try to find ways that you can use your talents most satisfyingly for yourself, and where you are not constantly feeling outclassed by unencumbered and eager males. Maybe setting up your own business or working as a freelance would suit. If you have chosen to put your career on hold while you give priority to caring for your children, let yourself feel strong in that decision.

• Perfectionism •

If you are driven to perfection it means that you probably set impossibly high standards for yourself and that your self esteem suffers an enormous blow every time you fail to meet them.

Perfectionists often end up being poor at their jobs because they take too long over details and so fail to complete work by the necessary deadline. Perfectionists are anxious lest they make a mistake because that equals complete failure. They are so fearful of failure that they may not begin some projects at all or daren't take on new challenges. Perfectionists are performance and achievement-oriented.

If there is something of the perfectionist in you, try looking at how this quality affects your life: make a list of the advantages and disadvantages of being a perfectionist; make a list of activities or chores that you don't excel at but that you enjoy (to show yourself that outstanding achievement isn't everything); and try to stop over-generalising from specifics. If someone criticises you for something, accept the criticism for what it is about instead of assuming it means you must be incompetent and worthless in every respect.

• Your working environment •

Where you work or the conditions you work in, may make you ill. Women working with dangerous substances in laboratories, factories, hospitals, etc, must take especial care to follow safety regulations and, if planning pregnancy, to know which substances might be harmful to a foetus. Anyone with any concerns can contact the London Hazards Centre for advice: see Useful Contacts. However, it is office environments which have particularly come under criticism in recent years for contributing to ill health (and the London Hazards Centre can offer plenty of information on this subject, as well).

Office workers, particularly women, who seem more sensitive, may suffer from office-induced symptoms such as nasal congestion, nose bleeds, eye problems, tightness in the chest, wheezing, shortness of breath, headaches, dry itchy skin or skin rashes and fatigue. Causes are various and include air-conditioning systems, humidifiers, new technology, inadequate lighting, overheating and chemical pollutants such as formaldehyde from wall insulation or furniture, chemicals used in furniture veneers which may give off a gas when hit by sunlight, carpet cleaning fluids, and ozone and nitrogen dioxide emitted from poorly maintained photocopiers.

Air-conditioning systems with humidifiers are risky because, if they are not operating correctly, bacteria can breed in the humidifier and be released into the air where they can spread infection. Flu epidemics and outbreaks of Legionnaire's Disease have started in this way.

Another big health problem is unsuitable work stations. Desks and chairs that are at the wrong height and computers that are uncomfortable to work at are the cause of much eye strain, backache, strained muscles and ligaments, and damage to nerves of the hands, wrists, arms and shoulders. The more general stress you are under at work, the more susceptible you are to muscle and bone injuries.

• Keeping fit for work •

You can do a lot to reduce the hazards of the work place.

I Improve a dry office or work atmosphere by introducing some large-leaved plants that give off moisture, putting bowls of water near central heating radiators, or installing ionisers.

2 Always get outside for some part of the day, whatever the weather. A good walk at lunchtime can help clear a head made muzzy by the workplace atmosphere.

3 Take regular exercise both inside and out of work. If your job is sedentary, you need to take exercise to keep your body functioning at peak. Too little exercise puts you at risk of injury from straining your hands, wrists and arms. If you spend much time sitting at a computer terminal, take regular breaks and do regular exercises that you can carry out right on the spot, such as circling the head, shoulders and ankles, shrugging the shoulders and reaching up with your arms.

4 Make sure that your desk and chair are comfortable and at a suitable height. Your desk should be large enough to hold all the documents you need to work from as well as larger equipment you require, such as a computer. Your chair should be adjustable and there should be adequate footrests.

5 Computer screens should be on a swivel and tilt mechanism so that you can move yours into the position that best suits you. Screens should have an anti-glare surface; not an additional anti-glare filter. If they do, it could mean the general office lighting is bad and needs attention. Light, natural or otherwise, should not shine directly on to the screen nor should the screen receive reflections from windows.

6 Try to remember to blink a lot if you have to look at a computer screen for much of the day. Computer users tend to stare and blink less than normal, whereas in fact they need to blink more because the fluids that lubricate the eyes evaporate more quickly when looking at a computer. Blinking replaces the fluids.

7 Health and safety directives, now law in the UK, mean that there are standards which office lighting, ventilation and computer equipment must meet. Check with whomever is responsible for health and safety that yours do.

8 Eat fruit if you hit an energy low, not crisps and chocolates.

9 Get yourself a view. Being able to look up and out at a park or green area is soothing for the eyes and the brain. American research shows that deskworkers are more enthusiastic about their jobs, less frustrated and take fewer days off sick if they have some natural scene to glance at from their office.

10 Remember the golden rules for keeping down stress: keep a sense of proportion, give in occasionally, go easy with criticism, take one thing at a time, learn to delegate, learn to ask for help and support when you need it and know when you need a break.

8

PROFESSIONAL HELP FOR HEALTH

HOWEVER healthy you are, you are likely to need the services of certain health professionals at various points in your life. Women are used to the idea of having to see doctors and nurses when healthy because we may have to do so in order to be prescribed contraception, to be monitored during pregnancy or be helped to achieve a pregnancy and be assisted during childbirth.

Women consult health professionals more often than men, not necessarily just because we suffer more illness but because we are in general more willing to recognise problems and seek help. More women than men will see their doctor because of emotional and psychological problems. Gynaecological conditions, common reasons for women to seek medical help, have no real equivalent for men.

Even if we don't need help for our own health, women are the ones who most commonly consult doctors on behalf of others they care for: children, elderly dependants and sometimes even reluctant partners.

It is important, therefore that we are comfortable about approaching and relating to health professionals, so that we can best help take care of ourselves and those we love.

• Talking to doctors •

Doctors used to be treated as godlike figures and some of us still feel awed by people in white coats, especially if we are feeling vulnerable and ill. However, nowadays we prefer our doctors to behave like humans and to talk to us as if we are equally valuable human beings. We are no longer quite so prepared to put up with unhelpful or patronising attitudes which leave us feeling as though we are stupid, time-wasting, neurotic or too inquisitive by half. Doctors, too, have learned that communication is a very important part of the medical armoury of skills, albeit one that used not to be taught in medical schools.

Inevitably, as doctors are only human, some will be better at communicating than others. Some came into medicine primarily because of an interest in treating diseases but are not so hot at handling the humans who have them. Others somehow create the time to give everyone sufficient attention and understanding, and this is what adds to their own job satisfaction. As we may not always be able to choose our own doctors, it is important to ensure that we try to get the best from whomever happens to treat us.

• Your GP •

Your general practitioner (GP) is your entry point to the health service. It is your GP who makes a diagnosis or judgment about symptoms which are bothering you, and either treats you or refers you if necessary to another more appropriate health practitioner for further investigations, such as a specialist hospital doctor or a physiotherapist; or to a specialist hospital department, such as X-ray or ultrasound.

When you visit your GP because of ill health you will receive, on average, a four-minute consultation. This isn't long to get across what is concerning you and for your GP to make a diagnosis. So it makes sense to go as fully prepared as you can.

Note down your questions If you know that you tend to forget things or that you can become forgetful once you are with your doctor, note down beforehand all the questions you want to ask. Also note down everything you think might be relevant about your symptoms: how long you have had them, when they are worst (for example, at night or after eating), whether you have had them before but have not sought treatment.

It can be very useful to do this, even if you think you have a good memory. It is surprising how often an important point pops out of your head and only pops back in again once you have left the surgery.

Take someone with you You always have the right to take someone along with you to the consultation, whether a partner, family member or friend. You might choose to do this if you know you become easily daunted when in the doctor's surgery and don't say all you want to say; or if you can't think quickly enough of questions to ask arising from whatever your doctor tells you. Taking along someone you know who is quick-thinking and articulate may enable you to relax, knowing that there is double the chance of the right information getting conveyed.

Another benefit of taking someone with you is that you then have another pair of ears to help you remember what was said. It is very common for people to forget what doctors tell them, and not only if the news is frightening or bad.

Expect a discussion Unless you are someone who prefers to leave everything in the hands of your doctor, you should feel comfortable enough with your GP to be able to discuss the diagnosis that is made and the treatment that is suggested. It may be that you would prefer to try a remedy that does not entail taking drugs, if possible: such as relaxation therapy or counselling for anxiety. Or perhaps a drug that is suggested caused you unpleasant side-effects when prescribed once before. Although, clearly, it is your GP who must lead this discussion, you need to be happy with whatever course of action is recommended.

If you are not happy with whatever your GP suggests, ask why this is the necessary treatment. It may be that, once you have received a fuller explanation, you too will accept that this is the best approach to your problem. If you expect your GP to have an open mind, keep your own mind open as well.

Don't try to dictate   You may not always get a wonderful reception if you enter your doctor's surgery brandishing a copy of a newspaper or magazine containing an article that describes your symptoms or a condition you have and demanding to be put on the latest treatment for it. By all means, show your doctor the article and say you would be interested in giving the treatment a try if appropriate for you; however, give your doctor a chance to make up his or her mind too. He or she may not have heard of the treatment and may want to do some research before prescribing willy-nilly. Offer to collect the information yourself, if easier, or to track down the relevant medical journal. Don't be too pushy, otherwise your doctor may simply become defensive or resistant and reject the idea out of hand.

Question jargon   If your doctor tends to talk in medical terms that you don't understand, don't feel small and silly. There is no reason why you should understand, any more than your doctor may know the language used by accountants or car mechanics. Ask for an explanation whenever you need to, or jot down any words you don't follow and ask for explanations when the doctor has finished talking.

Don't always expect pills   A prescription may not always be the right answer for your problem. For example, if you have a cold, antibiotics are not going to help as these treat bacterial infections and colds are caused by viruses. A national survey has revealed, however, that doctors very often do give prescriptions when they are not warranted because they are uncertain what else to do, are tired, want to avoid conflict with a patient who feels cheated without one, find it a useful way to bring a consultation to an end or else prescribe as a means to show compassion. This clearly isn't best practice. We can help to minimise it by not expecting a prescription just for the sake of one, even if our doctor can't offer us any very useful alternative for some difficult conditions.

You can ask for a second opinion   You can ask for a second opinion from a specialist if you are not happy with whatever your GP is suggesting. A GP cannot reasonably refuse. (It would be reasonable to refuse, for example, if you always ask for a second opinion, whenever you attend the surgery and however minor the complaint.) This may be especially useful if, for example, your GP is adamant that your breast lump is nothing but you do not feel convinced or if you would like cosmetic surgery for what you see as an ugly nose and your GP tells you not to be so silly. However, you will still need a letter from your GP to give to the second doctor, whether an NHS or private one. It is not down to you to find the name of a second doctor to see, although you may prefer to find one yourself. If you really can't, because no one you know can recommend one, insist your GP helps you.

Don't forget complementary therapies If you think that an osteopath or homoeopath, for example, might be better able to offer a solution to your problem, you are entitled to ask your GP to refer you to one. However, you are only entitled to ask. A GP has the right to 'delegate' a patient, while still retaining overall responsibility, to be treated by a particular complementary practitioner if he or she thinks fit and if the money is there. (Fund-holding GPs can make their own decisions on this, others must receive permission from the local Family Health Service Authority or FHSA which controls GP spending.) Some GP practices now even offer sessions with complementary practitioners in their own surgeries. The therapies which find most favour with GPs are homoeopathy, acupuncture, osteopathy and chiropractic.

Your own GP may or may not approve of complementary therapies, of course, although there is a tendency for orthodox doctors to be less dismissive, particularly in conditions where orthodox medicine cannot offer much. The most recent survey found that 70 per cent of FHSAs and GP fund-holders are in favour of some or all complementary therapies being available on the NHS.

However, complementary therapies are generally viewed as a fairly low budget priority. Nevertheless, even if you think it is unlikely that you would be referred for such help, do ask. Only when more people ask will more doctors realise the degree of interest from patients. (For more on complementary therapies, see page 77.)

• Do you want to change your GP? •

You don't only have the right to change GP when you move house. You can change GP if you are unhappy with the service you are receiving, and this might be for many reasons. For example, you might want to transfer to a practice where there is a woman doctor or one where the doctors are sympathetic to complementary medicine. You do not have to give your reasons, and you don't even have to see your doctor to announce your intention. All you have to do is find another doctor who offers more of what you want and who is willing to take you on. You can get a list of doctors from your FHSA: look for the telephone number in your local phone directory. Then ring the surgeries' receptionists to ask what you need to know, or select a new practice by recommendation.

Whatever your reason for changing doctor, before signing on with a new one it is worthwhile thinking about all the aspects of care which are or might at some time be important to you. For example:

- Do you want a single-handed GP or someone who works within a group practice?
- Is there a walk-in service, an appointment system or both?
- Is the presence of one or more women doctors important?
- Does the surgery run well-woman clinics or provide contraceptive services?
- Do the doctors do home visits, if necessary, or might an unfamiliar locum visit instead?
- What is the policy on home births (if you might want one)?

It is a good idea to ring or call in on the receptionist(s) to ask about these things. From the manner and warmth (or lack of it), you can make some fairly accurate judgments about the GP or practice. After all, this is the person that the GP is happy to have giving the first impression of the surgery. You can even ask to 'interview' the GP before making your decision; if you do, the GP may choose to use the occasion to interview you too and decide whether you are desirable as a patient.

A GP doesn't have to take you, even if there is a vacancy. Once you have found one who will, bring your medical card to the surgery and the rest of the transfer is done for you. If you don't have a medical card (which gives your NHS number), just supply the name and address of your previous doctor: a card will be sent to you in the post.

This process works two ways. Your GP can choose to take you off his or her list without giving a reason too, although this happens rather rarely and is usually because of a series of problems that have arisen between you and the doctor.

• Hospital consultations •

It is very important to feel as comfortable as possible about consultations with hospital doctors, whether at the investigative stage or prior to and during treatment. There are two ways people may choose to cope with investigation or treatment for a serious condition: some prefer to know nothing and leave everything trustfully in their doctors' hands; others cope better by finding out all they can about the procedure they are to undergo and the likely outcomes. Either method can be successful, so ask for as much information as you can handle. Research has shown that, in general, the more informed we are, the more likely we are to feel in control of our bodies and able to relax, aiding recovery.

The first five suggestions in the earlier section on GPs (see pages 73–4) also apply to hospital consultations. It is particularly a good idea to take someone with you to a first hospital consultation if you are fearful about the condition or illness you may have. Remember to write down all your questions beforehand and encourage your partner or friend to take as active a part in the consultation as you choose. Some people like to take a tape recorder with them so that, if the news is bad and they fail to take in any more information through shock, they can play it back later.

Try not to let a doctor rush you. If a certain treatment is recommended that daunts you, ask how long it is reasonable for you to think about it before making a decision. If need be, ask if there is anyone in the hospital who offers counselling for someone in your position, or whether there is any self-help organisation that offers further information and moral support. If this doesn't yield anything helpful, contact the Patients Association (see Useful Contacts) to ask about self-help groups for specific conditions.

Again, it is particularly important not to let a doctor who is poor at communicating create a more comfortable emotional distance (for him or her) by using complex medical terms. Ask – or encourage your partner or friend to ask – for information to be explained in lay-person's terms.

Remember, too, the value of a second opinion. One surgeon may recommend removal of a breast for a particular breast cancer whereas another may recommend removing only the lump.

If you are told you have a serious illness, it is hard to be assertive when you are frightened or in shock. Don't blame yourself if you come away from a consultation feeling confused and anxious. Try to get the confusion sorted out as quickly as you can, either by having a word with the consultant on the telephone shortly afterwards (many are willing to come to the phone to reassure patients), by making another appointment to see your consultant quickly, if possible, or by arranging to speak to someone else who can talk through the implications of your illness and your options: your GP, a nurse, a counsellor, or a member of a self-help organisation. Do not be rushed into anything you may regret, unless emergency treatment is vital.

· Complementary Therapies ·

One of the reasons that increasing numbers of people are turning to complementary therapies is that the practitioners are especially likely to be sympathetic and understanding. The nature of most complementary therapies requires often an even fuller history-taking than conventional medicine, and there is plenty of time in every session to explore an individual's problem fully.

Complementary therapies take a holistic approach to health, viewing the person with the problem as a whole person rather than as a collection of symptoms. The aim in many will be to find the root cause of a problem, which may take quite some time and many sessions. In the holistic philosophy of health, the mind and body are viewed as inextricably linked and interconnected. Conditions which affect the body are seen as likely to affect mood and mental functioning, while depression or bottling up negative feelings can lead to physical ill-health.

Complementary therapies can be practised by people who are not medically qualified (but should be qualified in their own field) and usually take a gentler approach to the treatment of illnesses than conventional medicine. They used to be known as alternative therapies or alternative medicine. But this was a slight misnomer because, while some people may choose these therapies instead of those offered by conventional medicine, it is perfectly possible for most to be used alongside conventional medicine, to boost its benefits, as many complementary therapies are concerned with strengthening the body's immune system.

Some complementary therapies may be welcomed by medical doctors. They may recognise that some alternative approaches seem to help in certain conditions for which conventional medicine has little to offer. Some medically trained doctors also practise a complementary therapy, such as acupuncture or homoeopathy.

There are an enormous number of complementary therapies to choose from. As explained earlier, GPs can refer patients to a complementary practitioner if they think fit and if their budget will bear it, but most complementary therapies are paid for by the individuals who seek them. Not only, therefore, do you need to make decisions about which type of therapy might suit you and your complaint, but how long you might need to attend and whether you can afford it. You will also need to accept that there are no guarantees that a particular therapy will help you. Many people experience enormous benefit; others little or none. Alternatively, a particular therapy may help a person with one complaint but not someone else with a different one.

The following is a brief outline of some of the more commonly available therapies. It is vital that you choose only a therapist who is correctly trained or qualified in their own field. (See What Else to Choose and Who to Go To, page 80.)

• Acupuncture •

An ancient Chinese form of medicine in which special needles are inserted into specific points of the body. The theory is that life energy runs along lines or channels in the body called meridians, along which specific points correspond to different organs in the body. Ill health occurs when the balance between positive and negative energy is upset, affecting the flow of life energy and causing various symptoms. Stimulating the correct point for the affected part frees energy to flow fully again. Acupuncture can also stimulate the body to produce endorphins, its own natural pain-killing chemicals.

Acupuncture may be particularly useful for chronic conditions such as migraine and arthritis, addictions and pain relief.

The Council for Acupuncture (see Useful Contacts), has a register of traditional acupuncturists. There is a charge for the directory but if you want the names of just one or two local practitioners the Council will provide this for free over the phone.

For the name of medical doctors who have trained in acupuncture contact the British Medical Acupuncture Society: see Useful Contacts.

• Aromatherapy •

One of the most popular complementary therapies, this is the use of essential oils, extracted from specific plants, which have the properties to affect physical and mental health. The oils can be massaged into the skin, added to the bath, inhaled, used as a compress and occasionally swallowed. Aromatherapy practitioners take a detailed history in order to create a combination of oils suitable for your needs. Oils for more general purposes are also available from health shops.

Aromatherapy is most commonly used to help relieve stress and stress-related conditions.

To find a correctly trained aromatherapist, send an A5 SAE to the Aromatherapy Organisations Council, which will provide a list of their member associations. You then need to contact the associations individually for a list of aromatherapists who trained with them. The council will also provide a booklet on aromatherapy, if you ask for it. See Useful Contacts.

• Homoeopathy •

Homoeopathy is based on the principle of like treats like. It comes from the findings of a German physician that substances which cause particular symptoms in a healthy person can cure those same symptoms when suffered by someone who is ill.

Homoeopathic remedies are diluted so many thousands of times that even plant substances which would normally be harmful if ingested are rendered perfectly safe. Conventional doctors who are sceptics claim homoeopathic solutions are so weak as to be useless whereas homoeopaths claim that the weaker the dilution, the more potent its ability to cure.

Homoeopaths take into account not only your symptoms but your full medical history, your personality, likes and dislikes when prescribing you a remedy. These come in various forms such as tablets, creams and drops. Homoeopathy may be particularly useful for chronic conditions, allergies, plus gynaecological and gastrointestinal problems.

For a list of homoeopaths registered with the Society of Homoeopaths, contact the society; for a list of medically qualified homoeopaths, contact the British Homoeopathic Association: see Useful Contacts.

• Osteopathy and chiropractic •

Both of these therapies are concerned with manipulation of the body to correct musculo-skeletal problems, but there are differences in their technique although these may seem subtle to the outsider. Osteopaths look particularly at how the function of a joint is affected, and use leverage, loosening and a stretching of the ligaments around the joint to recover movement. Chiropractors look especially at the spine's structure, usually taking X-rays first, and aim to reposition particular bones with thrusting movements. The two techniques overlap and even vary according to individual practice and experience.

These therapies are usually sought for relief from back and neck pains, sports injuries and arthritis, but may also help with asthma, discomforts of pregnancy, period problems, gastrointestinal problems and migraine.

To find a properly qualified osteopath in your area, contact the General Council and Register of Osteopaths: see Useful Contacts. When the 1993 Osteopathy Act comes into force (this is expected to be in 1997) practitioners will only be able to use the title of osteopath if they are registered with the General Osteopathic Council (GOsC), which will be the new regulating body for the profession.

To find a properly qualified chiropractor in your area, contact the British Chiropractic Association: see Useful Contacts. Chiropractors now also have to be registered.

• Shiatsu •

This increasingly popular therapy is a form of massage that focuses on the acupuncture points. Fingers, elbows, knees and feet may be used to put pressure on the requisite acupuncture points (see Acupuncture, page 78), with the aim of freeing blocked energy and dealing with the resultant symptoms of ill health. For the recipient it is like having a very vigorous massage but at the end of it you should feel relaxed. It may be particularly useful for stress and stress-related conditions.

To find a properly qualified practitioner contact the Shiatsu Society: see Useful Contacts.

• What else to choose and who to go to •

An excellent little paperback which describes very clearly and vividly all the available complementary therapies, what to expect from a session and the conditions for which they are thought to work best is the *HEA Guide to Complementary Medicine and Therapies* (see Further Reading).

This book also gives details of how to find a qualified practitioner for each of the therapies included. Alternatively, you can send a large sae to the Institute for Complementary Medicine (see Useful Contacts), asking for a list of local approved practitioners of the therapy you are seeking.

9

....

HAIR

THE HAIR on the face and body is made up of two types. Vellus hairs are the fine, soft, very short and colourless hairs that babies have on their bodies from birth and which stay with us as downy hair on many parts of the body. Terminal hairs develop after puberty and are coarse, pigmented and often curly. They are dependent upon the male hormone testosterone, produced by both men and women, for their growth. In women terminal hairs are usually absent or sparse on areas such as the upper lip, tip of the nose, chin, cheeks, ear lobes, upper pubic triangle, chest, abdomen and thighs, compared with male hair in these places.

However, it is certainly not abnormal for women to have quite a lot of hair on various parts of their faces and bodies as well as their heads. According to studies, about one in ten women when young has clearly visible hair on the face, particularly the upper lip, but probably as many as a quarter have at least some noticeable facial hair. After the menopause, facial hair growth increases. One in ten women by the age of 65 has hair on the chin and nearly half have a moustache that is easy to see.

About 15 per cent of younger women have hair around the nipples and on the lower back; 30 per cent have it along the mid-line on the lower abdomen, and in 10 per cent the pubic triangle extends upwards and probably downwards too. Over a third of women have hair on the thighs and almost all have hair on the lower leg. All this hair increases until the menopause and then starts to diminish or disappear.

· Too much hair? ·

Whether we consider we have too much hair is often a matter of fashion and cultural norms. Most women who consult their doctors because they are anxious about excess body hair do not have any abnormality or illness, although, alas, that is unlikely to lessen their embarrassment and anxiety about their appearance.

If your menstrual cycle is normal, you are ovulating normally or you have been pregnant at some time, you are unlikely to have a medical condition to account for your hair growth or distribution. Irregular periods and inability to get pregnant may, however, indicate a problem.

Certain drugs can sometimes increase body hair. These include:

- Some kinds of the contraceptive pill (see page 404).
- Danazol, used to treat endometriosis and breast cysts amongst other things, if given at a high dose. Only a very small proportion of women are affected but the hair growth is not always reversible.
- The steroids cortisol and prednisolone if given for long periods at a high dose.
- Anabolic steroids.
- Cyclosporin, used to help prevent organ rejection in transplant patients. The hair growth is not always reversible.
- Minoxidil, used to treat high blood pressure, which can cause such a marked increase in hair growth that it is now often tried as a treatment for baldness. However, its effects disappear once the drug is stopped.

• Drug Treatments •

If you are very unhappy about your amount of body hair, even if there is nothing technically abnormal, and hair removal methods such as shaving, waxing, bleaching or electrolysis are not a solution, you might want to ask your doctor whether you would be a suitable candidate for drugs that can reduce hair growth.

The drugs most commonly used are different forms of the contraceptive pill (see pages 399–404) which either have the effect of reducing the amount of testosterone circulating in the body and/or reducing the body cells' own degree of sensitivity to testosterone; the factors which decide how much hair we each have and where. However, they may take a few months to start working and after a year they will have achieved their maximum effect. Reducing hair on the legs is the most marked in improvement whereas there is usually little impact on facial hair.

The biggest negative, however, is that hair growth will probably return to previous levels within several months of having stopped taking the drugs. You might rightly ask, why bother to take them then? The answer is that, for a minority of women, these drugs reduce the amount of hair that regrows and persists. Unless you try taking the drugs you can't know if you will be one of the women for whom they work. It is therefore a case of weighing up for yourself the pros and cons of giving it a go.

Which drugs?   Certain types of the combined, oral contraceptive pill, containing both the female hormones oestrogen, and progestogen (the synthetic, artificial form of progesterone), may be tried. Those containing the progestogens norethisterone or ethynodiol have been found to be most effective. Some progestogens themselves promote male hormone activity and worsen the problem. Those progestogens perhaps best avoided if you think you have too much hair are norgestrel, norethisterone acetate and levonorgestren. Over half of women who try the advised brands find a marked reduction in hair growth. However, those who have high blood pressure, are at risk of heart disease or who smoke should not use the contraceptive pill.

Cyproterone acetate (brand name Dianette) is an oral contraceptive containing an anti-male hormone and oestrogen which is used for severe acne and excess hairiness. It is essential not to get pregnant while taking this as feminisation of a male foetus would very probably occur. The drug needs to be taken for between six months and a year for full results to be noticeable because it takes time to deplete the male hormone levels in tissues. However, after treatment is over, hair growth is quite likely to return to pre-treatment levels after several months. Again, those with high blood pressure, raised heart disease risk and smokers should not use Dianette.

Another drug which may in the past have been prescribed in combination with an oral contraceptive is the diuretic (a drug that increases the flow of urine) called spironolactone, which also has the effect of decreasing levels and effectiveness of testosterone. However, its use has now been discouraged by the Committee on Safety of Medicines after reports of carcinogenic effects found in animal studies.

• Hirsutism •

Women who have clearly excessive hair, particularly on the upper back and shoulders, on the upper abdomen other than on the midline and a lot on their faces, particularly the cheeks and neck, are said to be suffering from hirsutism (meaning excess hair), a condition usually caused by a hormonal problem.

The most common cause of hirsutism is polycystic ovarian syndrome: multiple, benign fluid-filled cysts on the ovaries. Symptoms are various (sometimes even non-existent) and include all or any of obesity, irregular periods, loss of periods, infertility, excess body hair and acne. The treatments described above may be useful for reducing hairiness and acne. To restore fertility, different treatment is required (see Polycystic Ovarian Syndrome, page 249).

Other causes of hirsutism are extremely rare. An ovarian or adrenal cortical tumour is one. Another is Cushing's syndrome which is an excess of steroids in the blood, usually caused by taking high doses for another illness such as rheumatoid arthritis or asthma, or in very rare cases a tumour affecting the adrenal glands. If the tumour is in the pituitary gland, the condition is known as Cushing's disease, an extremely uncommon disease affecting mainly young and middle-aged women. First symptoms of Cushing's are a fattening and reddening of the face and an appearance of round shoulders. Later, a deep voice develops, plus more body hair, loss of periods, purpling of the skin and bruising, tiredness and bone thinning.

If excess steroids taken for another illness are the cause, do not stop taking them. Your doctor will reduce them slowly and change you to another treatment. Tumours are treated by surgery or radiotherapy.

• Temporary hair loss •

Hair goes through a growing phase and a resting phase, after which it falls out to be replaced by new hair. Different hairs are at different stages in this cycle so, although it is normal to lose up to 150 hairs a day, we don't notice because we have plenty left. Losses greater than that start to be noticeable to you. Reasons for abnormal temporary hair loss are numerous and the degree of the problem variable. Possible causes are:

Shocks to the system Severe stress, a physical illness which severely weakens the body, crash dieting, a major operation or fever can force hair follicles from the growing phase into the resting phase, the result of which is a considerable fall of hair a couple of months later.

Pregnancy and after Hair loss during pregnancy is common because more hairs than usual go into the resting phase at this time. Natural hair growth normally returns about three months after the end of pregnancy but in some women may be delayed for up to two years. Sometimes hair is not lost during pregnancy but about three months afterwards for a few months. It may even occur for the first time after a second or third child. Some women also notice hair loss a few months after stopping the contraceptive pill.

Iron deficiency Most women do not know when they are deficient in iron, which is very common. Hair loss in pregnancy is exacerbated by low iron levels.

Hair styles and fashion Pulling the hair back into a pony tail and securing it with a tight elastic band, putting hair into tight braids and too tight rollers all put pressure on the hair and lead to the beleaguered hairs falling out. Hair bands, wigs or hats that are too tight can cause friction and make hair break.

Alopecia areata Sudden complete loss of hair in round patches which may be minor or extensive (see next page). In a third to two-thirds of cases, hair growth eventually returns to normal.

• Permanent hair loss •

Bald patches can be caused by improperly applied perming agents, radiation and certain illnesses such as extremely severe shingles or ringworm. *Alopecia areata* may be permanent in 20 per cent of cases (see below).

• Alopecia areata •

This is a scalp disease with no known cause that is thought to affect up to one in 100 people. It is a sudden dramatic hair loss which can occur in one, two or three round patches on the scalp or can lead to total baldness and loss of all body hair, including hair from the eyebrows, eyelashes, armpits and pubic area as well. Nails can also become pitted and ridged, according to the severity of the hair loss. Clearly, it can be a devastating condition. Doctors

WHY A SHOCK MAY SEEM TO TURN HAIR WHITE

If your hair turns white overnight the cause may be a form of *alopecia areata*. On rare occasions, a severe and sudden shock can cause the immune system to turn on itself and see a particular part of the body as a foreign invader; in this case the pigment cells which give the hair its colour. The effect is that the dark hairs drop out and the white hairs are all that will remain. As new hairs grow through, these too will be white.

believe that it is an auto-immune disease, meaning that the the body's own immune system attacks the hair follicles as if they were foreign bodies.

According to experts there has been a marked increase in the incidence of this disease over the last 30 years which has posed the question of a link with use of the contraceptive pill. Although experts disagree among themselves, it would seem that the two main progestogens in the combined pill which can cause excess hairiness (norgestrel and norethisterone acetate) can also, in other women, cause hair loss in the form of male pattern baldness. Dr Katherina Dalton, an authority on progesterone, believes there is a simple reason for progestogens causing hair loss: hair follicles need natural progesterone for their development but when a woman is on the pill, the hair receives only the artificial version, progestogen, which can't meet the need. Some endocrinologists now advise women to change pills or stop taking them altogether.

Stress may also play a part in some cases of *Alopecia areata* and some women are certain that the menopause was a trigger.

• Treatment •

1 Minoxidil: a treatment for high blood pressure which has the side-effect of making hair grow. A topical solution applied to the bald patches may be helpful where hair loss is not excessive, but only one in three users notices any real benefit. It is probably necessary to keep on using it, where it works, until any spontaneous, good regrowth occurs. A doctor can prescribe minoxidil but it is an expensive treatment.
2 Steroid creams. These need to be rubbed into the bald patches every night. May be helpful for less severe cases.
3 Dithranol. A cream rather like tar, usually used to treat psoriasis. It is rubbed into the patches and left for a few hours before being washed off but has the disadvantage of being messy and not smelling very pleasant.
4 Monthly injections of corticosteroids into the bald patches. Most successful when only small areas are affected.
5 Natural progesterone. Dr Dalton believes that natural progesterone given at high doses may help reverse hair loss. The body cannot absorb it orally so treatments must be in the form of suppositories or pessaries.

• Further help •

Hairline International is an information and support group for sufferers from *Alopecia areata*: see Useful Contacts. Also see Further Reading for helpful books.

10

EYES

UNLIKE other parts of the body, eyes don't need cleaning, washing or brushing. For the most part they can look after themselves, but only if they are treated properly.

• General tips for eyes •

1 Some people swear by splashing their eyes with cold water first thing in the morning. This is fine, if your eyes are shut, but it is not necessary for health or hygiene. You may just feel a bit more alert and ready to start the day, say eye experts. However, practitioners of the Bates Method (see page 91) believe splashing can help strengthen the eyes.

2 If your eyes feel tired and irritated, perhaps from being subjected to smoky atmospheres or not getting enough sleep, don't rub them. You can easily transfer bacteria from the hand to the eye. Getting sufficient sleep or quickly making up on lost sleep is the best solution, as corneal cells then regenerate quickly.

3 If you want to refresh tired or irritated eyes, a salt eye-bath is as good as a commercial preparation. Make a solution of 5ml (1 level tsp) salt to 600ml (1 pint) of purified water.

4 Avoid wearing eye liner inside the lashes as this can clog up tiny glands and lead to an infection. Too thick an application of mascara or using metallic-coloured eye shadow too close to the eyeball can make the eyes red and sore, because bits drop off on to the eyeball.

5 Your eyes may look less red after using a commercial eye preparation because they usually contain a substance that constricts the blood vessels around the eye, making them appear paler. Don't over-use them because blood vessels when constricted can carry less oxygen to the eye and your eyes need oxygen to stay healthy.

6 If your eyes remain red and irritated when you don't use drops or eye washes, find out the cause. If it isn't make-up, too little sleep, etc, you may have an infection or allergy which needs medical attention. (You may even become allergic to eye washes.)

7 If you do use a commercial eye wash, it may seem to make economic sense to keep the plastic eye cup that comes with it and just buy refill bottles but this is not such a good solution for your eyes, as plastic can quickly become contaminated if not kept scrupulously clean. You are safer using a new bottle with a new cup.

8 You cannot damage your sight by reading in a bad light, sitting under fluorescent lighting or sitting very close to a television.

9 You cannot protect your eyesight by trying not to read too much or avoiding too much close work.

10 Don't rub your eye to try to remove a speck of dust, an eyelash or any other foreign body that has fallen into it. Let your eyes fill with tears, as they will do, to try to remove it for themselves. If the foreign body can't be dislodged in this way, carefully use a clean tissue.

11 Avoid looking directly into bright sunlight for any extended period and always wear goggles if you use a sunbed. Intense ultraviolet light shining directly into the eye increases the risk of cataracts (clouding over of the eye).

12 If you use a visual display unit (VDU), try to remember to blink more than usual. Japanese researchers found that people using VDUs tend to blink just seven times a minute instead of their normal 22 times a minute, reducing tear production. We need to blink more to replace tears lost in evaporation. Because the surface of the eye is exposed more when looking at a VDU than when looking down to read or write, the evaporation rate of tears is higher, compounding the problem. So this is why VDU users often complain of dry and tired eyes. One solution that the researchers suggest is to place the VDU screen below eye level and tilt the screen upwards.

• Common eye infections •

Conjunctivitis This is quite a common complaint in which the eyes feel red and sore and have a sticky discharge. It is also sometimes called red eye. It can be caused by bacteria or a virus, but a viral infection is more common in adults and is usually preceded by a cold. Conjunctivitis is very contagious, so you should take care to keep your hands clean and touch your eye only with a clean tissue, to avoid passing it from one eye to the other or to anyone else. Bacterial conjunctivitis can be cleared with antibiotic drops or ointment but viral conjunctivitis has to clear up by itself, although eye drops may help reduce the discomfort.

A nasty conjunctivitis can be caused by the herpes virus that causes cold sores, if you touch the cold sore and then touch the eye. Should you seek a doctor's help for conjunctivitis, always say if you are a sufferer from cold sores. When the inflammation is caused by herpes any steroids or ointment prescribed can permanently scar the eye and damage your vision unless you are on antiviral medication at the same time. You may need to see an ophthalmologist for a reliable diagnosis of conjunctivitis caused by herpes.

Allergic conjunctivitis Another common complaint. Usual causes are allergy to the house-dust mite, pollen and animals, but you can develop an allergy to anything which touches the eye, including drugs to treat an eye infection, make-up, or any substance that gives you itchy hands when you touch it and which may make your eyes red and itchy too if you then proceed to rub them.

Styes   The most common problem for the eyelids, caused by a bacterial infection at the root of the eyelash. The lid gets red, swells and a boil develops which eventually bursts. Treatment for styes is 'don'ts' rather than 'dos': don't rub the eye; don't remove the affected eyelash (unless it is loose, in which case removing it will release the pus); don't burst the boil. When the pus emerges, wipe it away with a clean tissue. Styes are more common in children but adults can get them particularly when run down physically or if they have diabetes. See your doctor for a urine test to rule out diabetes if you are not already a sufferer.

• Problems with eyesight •

The most common problems with sight are those of focusing the eye to see clearly.

Short-sighted   You are short-sighted if your eyeball is longer than normal, making distant objects appear blurred. Glasses or contact lenses can correct the problem.

Long-sighted   You are long-sighted if your eyeball is shorter than normal, but before middle age it is usually possible to compensate by refocusing to make both distant and near objects clear. After middle age, it becomes more difficult to do this and you will probably need glasses for near work and, eventually, glasses or lenses for distant vision too, or bifocal glasses or contact lenses.

Astigmatism   The name for the condition if your eye is irregularly shaped. Refocusing is not possible but glasses or contact lenses can correct the problem.

Presbyopia   With age the eye muscle works less efficiently and it becomes harder to see close objects.

Mild defects   Sometimes short sight, long sight or astigmatism can occur so mildly that you notice no problem except in sunlight, when you find your eyes are more sensitive. This could be the case if you find you need sunglasses even on cloudy days, or if you find night driving uncomfortable. A weak prescription for glasses to use solely when driving at night is an easy solution to this sort of problem.

Improving eyesight   Most ophthalmologists and optometrists would maintain that you cannot alter your eyesight yourself and that wearing glasses or contact lenses will not make your eyes weaker, nor will not wearing them help them work better. However, practitioners of the Bates Method believe

---

IMPORTANT

If you have any other visual disturbance, such as gradual loss of vision, blurring at the centre or sides of your visual field, loss of half your field of vision in one or both eyes, double vision, flashing lights or deep pain, see your   doctor as this can be a symptom of an eye injury or eye disease or of another disease: flashing lights, for example, may occur in migraine, and double vision can occur with diabetes, multiple sclerosis, high blood pressure and stroke.

that you can strengthen your eyes and your sight, and recommend specific exercises and a healthy diet: see page 91.

• Contact lenses •

The first contact lenses were hard lenses which were made of a material that didn't allow oxygen to pass through to the cornea. Nowadays, lenses are made from materials which do let oxygen pass freely to the eye, so it is very unlikely a new wearer would ever be prescribed a hard lens. The choice today is between soft lenses and rigid, gas-permeable lenses.

Soft lenses Made from oxygen-permeable plastics which can contain up to 80 per cent water. They are comfortable, easy to get used to and can correct many types of astigmatism and presbyopia. However, they have to be looked after very carefully, with daily cleaning, daily disinfecting and regular protein removal, because of the considerable risk of infection and other problems. They should be changed yearly.

A newer option is disposable (soft) lenses, which are thrown away after a week. They also must be cleaned daily but protein removal is not necessary. Claims that they carry less risk of infection because they are changed so often have not been proved, however. Even newer are daily disposable lenses. They are more expensive but, of course, need no cleaning at all. Don't be tempted to use either for longer than they are designed for.

Rigid gas permeable lenses Flexible hard lenses made from oxygen-permeable plastics. They usually last longer than soft lenses, have a lower risk of infection and require less extensive cleaning procedures.

• Tips for contact-lens wear and care •

I Don't skimp on sterilisation procedures for soft lenses, as the corneal infections which can otherwise occur may, in severe cases, even cause blindness. Home-made saline solutions should be avoided as these may harbour an organism called acanthamoeba which can cause severe eye pain, impair vision and even threaten sight.

2 Put on eye make-up after inserting your lenses. If you have problems with eye irritation, ask your contact-lens specialist about special cosmetics which are least likely to cause allergy or irritation.

3 Hold contact lenses between finger tips, not finger nails.

4 Some women sometimes find they cannot tolerate wearing their lenses at certain times in their menstrual cycle, but this usually occurs irregularly and for only one or two days. During pregnancy, hormonal changes can affect tears, leaving the eye drier and less comfortable in lenses, in which case it may be difficult to carry on wearing them. One in ten women on the contraceptive pill find the same problem.

5 Keep your lens case really clean. Give it a weekly wash with hot water (but no soap or harsh detergent) and a very small brush such as a child's toothbrush. Rinse the case with tap water, shake to remove excess water and then blot the outside with a tissue but leave the inside to dry in the air. Buy a new case whenever an old one becomes discoloured.

• Laser treatment of short sight •

Lasers can now be used to correct short or even long sight permanently by cutting away a minute piece of the cornea. The procedure is called photorefractive keratectomy or PRK. The laser used doesn't burn or ionise. It works by breaking chemical bonds, and can remove tissue to the accuracy of a quarter of a thousandth of a millimetre. However, the method has its critics, who claim that a large minority of people still need glasses after surgery; the majority suffer from glare at least some of the time, especially when driving at night; and some suffer from double vision.

There are at least 30 centres in the UK that offer PRK and it will probably become even more widely available in the future. Until then, contact the pioneering Corneal Laser Centre which at present has two clinics: one in Leeds and the other in Wirral. Or contact the Royal College of Ophthalmologists for a leaflet about PRK laser surgery: see Useful Contacts.

• Problems of the older eye •

As we age, not surprisingly eyes become more susceptible to problems. The following are the most common.

• Glaucoma •

The most common form of this condition is chronic glaucoma, a rise in the pressure of the fluid in the eye caused when the fluid ceases to be able to drain away naturally. It builds up slowly and can affect vision if not caught and treated early, but it cannot be completely cured.

One per cent of the population over 40 years of age is affected, with those

THE BATES METHOD

Practitioners and followers of the Bates Method believe that eye exercises can help the eyes stay strong and healthy, and that the method is useful for anyone with healthy eyes, whatever the condition of their sight. (It is not a means of curing disease.) It was devised by a New York ophthalmologist, Dr William Horatio Bates, who found that certain simple exercises not only removed eye strain but made objects seem clearer. Bates Method exercises include:

Splashing First thing in the morning, splash your closed eyes 20 times with warm water and 20 times with cold water, to stimulate circulation. At night, repeat, but splash first with cold and then with warm water. If your eyesight is very bad, bathe the closed eyelids with a sponge or flannel instead.

Blinking Blink often, sometimes quickly and sometimes really squeeze your eyes shut slowly. This is to clean the eyes and encourage tears to lubricate them.

Palming Relax and sit in a comfortable position at a desk or table. Rest your elbows on cushions on the desk or table top with your back straight and your head not tilted. Close your eyes, then cover them with your hands slightly cupped so that you don't actually touch your eyes. The aim is to rest the eyes.

Remembering While palming, try to remember some strong visual experience. 'See' a familiar object in all its detail, or visualise a scene in which you are conscious not just of the visual impact but the accompanying noises and smells, etc. Seeing more clearly in the imagination is meant to increase the clarity of your eyesight. Concentrating on the other senses helps to take some strain off the eyes and stop you putting in too much effort to see clearly.

Shifting Move your gaze about from one thing to another, instead of staring at any particular object, so that your eyes relax more.

Swinging In the standing position with feet apart, sway gently from side to side and let your eyes swing along with you, to help eye relaxation and flexibility.

Focusing Hold your index fingers in front of your face: one hand about 7.5cm (3in) from your eyes, the other at arm's length. Look first at one finger, blink, then look at the other. Do this several times to help your near and distant focusing.

If you would like to find a practitioner in the Bates Method, write with an sae to the Bates Association of Great Britain, or contact the Institute for Complementary Medicine: see Useful Contacts.

who have a family member with the disease or who have diabetes at most risk. It is usually diagnosed during routine eye tests, which is why it is important to have checks once a year after 40. (If you have a parent, child, brother or sister who is affected, you are entitled to eye tests free.) Treatment is to lower the pressure in the eye, by the use of drugs, eye drops, or in some cases surgery.

• Cataracts •

A cloudiness in the eye caused by a change in lens protein which becomes quite common between the ages of 50 and 60, with over half of women and men suffering some degree of cataract by that time. Whether sight is affected depends upon the location of the cataract in the eye. Some cataracts cause blurring, others double vision.

Most people can learn to live with their cataracts, by shielding eyes from the light outdoors, protecting eyes from direct light indoors by careful arrangement of lighting and reading with light shining on to the book or newspaper, not the face. An operation, currently the only treatment, is usually only thought necessary if the cataract develops to the point where it seriously interferes with or prevents ordinary life. The cloudy lens is removed and vision is restored by the use of cataract glasses, contact lenses or a lens inserted within the eye.

• Macular degeneration •

The macula is the part of the retina used for reading and close work and its degeneration is an inevitable consequence of ageing. One in four people over 65 are affected, but the degree varies. One eye is affected before the other and it becomes harder to see what you are looking at directly, although side vision is unaffected. Colours seem slightly different and objects seem smaller.

Shutting one eye can help when reading, if only one eye is affected. (It can be over ten years before the second eye goes too.) Good lighting and a magnifying glass can help. So too can changing the way you use your eyes when you read. Researchers have found that in different people different parts of the retina will still function properly and it is a case of finding the bit that is working for you. Instead of looking at the letters and following them with your eyes, look off to the side – left, right, up and down – until you find a position that lets you see the words.

11

TEETH

FAR FROM expecting to face the latter part of our lives with missing teeth or dentures, it is now usual to keep our own teeth for life. Better health, better dental care and fluoride have all contributed to a significant reduction in dental caries. However, we still need to take good care of our mouths because the big problem these days is gum disease, which threatens the life of our teeth.

• Tooth decay •

We all have a sticky layer of bacteria, called plaque, that lives on our teeth and gums. It can be brushed away, but the bacteria immediately set about growing again. There are various different kinds of bacteria in plaque but those responsible for tooth decay turn sugar consumed in the diet into acid. The acid starts to destroy the enamel on our teeth almost instantly and keeps on working for at least 30 minutes after eating or drinking something sugary. After brushing our teeth to remove plaque, it is the sugar-converting bacteria which grow again particularly quickly. Fluoride in toothpaste and in water can help repair the enamel and so does calcium in saliva, unless damage is particularly severe and continual because of very frequent consumption of sugary drinks and foods.

• Treatment •

Where holes do form in teeth and need to be filled, often the filling materials used can be less unsightly than the old grey-black amalgam variety which was made up of copper, silver and tin alloyed with mercury. (See Cosmetic Dentistry, page 91.) However, this is only possible on the NHS when the teeth to be treated are at the front of the mouth.

Currently, teeth are filled by drilling the cavity so that it is bigger than its opening. This prevents the filling from falling out. Some time in the not-too-distant future, lasers are likely to be commonly used in a painless procedure to make a small hole in a decayed tooth, kill the bacteria causing the problem and fill the hole with a thin bactericidal material.

• Gum disease •

Gum disease occurs when the bacteria which form plaque get a chance to grow at the join between gum and teeth. Those which cause the problem are

MERCURY IN FILLINGS

There is still controversy over the safety of the mercury content of amalgam fillings. There have been reports claiming that mercury slowly leaks out of fillings, causing damage to the central nervous system and the immune system. Most dentists do not feel the evidence is satisfactory, particularly as dentists handle amalgam every day and have no higher incidence of health problems than the general population.

Even if mercury leakage does cause problems for particularly susceptible individuals, there is, alas, no easy solution as removing amalgam fillings itself releases a great deal of mercury. Special precautions have to be taken, along with detoxification pills. For further information and to find out about testing for mercury sensitivity contact the British Society for Mercury-free Dentistry: see Useful Contacts.

different bacteria from those which cause tooth decay. The gum support for the teeth can be destroyed by poisons made by these bacteria but, unlike those which cause tooth decay, they are very slow-growing and don't manage to reach numbers significant to do damage until about 48 hours after the plaque first forms. So careful cleaning can eliminate this problem altogether.

However, brushing of the teeth is not usually enough (see Looking After Your Mouth, page 97). Also, if you have any rough areas on your teeth near your gums (commonly caused by decay), tartar or poor fillings, plaque can more easily cause you gum problems. Tartar (or calculus) is the hard substance that can build up on teeth and is made up of old plaque and the calcium salts deposited on it from saliva. Although not directly harmful itself as it has been neutralised by the calcium salts, it is a place to which plaque can conveniently stick and inconveniently be hard to budge from.

Most adults have some degree of gum disease. Over three quarters of young men and women aged between 16 and 24 have some, and 81 per cent have it by the age of 44. Women and men are equally affected, although women are especially prone to gum disease during pregnancy. In its very early stages it is called gingivitis.

• The consequences •

Your gums will bleed when you brush them and will also be inflamed and red, although you may not know that. If the gum disease is allowed to worsen, the gums will separate from the teeth, forming a space or pocket which will quickly fill with plaque. Eventually, bone is lost and the tooth will loosen in its socket or even fall out. It may take many years for the damage to progress to this degree, but because you are unlikely to feel pain you may not know anything is happening. The main cause of tooth loss today is gum disease. Flossing is vital to preserve the health of gums. (See Looking After Your Mouth, page 97.)

• Infections •

Sometimes dental decay, gum disease or an injury to the teeth can cause infection in the pulp, the nerves inside the tooth which contain blood vessels. The infection, if untreated, can spread along the whole root canal of the teeth and form an abscess which may then ooze pus and cause bad breath. Even if, as in some cases, the problem does seem to settle on its own, bone may be lost and the affected tooth may loosen, fall out or have to be taken out because pulp destroyed by infection cannot grow again. Root canal treatment is necessary: the dentist removes the infection, drains any abscess and then fills the canal again.

• Oral cancer •

Oral cancers are those affecting the lips, tongue, gums and lining of the mouth. They affect almost 2000 people in the UK every year and, at present, over half will die within five years, usually because of not seeking help until tumours are quite large. If tumours are treated when less than 2cm (¾in) in diameter, success rates are very good and two thirds of sufferers will recover.

No one knows why oral cancers occur but it is known that smoking, particularly if combined with heavy drinking, significantly increases risk. The disease is unusual before the age of 40 and men are currently affected more than women. However, the incidence in women is rising because we now drink and smoke more; a startling increase of 40 per cent in these cancers has been logged in women over the last 30 years.

The first pre-cancerous signs may be a red or white patch somewhere in the mouth or on the tongue, although this can and does usually have other, far less serious causes. Most often, there is a painless ulcer in the mouth which doesn't clear up. A good reason for going for at least yearly dental check-ups, particularly after the age of 40, is that dentists are now recommended to look for early signs of problems. However, diagnosis is not always easy even for dentists, so do go back for a second check if symptoms persist or if you are not reassured that any symptoms you have are insignificant .

Surgery or chemotherapy and radiotherapy are currently the common treatments but a promising technique for small tumours is called photo-dynamic therapy, in which a special dye is used to sensitise cancer cells to laser light. When the laser beam is directed at the tumour, only the cancer cells are killed. Such a treatment is obviously far less traumatic to a patient; but if tumours are not discovered until they are very large, radical surgery is usually required and this is, inevitably, enormously upsetting because of resulting facial disfigurement and disability.

• Jaw problems •

The temporomandibular joint (TMJ) is the joint between the lower jaw and the skull which lets you open and close your mouth and chew. If your teeth don't fit together properly (perhaps because of heavily worn teeth, broken fillings or lost teeth) you can get various problems, collectively known as the TMJ syndrome.

Grinding or clenching of teeth, clicking or pain in the jaw joints, ringing or buzzing in the ears and difficulty opening and closing your mouth can all be due to teeth not meeting properly. If your jaw is pushed out of position by an incorrect bite, the jaw muscles get overworked and can go into spasm, causing headaches and migraine, especially when you wake up; discomfort in the face; sinus pain; pain behind the eyes; and even pain in the neck, shoulders and back. If this is your problem, you may need to be referred to a specialist for a brace and/or replacement of missing teeth.

• Stress •

Thousands of people suffer from severe facial pain for which there appears to be no organic cause. Commonly cited symptoms are a dull ache in the face; a sticking and clicking feeling in the jaw; a pain like toothache; a burning pain in the gums, tongue and lips; the sensation of a dry mouth despite plenty of saliva; distorted taste; and discomfort in the way teeth meet together.

Stress appears to be the main trigger for this kind of facial pain, which makes the pain none the less real but means a different approach is needed to deal with it successfully. Antidepressants have been found helpful, as an analgesic. One of the reasons these work may be lowered levels of a chemical called conjugated tyramine sulphate, a metabolic defect found in people with stress-related facial pain as well as people who are clinically depressed. When not used as a treatment for depression, however, antidepressants can work quickly, in small doses, and can be effective even when used intermittently.

Lifestyle changes are important too. It is necessary to learn how to reduce stress levels, handle them more effectively and think differently about the pain: using relaxation or distraction methods to lessen its impact.

• Hypodontia •

Hypodontia means developmentally missing teeth. Not counting wisdom teeth, up to two and a half million people fail to develop at least one adult tooth while a quarter of a million people are missing at least six. There is often a genetic component, although sometimes a generation is skipped and severity of the condition will vary.

_____WISDOM TEETH_____

One in five people in their thirties have at least one unerupted third molar or wisdom tooth, and numbers of people with this condition are likely to increase as improved dental health leads to the extraction of fewer teeth and therefore there being less space for wisdom teeth to erupt into. The removal of unerupted wisdom teeth accounts for nearly three quarters of all surgery for the removal of teeth, yet experts now claim this is an absolutely unnecessary operation if the unerupted teeth are causing no problem. Unerupted wisdom teeth can remain in place and continue to be problem-free for the whole of most people's lives, whereas surgery can often cause nerve damage to the mouth and tongue.

When many teeth are missing, skilled specialists can rearrange existing teeth and replace missing ones in a special treatment programme, but it can be a lengthy business, stretching over a couple of years. Usually the condition is treated in the teenage years but adults who have not sought treatment before can be treated too. There are just a few dental clinics specialising in missing teeth. The oldest and largest is at the Eastman Dental Hospital in London: see Useful Contacts.

· Looking after your mouth ·

Brush your teeth properly Brushing should be done every day for at least three minutes. To avoid dental decay, it is actually better to brush teeth before a meal, because a thorough clean will remove all plaque from the teeth, eliminating briefly the bacteria that turn sugar into acid and start off the problems. For gum health it doesn't make any difference when you brush, as different bacteria are responsible for any damage.

Avoid too much sugar There is no evidence that foods or drinks that don't contain sugar can do any damage to the teeth at all. The worst harm is done by eating or drinking sugary things very frequently throughout the day, because the calcium in saliva doesn't have a chance to repair damage to the tooth enamel before the next onslaught of sugar. It is better to eat a packet of sweets in one go, therefore, rather than suck one at odd hours throughout the day.

Use a fluoride toothpaste and floss regularly Your dentist or hygienist can show you how to floss correctly to remove plaque from otherwise inaccessible places between the teeth. This needs to be done daily, particularly if you have crowns and want to preserve the life of them. If you can't get the hang of flossing with long bits of thread or put it off because of the nuisance, try Flossette dental flossers, an ingenious simple little device that takes the trouble out of flossing, but at a higher price, of course.

Change your toothbrush Buy a new toothbrush at least every two months. A small toothbrush head is easier to manipulate inside the mouth and nylon is preferable to bristle because it lasts longer and doesn't get soft. Always go for those labelled as medium or hard. If an electric toothbrush appeals, remember you still have to brush properly and in the right places to find plaque. Don't rely on tooth picks or home-use water jets for getting rid of plaque: they are designed only to dislodge trapped food.

End a meal with cheese This can help reduce plaque damage. Also, chewing sugarless gum after meals can be helpful as this stimulates saliva.

See your dentist and hygienist regularly This will ensure your mouth remains healthy.

• Cosmetic dentistry •

Cosmetic dentistry is anything which improves the appearance of teeth. Here is a guide to the range of services on offer at present.

• White fillings •

For front teeth unobtrusive white fillings can now be used, with the advantage not only of being less obvious but of not requiring much drilling because the filling material is glued into place with special techniques and materials. The tooth surface is treated with specific conditioners and an adhesive is applied. A dentist can either use 'composite' (plastic) materials moulded into the shape of the tooth which set when a particular blue light is shone on them, or bond into place a piece of porcelain that has been shaped from a model of the tooth.

White fillings for front teeth are available on the NHS. Not so white fillings for back teeth, where there is more wear and tear on the teeth. Opinions vary as to whether white fillings made from composite materials are as strong as amalgam.

• Porcelain onlays or inlays •

These are porcelain fillings which are bonded to the teeth. They are a more attractive option than amalgam for filling back teeth, although not available on the NHS. Inlays can be particularly useful to prevent fractures in teeth with very large fillings. Onlays can replace biting surfaces that have been ground down. Both are very long-lasting but probably pricey, because a lot of dentist's and dental technician's time is involved.

• Glass ionomer cements •

A strong glass-like material that can be bonded on to back teeth where the surface has suffered wear and tear as a result of enthusiastic use of the toothbrush. If this procedure is used to fill a cavity caused by overbrushing around the neck of the tooth, it may be available on the NHS. Sometimes, white composites may be bonded to their surface to improve appearance, as the cements are not quite invisible. As well, sometimes the cements are applied under a white filling in a back tooth to help prevent decay, as the material contains fluoride and sticks to the tooth, but this is not available on the NHS.

• Repairing chipped teeth •

For small chips and breaks in front teeth white composite fillings or porcelain may be used. The surface of the tooth is etched with acid and adhesive applied: on the spot, in the case of composites, whereas porcelain has to be moulded from a tooth model by a dental technician. Modern adhesives are now so sophisticated that sometimes broken teeth can just be stuck back together again.

• Closing the gap •

If you don't find a gap between your front teeth attractive, you can have it closed up with little problem using white, composite materials. Your teeth will look just slightly wider than before. The white plastics used may need repolishing after some time as they can stain, but they give a very lifelike appearance. Another option, not available on the NHS, is a porcelain tooth corner but as this might involve some adjustment of the teeth and require two visits it could be correspondingly more expensive. However it will last longer.

• Veneers •

These are intended to improve the appearance of front teeth which are dis-coloured, either naturally or through wear and tear, or because an old dis-coloured filling is showing through. They work rather like false fingernails in that they are placed over the natural tooth, but the tooth does need a little preparation first. White composites can be glued to the whole of the visible surface of the tooth. They look good but may discolour and wear away after a few months. Porcelain lasts longer but requires two visits because a mould must be taken of the tooth for shaping by a dental technician. Neither is available on the NHS.

• Crowns •

A broken tooth, a tooth that has been so heavily filled that it is both weak and ugly or a tooth so decayed that it cannot be filled can be made to look good again with a crown. The tooth is filed down to a peg on to which the crown is cemented. Crowns can be made of porcelain, porcelain bonded to metal alloy, gold or non-precious metal alloy and, most recently, castable glass. Gold or other metal alloy would only be used at the back of the mouth where the teeth cannot easily be seen. Porcelain alone may be suitable for front teeth but, if used on teeth needed for chewing, is more likely to be combined with metal. Castable glass is very lifelike, and in strength lies between porcelain and porcelain bonded to metal. It is not yet available on the NHS.

• Bridges •

Bridges are usually fitted when a tooth is lost. It is important to have something in the place where a tooth used to be because teeth opposite or next to a gap can move into it, increasing risk of tooth decay and gum disease. Conventional bridges require the teeth on either side to be filed down for crowns, necessarily destroying much of the tooth structure, and then two crowns are made with an extra tooth between them. The problem with this is that healthy teeth are filed down for no good reason.

Newer, adhesive bridges avoid this big drawback; there are a number of techniques which require very little reduction of the supporting teeth. Although specific techniques vary, the basic principle is that the false tooth is prepared with metal tags on either side and these are bonded to the adjacent teeth. Adhesive bridges are available on the NHS, and are now cheaper than the conventional kind.

• Dentures •

If your teeth are not strong enough to support a bridge, you may need a partial denture. This consists of false teeth fixed to a plate and held in place by clasps that fit around some of the remaining teeth. The disadvantage is that these clasps can sometimes be visible. Dentures are usually made of acrylics (plastics) with plastic or porcelain teeth, or are metal based with plastic gum and teeth attached. Metal dentures can be made more accurately and can have a smaller, thinner plate as the material is stronger; but they are also considerably more expensive. Your dentist should advise on which to go for.

There are even magnetic dentures available now. Magnets are placed in the plastic denture base and in the top of retained tooth roots. Once the denture is in position over the roots, the magnets help keep it in place. Magnetic dentures can be particularly helpful when a lot of teeth are missing or if worry about the denture becoming dislodged is a major concern.

• Implants •

Implants are a means of anchoring dentures that eliminates all need to remove them for cleaning or sleeping. Any feeling of looseness when talking, laughing or eating becomes a thing of the past. They are, however, a lengthy and expensive business and need to be performed by an expert specially trained in the technique. The implant itself is a metal device which is placed in the jawbone by surgery, leaving special parts protruding through the gum as anchors for full or partial dentures, or even for a crown. The metal most commonly used is titanium which can bond well to bone but other metals are still being experimented with.

It takes about three months for the implants to bond with bone in the lower jaw and six months in the upper jaw (during which time ordinary dentures can be worn). Then, false teeth are attached to the implants. Between 12 and 15 visits to the dentist will be required for the whole process, and treatment is likely to take, in total, five months for the lower jaw and eight months for the upper jaw. Once in place, teeth are cleaned and cared for in the same way as natural teeth.

There is scientific evidence that implants in the lower jaw are 90 per cent successful over a 15-year period but figures for the upper jaw are not yet available. Not everyone can have an implant, however. There has to be sufficient healthy bone in the jaw to make the procedure possible.

• Fear of the dentist •

Some people are frightened of going to the dentist, often because of some bad experience in the past or the uncaring attitude of one specific dentist. To try to find one who makes a point of being understanding with anxious patients, ask friends if they know anyone they would recommend or phone a few dental surgeries and ask if they are prepared to help anxious patients and how they go about it. (If you get an off-hand response, it is an indication that this surgery is not for you.) You can get a list of local dental practitioners from your Family Health Services Authority, which is listed in your local telephone directory.

There are many ways that a dentist can help reduce anxiety. For some people, it helps if dentists explain before each step of the treatment exactly what they are going to do next. Or being invited to raise your hand if you need treatment to stop for a moment because of discomfort or a need to swallow can make many people feel sufficiently in control to relax more.

A caring dentist will try to help you relax. Some are trained to offer hypnosis, that is, they will put you into a relaxed state by taking you through a gradual relaxation process, so that you will not be anxious although you will still be aware of what is going on during treatment.

Another helpful technique is relative analgesia. You breathe, through a nosepiece, a mixture of nitrous oxide and oxygen which quickly makes you feel relaxed and comfortable. You are conscious but a little drowsy during treatment and do not feel any pain. After the treatment is over, the effects are quickly reversed by breathing pure oxygen. Fifteen minutes later you can drive a car home. Your dentist will advise whether this method is suitable for you.

Sedation – sedative medicines which can be given orally or be injected in the arm – is another alternative, but this is not suitable for everyone. You become drowsy but you stay conscious and know what is going on, although whatever it is doesn't bother you. Time seems to pass extremely quickly, so this method can be useful for any lengthy procedures. It takes some time for effects to wear off, however, so you must be collected from the surgery and will probably need an hour's nap once home. Your dentist will tell you how long you should avoid driving, operating any machinery or drinking alcohol. It will depend upon your dentist whether he or she carries out this procedure on the NHS.

For further information or specific questions about overcoming fear of the dentist, send an SAE to the British Dental Health Foundation: see Useful Contacts.

• NHS treatment •

Dentists are not obliged to offer NHS treatment and a number of those who used to no longer do, claiming they cannot make a reasonable living and offer their patients a good enough service at the same time. It is more difficult in the south than in the north to find a dentist who does do NHS work, and some will only treat existing NHS patients on the NHS, refusing to take on new ones. Many others are considering reducing their NHS commitment, so if you want to find an NHS dentist, you may have to be prepared to search long and hard.

Ask your local Family Health Service Authority (number in telephone directory) for a list of NHS dentists in your area. If you cannot find a dentist from this list (some may have given up NHS work since the list was compiled), go back to the Family Health Service Authority and ask about dentists employed directly by themselves. You may be able to be referred to one for treatment.

When you find an NHS dentist, you arrange a continuing care agreement which lasts normally for two years and you should receive three months' written notice of its termination. (However, at the time of writing, the continuing care system is being reviewed.) The dentist should tell you what treatments you need at the time of joining and which are available on the NHS. NHS and private treatments can be mixed but only with your specific agreement and you should be given an estimate of costs for any private work. All the treatment specified must be carried out before the end of the agreement.

NHS dentistry is far from cheap, although private work is still considerably more expensive. Many people are now turning to dental care insurance schemes, designed to provide comprehensive dental care at a more affordable cost. For a regular monthly payment, you can have preventive and emergency care as well as ordinary dental treatments. Arrangements and provisions for different treatments vary from scheme to scheme. Ask your dentist if he or she belongs to one of these schemes and can let you have a leaflet.

12

SKIN

NO ONE HAS a flawless skin despite what the pictures in advertise-ments would have us believe. We all have our share of freckles and moles which some may consider beautiful and others may consider blemish-es. Because the skin is so exposed, it is prey to various problems caused by the environment in which we live. It can burn in the sun; it can become inflamed or itchy if subjected to too many irritant chemicals. Skin diseases are also common, often occurring as a physical expression of stress or exacer-bated by it, and tend to concern us more than some other illnesses simply because the effects are so embarrassingly visible.

• Bumps and blemishes •

Most of the following imperfections of the skin are extremely common.

• Moles •

Most adults have 20 or 30 moles. They arise from cells which were originally intended to be pigment-forming cells (melanocytes) but which cluster together becoming what we term a mole. We have many of them from birth but we also carry on developing new ones, often right into early middle age. As the cells that form moles are sensitive to hormones, women are particularly likely to develop new ones during pregnancy or if taking the contraceptive pill.

A new mole is small, dark and flat and looks like a freckle. However, unlike freckles, they do not darken in the sun. As moles get older, they sink deeper into the skin leaving behind them fibrous scar tissue which is what creates the raised brown lump. As the years pass, the mole gradually gets lighter and lumpier; with the exception of moles on the palms, soles of the feet and genitals which usually stay mainly flat and dark.

Most moles are perfectly harmless. However, some can undergo specific changes which may be a sign of melanoma, a dangerous form of skin cancer. The signs to be alert to are moles which are:

- 1cm (⅜in) across or more
- gradually increasing in size
- irregularly or jaggedly edged
- mottled in colour

- inflamed
- itching
- bleeding or crusting.

If you have three or more of these signs you should see a doctor as soon as you can. The smaller the cancerous mole and the less deeply it has penetrated into the skin, the easier it is to treat successfully.

New moles are more likely to be risky than older ones, although most of course will be harmless. Of pre-existing moles, at highest risk of malignant change are those we are born with, although even these become cancerous in only about 1 per cent of Caucasians. At a particularly high risk are the rare giant congenital moles which can sometimes cover an entire limb. Dysplastic moles, those which are larger than average, irregularly coloured, with jagged edges and which tend to appear in clusters around the time of puberty, need to be monitored, particularly if there is a family history of melanoma. The sites most common for melanoma are the calves in women and upper back in men, but it is possible to find it anywhere.

Least likely to become malignant are hairy moles, although myth would have it that these are dangerous and never must you risk plucking the hair or removing it by electrolysis. It can actually be a good idea to remove the hair because this prevents the hair follicle from becoming infected, the resultant symptoms of which may be confused with the changes associated with melanoma and cause unnecessary anxiety.

If you don't like a particular mole it is easy to have it excised by a dermatologist or cosmetic surgeon. However, if you are doing this for aesthetic reasons only, do bear in mind that the scar you will be left with will be about three times as long as the original mole. A shorter scar would puff up at the edges and be even more unsightly.

• Boils •

If a hair follicle becomes infected with germs, the result may be a boil, a raised area filled with yellow pus which bursts to leave a scar. They are extremely painful and most common in adolescents and young adults. Common sites are the face, neck, arms, wrists, fingers and buttocks. Any item of clothing which repeatedly rubs or chafes is likely to increase the chance of getting a boil.

• Warts •

Warts are hard lumps that form on the skin as a result of an overgrowth of cells caused by a virus known as human wart virus. Most of us are exposed to it, yet relatively few people are susceptible to warts. They are most commonly seen on the backs of the hands or fingers and the soles of the feet, which makes walking painful. Usually they disappear by themselves. However, troublesome and intransigent warts can be frozen off with liquid nitrogen by a GP or dermatologist or burned off with a special chemical preparation that can be bought from pharmacies and must be very carefully applied.

Warts on the face and warts on the genitals should not be self-treated.

Seborrhoeic warts are brown raised areas often seen on the skin of the elderly. They are harmless, if unsightly, ranging in appearance from flat brown patches to small protruding lumps with a crust. They can be excised or frozen off.

• Spider naevi •

These are minor abnormalities of the blood vessels which look like little red spots from which tiny veins fan out. They usually appear on the upper part of the body and are seen first at any age. Caused by hormonal changes in pregnancy, the contraceptive pill or hormone replacement therapy, and liver damage, they usually can be removed by electrolysis.

• Vitiligo •

An often distressing loss of pigment from the skin caused by a malfunction in the immune system which leads it to attack its own pigment cells. It is often first noticed after exposure to the sun because the affected skin stays white, but it is not actually caused by the sun. Small or large areas of skin can be affected, usually in symmetrical patches. It cannot be cured and so camouflage with cosmetics is all that can be done to hide it.

• Pityriasis versicolor •

Another cause of loss of pigment, that can be cured, fortunately. It is caused by a fungus and appears as white patches where the pigment has gone, although sometimes the fungus over-stimulates the pigment cells instead and then the appearance is of brown blotches. Pityriasis versicolor usually best takes a hold when skin is greasy and sweaty, so it is seen more often in the summer.

Usual treatment is to cover the patches with a shampoo containing selenium sulphide (Selsun) and then wash it off after about five hours, repeating the procedure for a few consecutive days. A less appealing but more thorough version of the same procedure is to coat yourself up to the neck in the shampoo, sleep in it (bravely ignoring the bad-egg smell and preferably using an old sheet, as it stains) and then wash off thoroughly in the morning. This prevents spread of the fungus and happily only has to be done once. Another option is an anti-fungal cream obtained on prescription and applied three times a day for a fortnight. Whichever method is used, however, it can be months before lost pigment returns.

• Xanthoma •

Small fatty lumps which may be found on the eyelids, sometimes indicating a raised cholesterol level. The fat content can be removed surgically.

• Lentigo •

The proper name for liver spots, those harmless flat brown spots that often develop on the back of the hands of the elderly.

• Keloid •

An overgrowth of scar tissue, caused by the skin over-enthusiastically repairing itself at the site of a wound. It can be a large lumpy area, looking like a growth, and is most commonly seen on the chest, shoulder or upper back, with people of African and Asian origin most susceptible. Keloids cannot simply be removed because more are then likely to develop as a result of the new wound. Corticosteroid drugs can usually be injected into the keloid to shrink it.

• Skin tags •

Superficial tags of skin which look like warts and may develop most commonly around the neck, under the arms, under the breasts and in the groin. They are often found in plump women but some women are just prone to them, whatever their build. Many notice them on the neck when pregnant. They can be burned, frozen or snipped off by a doctor.

• Darkening of the skin •

Brown patches may appear on the skin when women are pregnant or taking the contraceptive pill and are obviously hormone-related. However, they do not always disappear, unfortunately, once the pregnancy is over or the pill stopped. During pregnancy the skin may darken a little altogether in those who are already of darker complexion. A line of dark skin may also run from the navel to the pubic region.

• Nervous flushes •

Redness spreading up over the chest and throat is a not uncommon response to embarrassment or anxiety. It may occur more often at the time of a period or it may be caused by rosacea (see page 108).

• Broken veins •

These are not really broken veins at all but blood vessels near the surface of the skin which are permanently dilated and therefore can be seen more easily. The correct name is telangiectasia. They can be caused by exposure to too much sun or too much cold, steroids or radiotherapy treatments. Sometimes they result because of naturally thin skin. Electrolysis can solve the problem.

• Sweat rash •

This comes about from getting too hot, usually in the sun, and might take the form of a red rash between or under the breasts or under the thighs, if these are generously proportioned, or tiny little blisters, caused by blocked sweat glands. Cover up until the rash disappears.

• Wrinkling •

Wrinkling of the skin only happens in sites that are exposed to the sun, usually the neck and face. The fairer complexioned you are, the stronger your chances of wrinkling, and the more you are out in the sun the more wrinkles you are likely to get. Wrinkling seems to be the result of an actual change that takes place in the skin after sun damage.

Smokers are particularly prone to wrinkling because the nicotine in cigarettes impedes the circulation of blood to the skin, depriving it of the full quota of the oxygen it needs to stay smooth and healthy.

• Skin problems •

Dermatitis (eczema), rosacea, acne and psoriasis are the most common chronic skin problems.

• Dermatitis or eczema •

In this condition the skin becomes red, sore, inflamed and itchy and sometimes blisters can develop, which weep and then crust over. This miserable condition can develop in childhood and persist into adulthood or develop for the first time in adulthood. For adults, the cause is often very frequent contact with particular chemicals that can irritate the skin (irritant contact dermatitis). Common offenders are perfumed soaps, shampoos, detergents, cleaning materials, etc, which wear down the skin's defences until, for some people, breaking point is reached.

Sometimes the problem is caused by an allergic response to a particular material (allergic contact dermatitis). Very common is allergy to nickel in jewellery (such as ear-rings), to zips, sticking plaster, rubber and glue. You might suddenly become allergic to a perfume or deodorant that you have worn without problem for years, because the body has at last reacted to a build-up of assaults which it has struggled to cope with up until then.

It may be easy to identify the cause of the reaction – a red rash around the ear lobe for nickel in an ear-ring, for example – but a rash on the hands could have many causes and you may have to have patch tests to find out what is affecting you. Sometimes creams used to treat other conditions can cause an allergic response. In fact, just about anything can cause an allergy in someone, somewhere.

Your doctor may call these conditions eczema, as the terms eczema and dermatitis are used fairly interchangeably, although traditionally eczema referred to inherited sensitive skin and dermatitis only to a reaction to external substances.

For skin that is dry and itchy, use a good moisturiser. For extreme dryness, an emollient – thicker and richer than ordinary moisturiser – may be helpful. As far as possible avoid the cause of the dermatitis. Wear plastic gloves when washing up, washing your hair or using abrasives, and always dry your hands thoroughly, particularly under rings.

The National Eczema Society provides valuable information on good skin management and on household products to seek out and avoid. See Useful Contacts.

• Rosacea •

This is a reddening of the face, especially the nose and cheeks, caused – it is thought – by a problem with the tiny blood vessels supplying the skin. Far from being relatively uncommon as once believed, one in ten middle-aged women suffers at least mild symptoms.

First symptoms usually occur in the teens, in the form of intense facial flushing when embarrassed, anxious or after eating hot and spicy foods or drinking alcohol. The flushing attacks (which often feel burning) tend to worsen in the twenties, covering more skin, often with a burning sensation. Usually the flushing subsides quickly but in some unlucky sufferers the face becomes permanently red, especially around the cheeks, nose and forehead. By the thirties, spots which look like bad acne start to come and go. In the most severe cases eye irritation, facial swelling and a thickening of the nose can also occur.

Rosacea can be kept down by avoiding foods and drinks that are either too hot or too cold, avoiding caffeine, cutting down or giving up alcohol, not using oil-based cosmetics, keeping out of strong winds and strong sun and trying to minimise stress and anxiety. Antibiotic tablets containing tetracycline may help with acne symptoms and a topical antibiotic gel containing metronidazole to apply directly to the skin is also available for the same purpose. If menopausal flushing makes the rosacea worse, hormone replacement therapy (see page 446) may be advised.

• Acne •

Acne is supposed to be a teenage complaint, but as very many women know, it can persist through life or even start for the first time in an adult. Acne is the overall term for pimples, blackheads, whiteheads and cysts, any or all of which can cover the face and back. The greasier your skin, the higher the risk of acne. Washing the face repeatedly, steaming the face and avoiding chocolate do not help.

For mild acne, benzoyl peroxide solutions, available from pharmacies, can be useful but can cause redness and peeling too. If so, start by using the lowest strength on alternate days and build up tolerance gradually. Topical antibiotics may also be worth a try; these can result in an 50 per cent reduction in symptoms after two or three months. Another option is a newer treatment, azelaic acid cream.

If acne is more severe and oral treatment is needed, it must be taken continuously for a few months before any real results can be expected. Tetracycline is the most often prescribed, being the cheapest, but its effectiveness is reduced if any milk or antacids are taken before it is absorbed.

If acne does not respond to oral antibiotics, an oral hormonal therapy (Dianette) is available which doubles as a contraceptive. This may bring results within two months. For extremely severe acne, dermatologists have a drug called isotretinoin which is very potent and very effective but has to be extremely carefully monitored because of possible side-effects.

Acne is supposed to get better during pregnancy. Experience shows sometimes it does, sometimes it doesn't and sometimes it worsens.

One not uncommon cause of adult acne is over-enthusiastic use of lip balms to keep the lips moist. Some women apply them almost constantly throughout the day and the result for those with particularly sensitive skin can be acne around the mouth. Stopping use of the lip balm or drastically cutting down is usually sufficient to reverse the problem. If not, benzoyl peroxide should help.

Another cause of what appear to be acne-like eruptions in adulthood is not acne at all but rosacea (see page 108).

• Psoriasis •

Psoriasis is a very common and distressing skin complaint taking the form of red scaly patches which, when scratched, show silvery scales beneath. The patches may affect just a few areas of the body or very many, are uncomfortable, itchy and, to the naturally self-conscious sufferer, extremely unsightly. About 2 per cent of the population of the UK are sufferers, with men and women affected equally but with onset usually earlier in women. It can start any time from birth up till old age and the causes are unknown.

A number of factors can trigger a first attack, including streptococcal throat infection, burns, sunburn, skin infection and a highly stressful life event. Stress can contribute to flare-ups.

There is no cure and the treatments have always been rather unpleasant: for example, coal tar and other smelly, messy substances which have to be applied to the body. Fortunately, vitamin D ointments and creams are now available which are not only effective in treating symptoms but are odourless and stain-free.

For further information on psoriasis contact The Psoriasis Association: see Useful Contacts.

• Skin cancers •

There are three kinds of skin cancers: basal cell carcinoma (rodent ulcers); squamous cell carcinoma; and melanoma. The first doesn't spread far, the second is slow-growing but can be lethal if allowed to spread and the third is quickly lethal.

A possible precursor of skin cancer, though not a serious one, is the solar keratosis: raised pink crusty warty areas that can appear on sun-exposed fair skin. It is fairly rare that this does turn malignant but the signs, if it does, are an increase in size and thickness.

• Basal cell carcinoma (rodent ulcers) •

This is the most common form of skin cancer but it is very slow growing and almost never spreads to other parts of the body. A rodent ulcer looks like a pearly, raised or flat lump, usually appearing next to the eye or nose and sometimes on the scalp or neck. It is more common in those who have been exposed to a lot of sun. If left untreated it can take over larger and larger areas of the skin and look extremely unsightly. Radiotherapy, cryosurgery and simple removal are all very effective.

• Squamous cell carcinoma •

This looks like a wart or an ulcer and tends to bleed easily. It usually appears on body parts that have been exposed to the sun. Where once this cancer was thought of as an older person's disease, it is now becoming more commonly seen in women as young as 40 who have spent a lot of time in the sun. Those with red hair and fair skin are especially at risk early. Squamous cell carcinoma can also surface around a leg ulcer.

This skin cancer can spread, although progress is slow, and it is important to catch it before it does as, once it has spread to other parts of the body it can be lethal. Most dangerous are the ones which manifest themselves on the lip or ear. Treatment can be by freezing, surgery, radiation or laser. For both this cancer and rodent ulcers, often treatment can be given under local anaesthetic.

• Malignant melanoma •

This, the most lethal form of skin cancer, is a cancer of the pigment-producing cells, the melanocytes, and is very much linked with over-exposure to the sun. Half start in moles but the rest in unblemished skin.

Although it is still a relatively rare cancer, it has one of the fastest rates of increase in white-skinned people of all cancers, especially among the young and middle-aged. More women than men get it: in the UK about 2300 a year compared with 1300 men. It kills about 1300 people a year, of men and women equally.

For signs of possible malignancy, see Moles (page 103). Those most at risk are people who have higher than average numbers of moles on their bodies (50 to 100), have red or fair hair, blue eyes and freckles, tan with difficulty and burn easily or have had two or more family members who suffered the disease.

Melanoma must be treated quickly as the depth to which it has invaded the skin has a bearing on success of treatment. Once it has penetrated the deepest layer of skin it can quickly spread through the bloodstream all over the body.

Caught early, however, there is a 90 per cent chance of cure. Treatment is with surgery and radiation or chemotherapy.

Women with melanoma appear to do significantly better than men, with a greater five-year survival rate. This might be because women tend to have melanoma on the leg, which has a generally better outcome than melanoma on the trunk where men are more likely to suffer it. Also, women are more aware of the early signs and are likely to seek medical help earlier. But even taking these factors into account, the disease in women has a better outlook than in men and it now seems, according to recent studies, that oestrogens may inhibit the growth of melanoma to some degree. However, there is no evidence that taking oestrogens in the form of the contraceptive pill confers any benefit in this respect.

• Safer sunning •

It should be apparent by now that the sun may be responsible for many ills connected with the skin. It is important, therefore, to be wise about suntanning, especially as, despite all attempts at making pale skin interesting, we still seem to value a tan. So follow these guidelines to stay safe.

1 Don't lie out in very hot sun between 11am and 2pm. Even better advice might be to check the sun's intensity by its shadow, as time of day isn't always a good indicator of the sun's strength because of seasonal changes and differences in longitude and latitude in different parts of the world. Quick check: if your shadow is shorter than your normal height, the sun is particularly likely to be burning.
2 Remember that shade is not totally protective. Water, sand and concrete can all reflect sunlight and increase your chances of burning.
3 Don't think that sunscreens, useful though they are, are fully protective. Sunlight can penetrate glass, cloud and water and fine hosiery such as tights.
4 Don't apply sunscreen once and forget about it. Re-apply every few hours or more often if you dry yourself on a towel after swimming.
5 Loose fitting clothing is better protection against the sun than tight clothing and dark colours are more protective than light ones. Linen, cheesecloth and flimsy see-through materials could increase your risk of burning. Lycra offers very good protection, even when wet.
6 Don't imagine that you can't get enough sun to burn in Britain. You can and, especially, so can children who have thinner skins than adults. Serious sunburn when young can increase risk of skin cancer when older. Keep children covered when in the sun and keep them out of the sun altogether at the most dangerous times.

• Sunscreens •

A tan may look good, but it is in fact the body's defence against sun damage. Ultraviolet light (UV) from the sun comes in three forms: UVA, UVB and

UVC. UVC doesn't penetrate our atmosphere. UVB burns but starts the tan. UVA can also tan but is weaker and so more is needed before any effect is seen, but it certainly is not harmless. It plays some part in the damage that may lead to skin cancer and it has a strong role to play in causing wrinkles. UVB is most damaging in mid-summer and at midday in hot climates; UVA is present all day, all year round.

Sunscreens nowadays have sun-protection factors (SPF) which measure protection against UVB. The sun-protection factor is based on your own estimate of how long you can stay in the sun without burning. If you can manage 10 minutes, for instance, an SPF of 15 will allow you to multiply that by 15, giving you 150 minutes or two and a half hours of suntanning without worrying about burning.

As your suntan develops, so does your sun protection, so you can reduce your sunscreen SPF accordingly and tan faster without burning. SPF 15 and above are high protection, 7-14 are medium and 2-6 low. UVA used not to be taken into account in sunscreens but now there is a star rating system for UVA. Three or four stars indicate a high protection against UVA damage. If you need a high SPF against UVB, look for a high star rating for UVA too. However, a high SPF factor is more important than more stars for UVA. Choose your sunscreen on the basis of UVB protection first, then as high UVA protection as you can get with it. Ask the pharmacist for help if you are confused.

• Sunbeds •

Sunbeds are not necessarily safer than the sun. Check that operators at any solarium you choose are properly trained and understand their equipment. Check what wavelengths (UVA only, plus UVA and UVB combined) are emitted. You should be told that certain medications, such as use of tetracycline antibiotics or certain tranquillisers, can cause a rash if you use a sunbed, and women on the contraceptive pill or women who are pregnant risk blotching, just as they would do from the sun.

Always wear goggles if using a sunbed and don't exceed your recommended time. Don't assume that mere use of a sunbed will help your skin tolerate the real thing better: if you don't get a tan from a sunbed, you are still at high risk from the sun.

One unexpected and fortunately unusual hazard of sunbed use is pityriasis versicolor (see page 105), a fungus which causes white patches on the skin and thrives in hot, sweaty conditions, usually on sunbathers in natural sunshine. However, cases have been reported where women have caught this fungus from a previous user of a sunbed when the bed wasn't properly sprayed and cleaned between customers.

13

NAILS

NAILS ARE made of the protein, keratin, which is also in skin, but have their hard appearance because the keratin here is much more tightly packed. For all their hardness, nails tend to reflect the body's state of health – mental or physical – and some illnesses may cause specific changes in the nails. Nails are also susceptible to fungal and bacterial infections but these may be minimised by good nail care.

• Taking care of your nails •

1 To help stop nails splitting, avoid prolonged or too-frequent contact with harsh detergents or other household chemicals. As most of us have to use such solutions every day, protect yourself with rubber gloves.
2 Don't let your hands be in prolonged contact with water, particularly if the water is soapy. Nails are part water and can absorb more when immersed. Wet, sodden nails are more susceptible to fungal infections.
3 Wear gloves in winter or at any time when your hands are very cold. Nails are more likely to split when circulation to the finger tips is poor; most notably in winter. If the nails do not receive sufficient blood supply, they do not grow as strongly.
4 Don't pay too much attention to cuticles, the protective part where nail meets skin at the base of the nail. Excessive manicuring or picking can weaken the cuticles and allow entry to bacteria and infection.

• Nail infections •

Fungal infections may make nails appear yellow, greeny brown or greeny black if the infection is under the nail, and there may be some pitting.

Thrush, more familiar as the fungus that causes white patches in the mouth of babies and discharge from the vagina, can also affect the sides of the nails. Antifungal treatment is necessary, and if the infection is severe, it may have to be used for several months while the affected nail grows out.

Ringworm infections of the skin can also affect the nails, making them look thick and discoloured, and break easily. Anti-ringworm tablets will work but the process is lengthy because the affected nail has to grow out before treatment can be stopped.

WHITE SPOTS

Contrary to popular belief, white spots on the nails do not signify calcium deficiency. White spots can occur as a result of a knock or bang to the nail, of cuticle damage caused by too much prodding and pressing or of illness. Sometimes they appear for no clear reason at all and disappear equally unpredictably. They also become more common as we get older.

Bacterial infections have sudden rather than gradual effects. The area around the nails becomes red and swells and whitlows, blisters filled with pus, may develop along the edges of nails. Your doctor can lance the blisters to relieve the pain.

• Abnormalities caused by illnesses •

Pitted nails If not caused by fungal infections, pitted nails can be a sign of psoriasis. The nail may also separate from the nail bed. Pitting may accompany hair loss. Tiny pits may signify liver disease.

Ridged nails Marked ridges that run right across the nail, horizontally, may occur if you have heart or lung disease but also may appear during a bout of pneumonia and, to a lesser extent, after any bad bout of illness. Even worry and anxiety can cause ridges. Tiny ridges often form if you regularly press your cuticles so far back that the nail root is affected.

Yellowed nails Can be a sign of heart or lung disease but alternatively could indicate an allergy, infection, increasing age or nicotine-staining.

Spoon-shaped nails Can be a sign of iron deficiency, commonly caused by eating too little iron in the diet and, in women, from heavy loss of blood during periods. Ask your doctor for a blood test to check.

Clubbed fingers A condition in which the ends of the fingers tend to enlarge and flatten and the nails grow in a curve around them. Clubbed fingers are very often a sign of lung disease, although it is not understood why. They can also be a feature of some other illnesses, for instance, the inflammatory bowel disease called Crohn's.

14

BACKS

A FIRST attack of backache is surprisingly more a problem of the young than the middle-aged or elderly, although of course, more than enough people of all ages suffer the misery of back pain for one reason or another. A *Which?* magazine survey a few years ago showed that 61 per cent of first-time sufferers are under 35 and 38 per cent are under 24. Also, four out of five of us will suffer back pain that is severe enough to keep us away from work. Women are slightly more likely to suffer back pain than men, perhaps because pregnancy, childbirth and the picking up and carrying of babies and toddlers eventually take their toll.

• Causes of back pain •

There are innumerable causes of back pain, including disc protrusion (so-called 'slipped disc'), compressed nerves, joint strain, muscular tension, poor posture, certain illnesses and injury to the neck and spine.

Muscle tension A staggering 90 per cent of back pain has muscular tension as its origin, caused by poor posture; bad seating at home, work or in the car; repetitive strain; or bending and lifting incorrectly.

Disc problems Disc problems are a fairly common cause of acute back pain. In younger people they are most likely the outcome of a violent injury to the back, perhaps while playing a vigorous sport, dancing energetically or bending or twisting suddenly while moving furniture or pulling up a particularly resistant weed in the garden. From middle age onwards, however, disc problems are more likely to be caused by the continued wear and tear on the disc casing.

A slipped disc is in fact a prolapsed, ruptured disc. Spinal discs are like boiled sweets with soft jelly centres: if there is a build-up of pressure inside the disc, the coating cracks and out oozes the centre, causing a deep, dull aching pain in the lower back, although you may also feel the pain in the groin and one buttock, thigh and hip. Moving at all may be very painful.

About half of sufferers recover within a fortnight to a month, regardless of what treatment is given. However exercises, manipulation and any procedure which lessens the pain and therefore helps you relax your muscles will speed things up. The more you tense your muscles, a natural reaction against the pain, the harder it is to get moving properly again.

Female hormones   These may be responsible for much of the backache suffered by women. Three days before a period, progesterone levels drop suddenly, with the immediate effect of making muscles looser and softer and easier to damage. Seventy per cent of women hurt their backs for the first time before a period, often while doing very normal daily activities such as bending down to pick up a bag, turning suddenly to get something from a shelf or even simply sneezing.

Backache during a period is common because of excessive activity by hormones called prostaglandins. The womb reacts by going into spasm, preventing blood circulation in the pelvic area and so causing cramps.

Pregnant women are at especial risk because they produce a hormone called relaxin which softens ligaments so that the pelvis can open more easily during the birth. Relaxin affects all ligaments, so sensible back care is essential. The extra weight of pregnancy also adds strain and may cause a swayed back posture, increasing the likelihood of backache.

Prolapse   Also known as pelvic relaxation, this is a condition which occurs when the pelvic muscles weaken and allow the womb, bladder, rectum or urethra to drop out of place, and is often first signalled by backache. The most common reason for a prolapse is damage to the pelvic floor during a labour that was either particularly fast or else too protracted. (See also page 251.)

Gynaecological conditions   Ovarian cysts, fibroids or a fallopian tube infection can cause constant low back pain.

Kidney infection   When back pain is accompanied by a fever and a burning sensation on urinating, the cause is likely to be a kidney infection.

Sex   This can cause a bad back if the position doesn't suit you. Positions which enable particularly deep penetration may be painful for some women's backs but even pelvic rocking while lying on one's back can sometimes put a strain on the spine and the pelvis. Certainly, sex on your back doesn't help a bad back if you already have one. Better to lie on your side, or put a pillow under your hips if you do lie on your back.

Fashion   This has a lot to answer for. High-heeled shoes throw the weight forward unnaturally on to the toes and can strain the back. Bras which don't support the breasts properly can contribute to back pain (as can hunching the shoulders to try to disguise big breasts). Apparently most women unwittingly buy bras that are too small: to be sure of buying the correct size, leave your bra off for half an hour to let the muscles relax, then take and hold a deep breath while measuring around the largest part of the breasts.

Even tight jeans can help cause backache because it is hard to bend from the knee while wearing them. Bending from the waist instead is one of the easiest ways to cause back damage.

Emotional stress   For those susceptible to back pain, a time of overwhelming demands or difficult life circumstances can leave them more vulnerable to pulling a muscle or doing some back injury. Suppressed emotions such as grief and anger may also be manifested as back or neck pain, muscular tension being the unconscious means of holding the feelings inside. The upper back, neck and shoulders are particularly vulnerable.

Sometimes massage or manipulation of the affected areas can lead to an outpouring of the suppressed emotional pain, which may be confusing or shocking at the time but is a sign that you might benefit from exploring some of your powerful hidden feelings with a therapist or a sensitive and sympathetic friend.

· Caring for your back ·

1 Always bend at the knees, not from the waist.
2 When getting out of bed, turn on to your side, swing your legs off the bed and then use your arms to push yourself up into a sitting position.
3 Check your bed if you tend to wake with backache. Put boards under a sagging mattress or put the mattress on the floor. A bed is right for you if you can fit your hand snugly between the small of your back and the bed when you are lying down. If you can't insert your hand easily, the bed is too soft, and if there is enough space to draw your hand in and out very easily, it is too hard.
4 Carry a heavy object as close to your body as possible: carrying with your arms outstretched strains your chest, shoulders and upper back. Always split loads such as shopping as evenly as possible between both hands, so that your body is balanced. If possible, don't carry heavy loads at all: use a trolley, wheel a suitcase, etc.
5 Don't regularly cradle a telephone under your chin to free your hands as this position causes strain and creates neck and shoulder problems.
6 If you must stand for long periods, try resting one foot on a stool if and when possible. This helps take the pressure off your spine.
7 If you work in an office make sure your work environment is suitable. An office chair should enable you to sit with your knees lower than your hips. Your desk height should not be too low, forcing you to bend your shoulders and neck. If you work at a VDU screen, the screen should be raised to eye-level height. Get up and take brief breaks frequently. If you can't get up often enough, periodically shake and circle your shoulders and move your neck up and down and from side to side.
8 When driving, make sure your knees are not bent up too high. The seat should offer full support and you should feel the headrest supporting your neck and head. You should be able to reach all of the controls comfortably.
9 When doing housework, kneel to do jobs such as making the bed and cleaning the bath, sit on a stool of comfortable height to do the ironing, squat down while removing heavy wet clothes from the washing machine and putting them into a basket beside you on the floor. When working at a kitchen counter, rest your back by supporting one foot on a low stool some of the time. (You could also try this option while ironing.)

10 Never swing a child up into your arms from arms length. Bend at the knees and gather the child in towards you. Use cots with a drop side for babies and put baby baths on a table to avoid strain on your back. If you have a back problem already, don't add to it by lifting the baby bath to empty it. Empty it out gradually with a bucket or jug or ask someone who is able to do it for you.

11 If you have a four-door car (much healthier for the back) get into the back seat with your child to strap them into their seat, rather than leaning in at the door.

12 In the garden, kneel down rather than bend whenever possible or use long-handled implements. Don't overdo the digging.

• Professional treatment •

For serious back problems or those with an unclear cause, see your doctor who may advise further investigation. For many muscular or spinal conditions, other professionals, conventional and alternative, often have something to offer and you should seek help as soon as possible to stop a problem from becoming chronic. Spinal surgery is usually a very last resort.

Physiotherapists   You can be referred to a hospital physiotherapy department by your GP. Physiotherapists are trained to treat musculo-skeletal problems by a variety of methods including massage, heat treatment, cold treatment, hydrotherapy, ultrasonic therapy (the application of high-frequency, sound waves to the affected area by means of special equipment), short-wave diathermy (application of high frequency electromagnetic waves to create heat), traction and exercise.

Osteopaths and chiropractors   Both of these professionals use manipulation to help backs and necks when the problem is mechanical. Neither can cure disease and a severely prolapsed disc may need surgery.

You may need a number of visits or only one, according to your problem. Expect a full history to be taken at your first visit and the appointment to last about half an hour. Later sessions may last about 15 minutes.

See Osteopathy and Chiropractic, page 79, for further information and how to find a properly qualified practitioner.

Acupuncture   Although often helpful in relieving the pain of backache it cannot provide a cure and should only be tried if the cause of the pain is known. Some NHS pain clinics offer acupuncture and many general practitioners have trained in the use of it.

See Acupuncture, page 78, for further information and how to find a properly qualified practitioner.

Acupressure or shiatsu   See Shiatsu, page 80, for further information and how to find a properly qualified practitioner.

Alexander Technique   A method of realigning the body to correct poor posture and movement which can cause strain. Can be helpful for backache and neck ache caused by tension. To find a properly qualified practitioner who has completed an approved course, contact the Society of Teachers of the Alexander Technique (STAT): see Useful Contacts.

• Dealing with acute back pain •

Acute back pain is usually experienced in one of two ways: sudden excruciating pain after a particular movement such as stretching or turning, or the pain may come on gradually and become more and more severe.

1 Lie down briefly to take the stress off your spine and lessen the pain. This will help you to relax which is important.
2 Lie on your back if you can. If you can't, lie on your side or stomach.
3 Put pillows wherever they may lessen the strain: in the small of the back and under the knees if lying on your back, or between your knees if lying on your side.
4 Try relieving the pain with heat from a wrapped hot water bottle. If you prefer, try numbing the pain with cold from a bag of crushed ice-cubes or frozen peas.
5 Don't take to your bed for any prolonged period. People recover from acute lower back pain more quickly if they stay active. Recent research has shown that those who keep mobile are suffering far less disability between seven and 28 days later than those who take to bed for 48 hours. The longer you rest up, the more your muscles start to waste, causing later problems.
6 Take pain killers as you need them, within the maximum recommended daily limit.
7 Call the doctor if the pain has not lessened after two or three days. If you have any other symptoms, however, such as difficulty passing urine, giddiness or pain somewhere else besides the back, call a doctor at once.

15

FEET

WE DON'T pay half as much attention to our feet as we do to our hands but just because they are tucked away from view most of the time doesn't mean that we can comfortably forget about them. All sorts of things can go wrong with feet, and from an early age too, because of lifestyle and fashion. If we don't take care, even if nothing dire has happened yet, we could unwittingly be storing up problems for the future.

For instance, to keep a court shoe on your foot you have to screw up your feet, otherwise it would fall off. As a result the big toe may move sideways, the second toe is forced upwards to lie on top and you have an ugly dislocated or hammer toe which, unlike a dislocated shoulder, won't obligingly pop back into place with expert manipulation. Court shoes also make the foot slide forward continuously which can increase the likelihood of calluses. Wearing shoes that are too tight at the toe can cause bunions while constant wearing of high heels leads the muscle in the calf to shorten, so that returning to flat heels can be a painful experience.

Fortunately, feet are flexible enough to recover, given time, from the tortures we entrap them in, if we are sensible about avoiding foot problems. Diabetics need to be particularly vigilant of their feet because diabetes increases susceptibility to foot problems.

• General foot care •

Washing and drying Feet should be very carefully dried to avoid fungal infections but if your skin tends to be moist anyway between the toes, use talcum powder or surgical spirit to help keep them dry. If your skin is too dry, use moisturising cream around the nails and heels and anywhere you tend to get hard skin.

Toenail cutting Never try to shape toes like fingernails. Toenails should have the slightest of curves to follow the top of the toe, or be cut straight across. Don't cut down the side of the toe nail. This, and peeling toenails instead of cutting them, can increase the risk of an ingrowing toenails.

Buying shoes If possible, always buy leather as only leather gives and stretches and allows the absorption of moisture, plenty of which is released in sweat from the feet each day. New leather shoes will become more comfortable as you start wearing them but if you buy synthetic shoes you need to make sure they are comfortable immediately you put them on because they won't change shape at all.

Feet swell a bit over a day so do your shoe-buying in the afternoons.

Changing shoes Wear different shoes every day if possible, to allow sweat absorbed into the leather time to evaporate and dry out. Don't put the shoes near heat, as the leather will crack and shrink.

Suit the occasion Keep wear of court shoes and/or high heels to a sensible minimum, for example, for a party or for an occasion when you must look smart or fashionable. Never wear them at home. For working shoes, if you have to look smart, try to find an attractive lace up or something with a T-bar or strap to help hold the foot in the shoe.

If you don't have to look smart all the time, keep a comfortable pair of shoes at work to change into whenever you can, but don't choose slip-on shoes, as they don't give support. Long pull-on boots also lack support.

For comfort, heels should be lower than two and a half inches. If you have been a wearer of very high heels and plan to change, come down gradually to allow your calf muscles to adjust.

For walking or hiking, ideally wear a shoe that gives good support, has adequate breadth, laces high up and has enough depth for the toes. Go shopping in trainers or Doc Martens. Sports shoes should leave you plenty of room for movement as well as provide your feet with good support but beware heel tabs. According to one leading sports physiotherapist, heel tabs mainly serve the purpose of displaying the manufacturer's name and on some sports shoes the tabs can damage the Achilles tendon.

• Foot problems •

• Callouses •

These are areas of hard skin that may form on the heels, the balls of the foot or the tips of the toes as a result of pressure or friction caused when shoes are too tight or too loose. Initially, the callous may protect against discomfort but if it deepens it can cause considerable pain. Rubbing hard patches very gently with a pumice stone and moisturising them can help but avoid a callous scraper and never use a razor blade or anything with a sharp edge. If the pain is bad, don't try to treat yourself. See a chiropodist and change your footwear.

• Corns •

Also caused by pressure, usually from new or poorly fitting shoes. The skin thickens where it is compressed between shoe and bone and a hard central core of dead skin develops to produce the corn. There are no roots to a corn, contrary to common belief. If the pressure goes on and on an ulcer may form, so it is wise to deal with the problem early. If very gentle rubbing with a pumice stone doesn't help, you need to see a chiropodist.

Some corns – usually between the toes – are soft. They feel rubbery because of the moisture there and can be very painful. Because of where they are located, a chiropodist's skill is essential for removing them.

• Bunions •

This means that the big toe has moved at a sharp angle towards the other toes, pushing the second toe out of position. The big toe joint becomes painful and prominent. Wearing shoes with high heels and pointed toes significantly increases the risk of developing a bunion and unfortunately once it is there it stays unless the deformity is so severe that surgery is needed to straighten the toe. There is a hereditary element to bunions. If either your mother or your father suffered, you are all the more likely to get one. Once the damage is done all you can do is make sure you find comfortable shoes with a lot of 'give'.

• Hammer toe •

A deformity and dislocation of a toe, usually the second, caused by the big toe joint becoming fixed in a sideways position and thus squashing the other toes. Eventually, the second toe gets pushed completely out of position and ends up lying on top of the big toe where it is particularly vulnerable to painful corns. If strapping or better footwear doesn't relieve the pain, surgery may be necessary to straighten both the first joint and the second toe and to prevent them from moving. Court shoes, in which you have to scrunch up your toes to keep them on, are common culprits for this condition.

• Hallux rigidus •

Loss of movement in the joint of the big toe. It may become inflamed as a result of arthritic changes caused by trauma. These sorts of arthritic changes can occur at any time in life and in fact are very commonly caused by some accident, not even remembered, in childhood. The problem, however, may not surface for another 10 or 15 years after the injury. Another possible cause is shoes, if the big toe is constantly being stubbed against the end of a shoe that is too short.

Ice packs to reduce the inflammation and strapping to reduce movement can be helpful in the acute stages and wearing flat-heeled shoes will definitely be more comfortable. Eventually, the joint may become fixed and immobile, ceasing to be painful but making walking more of an effort for the other joints and increasing the risk of callouses and corns. If you see an osteopath before things get this far, there is a possibility that mobility can be returned to the joint. (See Osteopaths and Chiropractic, page 79 for details of how to find an osteopath.)

• Ingrowing toenails •

These most often affect people in their teens and twenties, particularly if their nails are brittle. It is the penetration by the corner of a nail into the skin around it, causing infection, and often occurs as a result of cutting down the sides of the nails instead of straight across or cutting them too short. Removal of a section of the nail is necessary to allow the infection to heal. Sometimes corns and callouses which can appear down the sides of a nail are mistaken for an ingrowing toenail.

• Athlete's foot •

A fungal infection which most commonly manifests itself between the toes as itchy scaly areas. Often the surrounding skin may look white and spongy. Anti-fungal creams and lotions are effective treatments but need to be used as long as the instructions recommend to ensure the fungus is eradicated. Symptoms will disappear before that. The fungus likes damp, warm places so avoid synthetic fibres in socks, if possible, and put talcum powder or surgical spirit between the toes on a regular basis.

• Sweaty feet •

Sometimes what appears to be athlete's foot (see above) may be caused by excessive sweating. If you sweat a lot elsewhere as well, the problem may need medical attention. If not, your shoes may be your problem. You need to wear leather to allow sweat to be absorbed. Avoid patent leather, as this finish stops the leather from being able to do its job. Also, make sure that the shoes' lining is not nylon. Tights or socks should be wool or cotton, or at least a mixture of natural and synthetic fibres.

• Chilblains •

These are painful, itchy, red swellings caused by poor circulation and most commonly occur in winter. Dressing warmly and avoiding shoes that are too tight can help. It is not a good idea to come in from the cold and soak your feet in hot water or warm them in front of a fire or against a radiator as extreme changes in temperature help to cause them. You can buy chilblain creams and ointments at pharmacies.

• Blisters •

Blisters form on the feet when there is friction between skin and shoes. The layers of skin cells separate and fill with fluid. If the damage goes a bit deeper, causing bleeding, the result will be a blood blister. Usually blisters should be left alone because the body will take care of them. If you feel you have to do something, prick the sides of the blister with a needle which has been sterilised in boiling water and gently squeeze out the fluid. Don't remove the blister as this may lead to infection.

You can help protect against blisters by putting a thin plaster over the vulnerable area, by wearing two pairs of thin socks instead of one thick pair or shaking a little talcum powder into socks or tights.

• Moles •

It is not unusual to have moles on the foot. However, those on the foot and leg may be a little more likely to become malignant, so any changes in existing moles or oddly developing new moles should be watched. See your doctor if the mole suddenly grows, has jagged edges, is mottled in colour, bleeds, itches or seems to be getting larger. (See Moles, page 103.)

• Professional help for foot problems •

If you have any problem with your feet, see your GP or a chiropodist. Chiropody is only available on the National Health Service for pregnant women, the elderly, people with diabetes, handicapped people and children. If you go to a private chiropodist, make sure they are state registered, with SRCh after their name. The Society of Chiropodists can provide you with a list on receipt of a large SAE: see Useful Contacts.

Some chiropodists train as podiatrists which means that they are able to carry out all kinds of foot surgery. If you need foot surgery and don't want to wait in what might be a long queue for orthopaedic surgery, contact the Podiatry Association for a list of their members: see Useful Contacts. Fellows of their Association must, by law, be state-registered chiropodists but will have spent seven years studying and passing approved examinations in foot surgery. They have the letters FPodA after their name.

16

COSMETIC SURGERY

OPTING for cosmetic surgery is still seen as a somewhat shameful course of action in this country. We seem to think, collectively, that it smacks of vanity, self-absorption or a lack of serious mettle although probably very many people have secretly wished a part of their anatomy to be different from the way it is. As a result of cosmetic surgery's own poor image, many people who might genuinely benefit are too embarrassed to do anything about investigating it.

• Why cosmetic surgery? •

Self-consciousness is the most common reason for wanting cosmetic surgery. Far from its being an inadequate solution, research now shows that for those with both major and minor physical imperfections or abnormalities, cosmetic surgery can in many cases have a dramatically positive impact upon their lives. There are, however, many others whose problems are not genuinely physical but psychological or social, and for these cosmetic surgery is never the answer. It is important to be completely clear about your motivation and expectations if you are considering cosmetic surgery. All surgery carries risk, so putting oneself under the knife unnecessarily and with an unsatisfactory outcome to boot is to be avoided at all cost.

• The effects of self-consciousness •

No one would expect someone to suffer a severe facial or other disfigurement – for example of congenital origin or as a result of severe burns, scars or illness – if surgery could help get rid of it. It is a sad fact, research has shown, that people keep their distance, even though probably unconsciously, from someone who is severely disfigured. In one study a woman researcher sporting a prominent facial scar created by clever make-up stood at a pedestrian crossing. A fellow researcher stood at a discreet distance noting the reactions of pedestrians who joined her at the crossing. They found that those who came up to her on the side where the scar was visible stood further away from her than those who approached on her other side where the disfigurement was unnoticeable. It doesn't take much imagination to conjecture how much harder people who are genuinely so disfigured must work to make friends, get a job or generally make a favourable first impression.

• Minor abnormalities •

Far more difficult to appreciate for many, however, is the misery and self-consciousness caused by a comparatively minor abnormality of the body, seen as too small or too large. It is these that often bring forth from others exhortations to accept in good grace what nature has given, declarations that the bit in question is lovable, unremarkable or not worth being upset about, and criticisms of vanity, frivolousness and self-centredness.

Mr David Harris, a consultant plastic surgeon in Plymouth who has carried out much research into the adverse psychological effects arising from discomfort about a relatively minor imperfection, has found these have been very much underestimated. When he asked about the life experiences of 54 patients who had undergone surgery for conditions as various as bat ears, cleft lips, facial scars, baggy eyelids, problem noses, large breasts or loss of a breast through cancer, he found very similar feelings and experiences regardless of the degree of abnormality present and the age at which it became a problem.

• Effects on behaviour •

In general he found that, once people become uncomfortably aware that they look different from most others in some particular way – whether as child, adolescent or adult according to the problem – they tend to feel a severe self-consciousness that leads first to defence mechanisms, such as rounding the shoulders and hunching over to disguise very large breasts or never letting a large nose be seen in profile, and then to avoidance of activities which throw the abnormality into greater prominence. Women who are embarrassed about breasts for example may avoid swimming or sunbathing, going to shops where there are communal changing rooms and any sports or even dancing, where the breasts are likely to jiggle up and down.

• Effects on personality •

For anyone very severely affected, if doesn't take long for self-esteem and self confidence to take a sharp turn downward and they may start to feel inadequate, insecure, sexually unattractive and even unlovable. Close personal relationships may suffer or perhaps no intimate relationships are ever formed because of some offending part of the body which would then have to be revealed.

For many people, such intense fears and feelings may never actually be voiced because of the terrible shame and embarrassment. In fact they may make jokes about the offending part, trying in effect to get a comment in before anyone else does, or else appear to be calmly resigned to their appearance. But underneath there is misery and often also guilt that they cannot overcome such disabling self-consciousness, especially when, they tell themselves, others have obviously much greater problems.

• Why some and not others? •

Not everyone does develop such severe self-consciousness, of course. It may depend upon the reaction of others at the outset: the degree of teasing from other children or teenagers, or the misplaced solicitude from parents or partners who carefully avoid referring to the matter with the intention of being kind, but sometimes with the effect of preventing a person from expressing their fears and anxieties and therefore dealing with them. Also, some people are just generally more sensitive to criticism or to their appearance than others.

It is often thought by those unsympathetic to self-consciousness that the embarrassment is used as an excuse for failure: for example, 'everything would be different if only I had a little snub nose'. However, the experience of cosmetic surgeons is that most patients who have surgery for the right reasons become far more confident, happy and outgoing afterwards.

• Other reasons for cosmetic surgery •

Not everyone wants cosmetic surgery because of embarrassment or self-consciousness. Many women, of course, yearn for face-lifts in the hope of holding off the appearance of ageing, or want to remove from upper arms or thighs and buttocks the sag that inevitably comes with age. Increasingly, women think about having fat removed or about improving the appearance of their lips or cheeks. Life for them would certainly not be insupportable without surgery and, in fact, the results may be far from what they were hoping for. In such cases, therefore, the risks must be weighed up against the perceived benefits extremely carefully before deciding to go ahead.

• Don't have surgery if. . . •

1 No one else can see the problem. If friends, family, your GP and the cosmetic surgeon you consult can genuinely not see what it is that you are bothered about, you may have become unhealthily fixated on a physical feature. This is different from someone telling you that such and such a bit of you is not so unusual/fine/attractive to me/not worth making a fuss about, etc. These are the kinds of responses which most people do receive. But if you are really out on a limb, with no one able to acknowledge you have the remotest cause for concern, you may need help in overcoming the fixation and certainly do not need cosmetic surgery.

Dysmorphophobia – or imagined ugliness syndrome as it is now being termed – is a long known psychological disorder which appears to be markedly on the increase, affecting more women than men. Root causes may be similar to anorexia. Women are first affected usually as young adults, are most often those who have been particularly fastidious about appearance, are perfectionists in many areas of their lives and are especially susceptible to images of the perfect woman in magazines and other media. Drugs such as antidepressants can be helpful but more important is cognitive therapy, in which a woman is helped to think differently about herself.

2 Someone else sees the problem but not you. Don't have cosmetic surgery if it is someone else – a husband, lover or parent – who is dissatisfied with your appearance while you are perfectly happy with it. A parent may think you will get on better in life if you don't have your particular nose or ears, and a partner might like the idea of different breasts. Better to find someone who loves and accepts you as you are.

3 Life events are the problem. Cosmetic surgery is never the solution to unfortunate circumstances in our lives. Sometimes women seek face-lifts or breast enlargements if their husbands have left them for another woman or if they can't find a partner. It will be more helpful in the long run to experience and learn to handle the unhappiness, to do something that extends your social life or to take a course that teaches you to assert and express yourself more easily.

4 You have unrealistic expectations. You are likely to be unhappy with the results of cosmetic surgery if you think that you can point to an admired face or body in a magazine and ask a surgeon for those particular legs, that nose, that stomach, those cheeks. A surgeon can only work within the framework of what you have already got. Be wary too of unrealistic expectations about scars.

• Scars •

Cosmetic surgery is like any other surgery: the joins show, as scars. Sometimes the scars can be hidden, for example, inside the nose, or be kept small, but if large incisions have to be made because a large area is being dealt with, the scars will be large too. Scars on the trunk of the body tend to be particularly thick, and different scars vary in how quickly they fade, if at all; but none disappear.

Some people are unlucky and form particularly lumpy scars. Most unlucky however are those who develop keloid scars, a massive overgrowth of tissue which forms like a growth in the area of the cut as a result of the skin repairing itself excessively. (See Keloids, page 106.) The chest, shoulders and upper back are the most likely areas for these scars and those people of African and Asian origin are most at risk of developing them. There is some hope, however, that people who are known to scar badly may be helped by the application of silicone gel sheeting to the incision site once it has healed. If kept on for at least 12 hours a day for a fortnight, it can reduce the likelihood of red or raised scars forming. It may also be able to help improve existing bad scars.

• Finding a surgeon •

In theory, some kinds of cosmetic surgery are available on the NHS: for example, surgery for severe disfigurement caused by deformity, accident or illness, or for other conditions that are a very obvious cause for distress. The waiting time is likely to be at least a couple of years for adults. Conditions of this kind that arise through accident or illness may be covered by some health insurance policies, however, making private treatment not such a costly option. Private treatment can be carried out within, at the most, a few months and sometimes within days and is probably the only option for most cosmetic procedures sought. This means you have to find a surgeon yourself.

Don't take any short cuts to finding a cosmetic surgeon. You need to take all the steps you can to find a good and reliable one because some disastrous consequences of bad cosmetic surgery can never be put right. Alas, many people are too embarrassed to approach their GP with the problem, perhaps because of an unsympathetic response in the past, and so contact directly cosmetic surgery clinics or agencies for clinics that are advertised in newspapers and magazines. While many will be bona fide, others will not. In addition, surgeons may be inexperienced and not correctly trained.

You may feel safer if you go to a surgeon a friend has used and recommended. However, unless you are going for the same operation, this may not be a good guide to competence, as he or she may do a lot of one particular type of surgery and therefore do it well, but be less competent in a completely different area.

• Qualifications •

It is best to get a referral to a reliable cosmetic surgeon from your GP. If you do not have someone in mind you would like to be referred to (although your GP is not obliged to refer you to someone of your choice) and your GP doesn't know anyone, you could ask your GP to acquire a list of the members of the British Association of Aesthetic Plastic Surgeons (BAAPS), whose members all are or have been consultant plastic surgeons in an NHS hospital. The list is available to GPs but not to the public (because of rules on advertising) from BAAPS: see Useful Contacts. Or you could phone the plastic-surgery department at your nearest large hospital and ask if the consultant plastic surgeon(s) there undertake private work. They will probably be members of BAAPS or else BAPS, the British Association of Plastic Surgeons, membership of which is also only open to those who are or have been consultants in an NHS hospital.

BACS stands for British Association of Cosmetic Surgeons and the members of this are not and never have been consultant plastic surgeons within the NHS. They may not have received formal NHS training at all and they most usually work at the private clinics which advertise directly to the public. However, it could well be the case that a particular BACS member is extremely experienced because of doing cosmetic surgery all the time, while a particular consultant plastic surgeon who does not do much cosmetic work might not get such good results. You need to use your own judgment.

• Doing your homework •

You may think it would be useful to know a little about the operation you are seeking before you have a consultation with a surgeon, so that you have a framework within which to formulate questions. The private National Hospital for Aesthetic Plastic Surgery in Worcester, the only hospital in the UK which carries out nothing but cosmetic surgery, runs a telephone information service in the form of a recorded message on all the cosmetic procedures they offer. See Useful Contacts.

• Meeting your surgeon •

If you do contact a clinic direct, never agree to have surgery at any clinic where you do not meet your surgeon till the morning of the operation. (Many clinics use lay representatives who 'sell' the operation to you.) You should have a consultation with the surgeon beforehand so that he or she can consider your case, whether surgery is appropriate or possible and, if so, how best to carry it out. Never believe anyone who tells you there are no risks or possible complications. You should be told exactly what to expect from the operation: that is, you will end up with a nose or brow or thighs that will look such and such a shape or size. Be suspicious of someone who offers to fulfil your wildest dreams.

• Questions to ask •

Ask the surgeon about his or her training and what experience they have in the operation that will be performed on you.

Expect to be told about the operation itself:

- anything you need to do or stop doing to prepare for it
- the recovery period
- what you will and will not be able to do during that time
- what will happen if there are any complications.

Some surgeons charge an all-in price, others charge extra for any additional work. Find out the whole fee and never feel pressured to sign anything immediately. You should take time to go away and think about whether to go ahead. If you are pressured to sign immediately, that might be a clear sign that your choice of surgeon or clinic is not a good one.

• Facelifts •

As we age, our facial skin ceases to be as elastic as it was when we were younger, and it doesn't return so readily to place when we laugh, frown or make any other facial expression that stretches the skin. Creases form around the eyes, mouth, nose and forehead. Gravity pulls the skin downward too, causing the sagging of cheeks and the skin under the chin. A hefty exposure to ultraviolet light over the years, perhaps in pursuit of a tan, helps age the face prematurely, so that many women now seek facelifts before they are 40 instead of in their forties and fifties.

There are two main kinds of facelift: the classic one that improves the lower part of the face and neck; and the composite facelift, a newer procedure which treats the brow, eyes, cheeks, top lip, mouth and neck in one operation all at the same time.

• Classic facelift •

By removing excess sagging skin, tightening the underlying muscle and removing underlying fat, the face can be made to appear younger again. If well done, the effects can last for ten years and those who look best are those who have the procedure done earlier, in their forties, rather than in their fifties or sixties. In the classic facelift, however, the forehead and the eyelids don't alter in appearance at all, so wrinkles and creases on the upper part of the face will remain as they were, even though larger wrinkles on the lower part of the face disappear once the skin is tightened. A separate operation on the brow or eyelids can be carried out at the same time or later.

Facelifts don't do much for people who have very full faces and short necks. They do, however, have a very positive effect on people who have lost a great deal of weight which can result in saggy skin on the face as well as other parts of the body.

What to expect The classic facelift takes about three or four hours under general anaesthetic. You will end up with a scar that runs right round each ear and across part of the scalp, although these can mostly be covered by your hairstyle. Recovery afterwards takes a few weeks, although some facial stiffness may persist for up to six weeks. Bruising and swelling should subside after a fortnight. Any activity or sport which might put the skin of the face under pressure has to be avoided and usual activities, including work, should not be resumed before two or three weeks.

Complications Possible complications include post-operative bleeding and slow healing of the sensitive area behind the ear. The area may scab visibly and the skin underneath may be a different colour from the rest, temporarily or permanently. If healing is poor, sometimes there is a loss of hair around the scalp incision.

The greatest risk is nerve damage to the face during surgery, which can result in numbness, tingliness or a lopsided smile for one to two years, depending upon which nerves are damaged. Occasionally, there is nerve damage to the lower ear which causes permanent numbness. These risks are rare, however, with a competent experienced surgeon.

Many women are disappointed with the outcome of a facelift because they feel that they look as though they have had surgery, their skin looks as though it has been stretched and there may be a clear difference between the appearance of the upper and lower face. Also, signs of the skin starting to drop again may be apparent after only six months.

• Composite facelift •

This is a new technique, fully perfected only in 1990 by an American plastic surgeon. It lifts the brow, upper and lower eyelids, cheeks, corners of the mouth, jaw line and neck, removing pretty well all tell-tale lines of ageing in the process. Because deep layers of the skin are lifted and the fat and muscle underneath them are repositioned where they used to be when you were younger, the effect is supposed to be more natural, even if dramatic, because it literally does remove years from your appearance. Although the change is instant, it is quickly obscured again temporarily by major swelling and bruising. The composite looks best, say surgeons who like it, after at least six months when the face has fully settled down again. Critics of the technique say it is more difficult to manipulate the skin in the direction you want when everything is moved at once.

What to expect   The composite is not for everyone, however. It is very major surgery which can take up to seven hours and you certainly wouldn't want a surgeon who hadn't done a lot of them before. It is best if a prospective patient is very fit and healthy beforehand. Bruising and discomfort last for about six weeks and scarring is slightly greater than with the classic facelift, with a scar behind or in front of the hairline, very fine scars on the eyelids and one beneath the chin where an incision has to be made to gain access to the neck muscles. The potential problems afterwards are similar. Like the classic, the composite facelift does not last indefinitely. It is also about four to five times more expensive.

• Nose •

Very many people want cosmetic surgery to alter the shape of their noses (rhinoplasty). It is not a risky operation in terms of safety but it is risky in terms of outcome. You need to be very clear about what you want and what you expect. Minor adjustments may be difficult to make to your satisfaction and major changes may be out of the question because of the nature of your nose. A bent nose, for example, usually cannot be straightened. It is best to describe what you don't like about the existing version and specify exactly what you would like changed, and then let your surgeon come up with drawings that show how you will look if you go ahead. It may even be that your nose only looks prominent because of a weak chin and that, in the opinion of your surgeon, this should be altered rather than your nose.

It is advisable to make any changes to your nose well before you reach 40, as by this time it has become very set in its ways and far less willing to be worked with.

What to expect   An operation to alter the nose takes about one and a half hours. Recovery time is three weeks, which is how long it will take for the nose swelling to subside; your eyes should stop looking swollen after one week. The good news is that scarring isn't visible, as the incisions are made inside the nose, and complications are few: there may occasionally be a nosebleed, infection or little whiteheads developing on the nose which can be removed with soap and water.

• Brow •

This is an operation often done simultaneously with the classic facelift to remove furrows on the forehead and slightly lift the eyebrows and upper eyelids. If you are thinking of going the whole hog and having your upper eyelids done too, make sure you have the brow operation first. Some lifting of the eyelids inevitably occurs with it, so the outcome can be disastrous if you have already had the skin of your eyelids tightened: you may not be able fully to close your eyes or you may ever afterwards look as if you are staring.

What to expect   A brow lift performed alone takes about one and a half hours. Bruising will spread down your face and last about a week. You can resume normal activities after about ten days. There will be a long scar just above the hairline, stretching from ear to ear, which you will want to cover with an appropriate hairstyle, probably avoiding a parting.

Complications   Severe problems such as significant bleeding or infection are rare after this operation. However if the scalp is stretched too tightly, healing may not take place properly and there may be little bald patches around bits of the scar; usually easy to camouflage with hair. Also, the hair may thin around the scar because of the trauma the area has undergone and may not return to full thickness for a year.

A permanent effect, however, is a slight receding of your hair by a few centimetres, giving you a slightly higher brow than previously. Temporary nerve damage can occasionally leave part of the forehead numb and, very rarely, a crucial nerve may be damaged which affects the muscle that raises your brow or eyebrow, preventing you from doing either.

• Chin •

Enlargement, by moving bone or inserting an implant, firms up the chin. Reduction, by removal of bone, softens it. These procedures, not carried out by all cosmetic surgeons, take about an hour under general anaesthetic, or even under local if you can bear the hacking and grinding. Swelling will probably only last a week and you should be fully recovered within a fortnight. There is no visible scar if the incision is able to be made from inside your mouth. If it has to be made under the chin, the resultant scar will be 2.5 to 5cm (1 to 2in) long. Nerve damage is an occasional hazard, leaving the chin and maybe your teeth numb for up to a year. The likelihood of infection is greater if you are a smoker and if you have had an implant, as it is a foreign body. Sometimes an implant may slip and need adjusting. If you get a nasty bang it may leak.

• Cheeks •

Cheek implants can give more definition to your face but can't alter it dramatically. Silicone implants are inserted in an operation that takes about an hour under general anaesthetic. A week should be sufficient time for swelling to subside and recovery to be complete. Scars are on the inside of the mouth, infections are rare (though increased if you are a smoker) and any numbness of the cheeks or lips usually passes within weeks. The main hazard is that one of your implants may slip or a sharp bang could make one leak and gradually disappear.

• Eyelids •

Some women want their eyelids altered to disguise ageing, others because of naturally baggy or puffy eyelids which, they feel, adversely affect their appearance. Although eyelid surgery (blepharoplasty) can make you look younger, neither the upper or lower variety can remove crow's feet.

What to expect   Upper eyelid surgery takes about an hour under general or local anaesthetic. Lower eyelid surgery, which can remove bags, is harder for the surgeon to perform and therefore takes longer and carries more risks. Swelling lasts for about a week and you can go back to normal activities after that. If all has gone well, the scars will be hidden by the upper and/or lower creases of the eyelid.

Complications   When the operation is done well, complications with the upper eyelid are rare: mainly a possible thickening to your scar if you get a bang during the healing period. If the operation is not done well, there can be nasty effects such as being unable to close your eyes fully, leading to dry sore eyes, your eyelids looking different from each other because more fatty tissue has been removed from one than the other or a sunken-eyed look because too much has been removed from both.

In the case of surgery of the lower eyelid, sometimes the lid may appear dragged down, exposing the white of the eye. If too much skin is taken away, the lid can turn outward exposing the red inner lining. This may correct itself in time but if it doesn't a skin graft, with accompanying scarring, is the only remedial action that can be taken.

• Wrinkles, facial scars and blemishes •

A chemical face peel, in which a strong chemical solution is applied to the relevant areas of your face, can smooth skin and remove fine wrinkles and brown patches that accompany ageing. It may have to be repeated once or twice a year. Dermabrasion is a means of sandpapering the skin to make scars less noticeable but it cannot get rid of them altogether nor can it help the appearance of pitted acne scars which extend too deep into the skin. When it works, it is permanent. Collagen implants, given by injection with a fine needle, can fill out little pockets in the skin caused by superficial acne scars, chicken pox scars and large wrinkles. They cannot help pitted acne scars.

They have to be repeated once or twice a year but don't work very well if your skin is sun-damaged.

All three are best done on pale skin. For those with dark or sallow skin the risk of patchiness is considerable after a chemical peel or dermabrasion.

What to expect   The chemical peel hurts most because your face burns for a couple of days. As your face has to be covered with adhesive tape after the procedure, it will also hurt when you have to pull this off after 24 hours. You will probably need strong pain killers. Your skin will be very sensitive until it heals. Dermabrasion also leaves a burning feeling and your skin will weep and crust. Collagen implants cause a little tingling or burning but you can resume all normal activities at once, whereas the other two procedures take at least two weeks of healing.

You will need sunblock for at least six months if you are in the sun after a chemical peel or dermabrasion and thereafter you must religiously use a good high-factor sunscreen because your skin will burn more easily. You must also protect your skin from the sun after collagen implants.

• Port wine stains •

These are birthmarks which are found on the face and neck and may range from pale pink in colour to deep purple or red. Their colour comes from dilated blood vessels either just under the skin surface or deeper down. Most are flat but some are raised and swollen. Both kinds can be successfully removed with a pulse dye laser. Light from the laser passes through normal skin but is absorbed as heat by the dilated blood vessels causing the stain. For many people, one treatment is sufficient to create natural-coloured skin but the deeper the stain, the more laser treatments are necessary to remove it. A very deep stain may need eight treatments and total removal may not always be possible because the paler the stain becomes, the less laser energy can be absorbed.

Brown pigmentation, such as birthmarks, can also be treated by laser.

• Arms •

Excess flabby skin and fatty tissue can be removed from the upper arms by cosmetic surgery but at the high price of severe scarring. Surgery under general anaesthetic takes up to two hours and recovery takes up to a fortnight, although strenuous lifting must be avoided for longer. The scars will stretch from each armpit to each elbow and may be a quarter of an inch wide. They will probably be red and angry for some months but eventually settle down to pink.

Complications   The only major but fortunately rare risk is that lymph glands in the armpit may be injured if too much fat is removed. If the damage is minor, it may repair itself. If not, the upper arm will swell and a support bandage may be necessary for life (see Lymphoedema, page 340).

• Stomach •

The aim of this procedure, called abdominoplasty, is to remove stretched muscle and saggy skin caused by abdominal surgery (for example, to remove gallstones or ulcers, but you should wait at least until a year afterwards) or by a very drastic weight loss after obesity. It is not a replacement for dieting and, as for the arms, the high price is heavy scarring. Stretch marks only disappear if they are on the skin that is to be removed.

Abdominoplasty is major surgery and can take up to four hours. A hospital stay of a week is likely and you will not be able to do anything strenuous for six weeks. You should take at least three weeks off work. There will be a scar the length of the bikini line, one around the navel and, possibly, one running from the navel down to the bikini line and one crossing this line where your old navel used to be – the navel is moved in this operation. You will, however, have a flat stomach which will be permanent but only if you don't put on weight or have a baby.

• Thighs and buttocks •

You can have saggy skin removed from thighs and buttocks but the scarring is extensive.The operation takes two hours and recovery should take about three weeks. Sex is out until then, as is walking a lot and working. The buttocks' scars will fortunately be hidden by the buttock creases but the scars that run halfway down your inner thighs will show in all their glory if you wear shorts or a swimsuit, etc.

• Liposuction •

Although this is a means of removing fat, it is not suitable for those who are heavily overweight and who might most dearly like to benefit. It also doesn't remove the dimpled orange-peel look that the thighs and buttocks often get when there are hard lumps of fat underneath. It is in fact most suitable for those who are at a good weight and who haven't had their skin irreparably stretched by repeated weight gain and weight loss or repeated pregnancies. In liposuction only fat is removed, so the skin has to be supple enough to smooth out again instead of wrinkling over the area from which the fat has been taken. Therefore, the best candidates are not only not overweight but under 35 as well.

Liposuction may help if you have hard lumps of fat on the buttocks, hips, thighs, arms, stomach, ankles or under the knees that just won't shift by dieting. Only five pounds of the stuff can be removed at a time.

What to expect The procedure is carried out under general anaesthetic and lasts an hour or two. One small incision or more is made in each area that is being treated and then a suction tube is introduced to first break down the fat and then draw it out.

You must expect to feel pain afterwards. Women often say walking is difficult after any liposuction carried out below the waist and swelling and bruising are unlikely to subside in less than a month. Usual activities can be returned to after two or three weeks, maybe earlier if little fat has been suctioned. Scars 1cm (½in) long will show wherever you had incisions, except for the buttocks where scars can mostly be hidden in the creases.

Complications Apart from the inevitable but rare risks of infection and bleeding that accompany all surgical procedures, the main concerns are cosmetic. Sometimes you end up with a wavy outline to the thighs and buttocks or you may be disappointed to find that not as much fat has been removed as you had hoped; swelling during the procedure makes accurate estimation of how much to remove difficult. It is worth bearing in mind too that having undergone liposuction is no guarantee that fat will not return, although the fat cells removed are indeed gone forever. However relatively few will have been removed overall and existing fat cells can swell out nicely if required.

• Breasts •

For information about breast enlargement, breast reduction, breast lifts and breast reconstruction, please turn to All About Breasts, page 285.

Part II

....

EMOTIONAL
AND
MENTAL HEALTH

OUR emotional and mental state is an enormously important aspect of overall health.

Inevitably, we will all suffer our quota of stress, anxiety, sadness, grief, fear, depression, anger and frustration as we go through life, and have to manage the hand it deals us. But women are twice as likely as men to be recipients of mental health services and are statistically more often the ones to suffer from anxiety states and depression of a severity to warrant treatment. Is this because women are inherently less able to cope (unlikely), have more to cope with (certainly sometimes) or are just more willing to acknowledge their feelings and admit a need for help, rather than retreat into something that will mask the problem, such as drink, sport or workaholism?

Whatever the reasons, it is important to face the strong negative feelings or fears that may put a damper on our lives. Emotional ill-health affects the immune system and in turn our physical health. Of course it isn't always possible to change the circumstance – such as poverty, chronic pain or a history of sexual abuse – that may be at the root of a problem, but in many instances we can learn how to change our responses sufficiently to help ourselves. At other times, unwittingly we are our own worst enemies, putting ourselves down, not daring to speak up for ourselves, lying down as doormats for others to tread on, and don't realise we could make things very different, if we only knew how.

This section explains common mental health problems and how to cope with them by yourself or with the aid of professionals. It also looks at tried-and-tested techniques for changing unhelpful mental 'habits' and better handling of situations, whatever happens to us all in our lives.

17

STRESS AND ANXIETY

STRESS is the word commonly used to describe being under pressure. But when we talk of stress being bad for our health it means being under more pressure in life than we can comfortably tolerate and the physical and psychological changes in us which may occur in consequence.

Stress can take many forms. Seemingly good or pleasant things, such as getting married, going on the holiday of a lifetime or having a baby, can be stressful as well as bad things, depending upon how we approach and face them. If we get into a panic trying to organise everything or are extremely anxious about the effects on us of major life-changing events, however positive, we may be suffering stress.

Most of us suffer from stresses from a combination of sources and accept them as a normal part of our lives, although, without our knowing it, dealing with them every day may lower our tolerance for handling other stresses on top. Women who have jobs outside the home, for example, often have to organise and deliver their children to wherever they spend their day before setting off for their own work, spend their lunch break shopping, getting shoes repaired, etc, then return home to cook, bath and bed the children before starting the cleaning.

The journey to work may be frustrating for many of us on many days of the week, when we are caught in traffic jams or wait for trains or buses that don't come. We may also be subjected to a great deal of wearing background noise from neighbours, busy streets, roadworks, machinery and aeroplanes.

In addition there are big 'life stresses'. We may have worries at work (see Stress at Work, page 65) and worries at home. Relationships and marriages that have run into problems, bringing up children, looking after seriously sick or dying family members, divorce, redundancy, loneliness, chronic pain from disability: all of these can cause stress and take a physical toll on our bodies, even though the stress is more mental than physical.

• Fight-or-flight response •

Our physical response to stress is in-built. When we were still in the wild, the concerns we had were mainly survival-oriented. We had to know how to behave if a wild boar suddenly loomed into view, so built into our bodies was the fight-or-flight response. This means that when under attack of any kind, the body gets into a state of readiness to deal with it: heart rate goes up, blood flow to the muscles increases to mobilise them faster (to run or strike), blood pressure goes up, more adrenalin is released, we sweat and our metabolism speeds up. Digestion slows down (the blood flow normally required for digestion is diverted to the muscles), blood flow to the skin decreases to minimise bleeding if there is a wound and platelets in the blood increase to ensure clotting, in case we need to prevent a haemorrhage.

When all this happens, the body is ready to flee or to fight. Unfortunately, this is what occurs every time we are under severe stress, even if it is nowadays more likely to be the emotional variety rather than the physical, and even though we are unlikely either to fight or flee. Consequently, unlike of old, the physical responses in the body are not resolved by action and so the blood pressure keeps on pumping, the heart carries on speeding and the muscles stay tense far longer than is healthy. Physical illnesses now known to be associated with unresolved stress include heart disease, stomach ulcers, irritable bowel, migraine and some skin diseases.

• Good and bad stress •

Stress reactions are not in themselves bad. In fact, life would hardly be worth living without some pressures and excitements, anticipation of a challenge or nervous expectancy about something potentially good. Stress becomes damaging only when we cease to be able to handle it; when the pressures are too much all at once; when we are out of our depth or feel defeated. When we feel fearful or angry over a long period but suppress those feelings, perhaps even unconsciously, the body is again in a state of unresolved flight or fight, with all the accompanying risks of illness.

It is not necessarily the big life crises that affect health most. Sometimes, of course, it is at precisely those times that we rise to the occasion and are most effective. American research has shown that what the Americans call daily hassles – everyday types of annoyances such as missing the bus, losing a key, irritations within the family – are often what lead to a lowering of the body's defences and a higher risk of infections.

• Symptoms of stress •

There are many possible symptoms of stress, which may occur in any combination. These include:

- palpitations
- ache or pain in the chest
- indigestion
- nausea
- diarrhoea
- need to urinate frequently
- fatigue
- insomnia or change in sleep patterns
- twitching
- feeling pain (such as headaches) more

- becoming easily irritated
- anxiety and edginess.

Of course, all these symptoms can be caused by other disorders, and in fact many people who are suffering stress actually fear that they are seriously physically ill. Such symptoms shouldn't automatically be put down to stress, unless you are pretty certain you know the cause.

Because stress can indeed lead to physical illnesses, it is important to do all we can to keep it in check. This may mean making lifestyle changes that allow us to slow down or spread our load more widely, learning to relax (see page 41), learning to face and deal with emotional difficulties and needs (see page 190) and getting sufficient support for ourselves during life crises such as divorce, job loss and bereavement (see page 206).

· Anxiety ·

Anxiety is a normal feeling. It would be unusual never to feel anxiety and most people feel varying amounts before events such as taking an exam, giving a speech, starting a new job, going on a first date, etc. When we are anxious our hearts beat a little faster, our breathing quickens, we may sweat, feel a tightness in the chest or butterflies in the stomach. This is a less intense version of what happens when we feel fear. In fact, anxiety and fear are simply different grades of the same bodily responses to stress.

When the stress is caused by something such as losing a job, having problems within a marriage or financial concerns, we call the feelings anxiety or worry. When the feelings are stirred up in response to an immediate threat, such as a potential assailant or a mad dog, we call them fear. The difference is that whereas fear always relates to something specific and something possible, anxiety may be vague, difficult to pin down the source of or not have a realistic cause.

· Abnormal anxiety ·

Anxiety starts to become abnormal when the anxiety symptoms begin to impinge on our everyday lives, affecting how we work, what we do and how we feel about ourselves. For example, while we all have concerns that worry us, it is not productive to worry incessantly for months on end in an incapacitating sort of way that merely exacerbates the problems.

Sometimes strong feelings of anxiety come seemingly out of the blue, with no apparent cause, and this is known as free-floating anxiety. When this sort of anxiety has extremely strong symptoms and includes a number of frightening feelings such as difficulty in breathing, dizziness, feeling detached, sweating, trembling, shaking and choking, it is called a spontaneous panic attack. For some people, panic attacks may occur not out of the blue but in some specific situation only. (See Panic Attacks, page 147.)

Sometimes anxiety is produced by circumstances or objects which aren't normally seen as threatening, such as going shopping or seeing a cat, and this is called phobic anxiety. If you feel so bad that you eventually avoid the feared circumstance or objects altogether, this is a phobia. Agoraphobia, a fear usually of crowded large or confined public places, is the most common phobia and can in fact arise from once having had a panic attack in such a situation. Fear of another one in a similar circumstance then causes the phobia. Other common types are social phobias, in which there is fear of public humiliation and embarrassment, and so-called simple phobias, where just one specific object or circumstance, such as spiders or dental treatment, causes the fear. (See Phobias, page 154.)

Another disabling form of anxiety is obsessive-compulsive anxiety. Irrational obsessive thoughts and ideas develop, such as a fear of serious disease from household germs. Compulsive acts, such as repeated hand-washing, then have to be carried out to dispel the obsessive anxiety. (See Obsessive-compulsive Disorder, page 160.)

Post-traumatic stress disorder is now recognised as a significant cause of disabling, but far from irrational, anxiety, in which disruptive or even terrifying psychological symptoms occur for up to years after a traumatic experience such as a serious accident or rape. (See page 165.)

Finally, anxiety very often co-exists with depression.

• Causes of anxiety states •

Why are some people more prone to severe anxiety or abnormal anxieties than others? There are no nice, easy answers and probably for most people there is a combination of factors which contribute. For example, having a more excitable personality type can mean a higher likelihood of anxiety, and to a certain extent this personality type can be inherited.

Upbringing can play a part: children of parents who are overly protective, overly critical, overly authoritarian or who don't give much encouragement or praise may be less confident about themselves and their abilities in the world as adults. Also, we learn from what we see. If one parent is or was a worrier, we may be more likely to learn this way of reacting to situations ourselves.

Stress, both cumulative over time or a major event in the present or immediate past, can very commonly help to trigger anxiety states. Significant stresses might be the loss of someone much loved, serious illness, moving home, changing job, etc. There may even be physiological imbalances in the body or brain which have some bearing on the development of particular anxiety states.

Caffeine, sudden caffeine withdrawal and withdrawal from alcohol and tranquillisers can all cause edginess, at the least, or severe anxiety.

Whatever the reason or collection of reasons for abnormal anxiety, the good news is that you don't have to ferret them out before you can do anything about handling the adverse effects of anxiety on your life. The sections that follow offer self-help advice for dealing with excessive anxiety of specific

_____ **IMPORTANT** _____

In a small number of cases, anxiety symptoms, particularly panic attacks, may be caused by an underlying physical condition such as thyroid disorder, heart and lung irregularities, epilepsy, and inner ear disturbances. See a doctor if you are concerned.

kinds. However, for all kinds of anxiety that seem to be even slightly excessive, it is also important to take a look at our usual coping styles in life because, without knowing it, we often behave in ways which keep our anxieties going. Learning to change our usual ways of thinking and to express and value ourselves more fully can help a lot. (See Handling Thoughts, Feelings and Needs, page 190.)

• Worry •

Worry is a natural part of life – in small doses. These small amounts can even be helpful, according to some experts, as it is, in effect, a rehearsal of the possibilities which may result from the feared or worried-about event, which could prove useful if one of them does occur.

Worry is not useful when it is unproductive, nebulous and continual. Doctors often term this version Generalised Anxiety Disorder. To get given this diagnosis you would probably have been worrying for at least six months about two or more specific stressful events in your life (for example, your marriage, redundancy, inability to get a job) and you would also have been experiencing anxiety symptoms such as feeling agitated, unable to concentrate, irritable and unable to sleep properly, tension in your muscles, inability to relax and some general fluttery feelings.

A person with generalised anxiety does not have panic attacks or phobic anxieties. There is fear, but in a less concrete form, such as worry about your ability to cope or a fear of being left, dying or failing.

For severe generalised anxiety disorders some doctors may prescribe an antidepressant, particularly imipramine. However, it is better, of course, if you can help yourself. If you worry too much and feel your life is adversely affected by worry, try the following tips.

• Self-help for worry •

Make worry productive   Whenever you catch yourself worrying incessantly, repeating your worries to yourself and reliving the various unsettling scenarios you have imagined, try to set yourself the goal of one or more specific steps you can take to deal productively with your worry. For example, if you are worrying about whether you are ill, accept your worry is real (even if unfounded) and make an appointment to see a doctor. If you are worried that some work you have produced is not right, work out how to make specific changes that will improve it, or arrange to see your superior to explain your concern. Worry loses its power once practical steps have been taken, even if the outcome is still uncertain.

Get information   If your worries tend to be of the 'what if?' variety, you could reduce many of them by finding out the facts about whatever is concerning you. For example, if you are having an operation, find out what needs to be done and what the recovery process is usually like, before you go ahead, so that you can make useful plans to help yourself instead of worrying unnecessarily. As for nuclear war and plagues, you can't prevent them, so try to accept that worrying will not help.

Question yourself   If you worry about unlikely eventualities, for example an accident while in public such as your skirt catching on something just as you rise from your chair, question yourself mercilessly. Ask why you think it would happen, has it ever happened, is it really likely to happen? Realising how unrealistic or pointless your worry is may help you to snap out of it.

Imagine the good and the bad   If you are worrying about a specific event such as a speech, a driving test, a ferry trip, a dinner party you are giving, try to visualise the occasion in two ways: first, going really well, and then going really badly but yourself managing to cope effectively with each set-back or disaster.

Set a time limit   Whatever you worry about, if you do too much of it try rationing yourself. Set aside a specific half hour every day, preferably in the latter part of the day, into which you must cram all your worries big and small. Do not allow yourself to dwell on these worries when they occur to you at other times in the day; simply note down what they are if you don't think you will remember them. When your worry time comes round, either try to think of ways to deal with your worries or just sit and worry. You'll benefit even from the unproductive worry because you will have cut down the time spent on it at other times of day.

18

PANIC ATTACKS

THERE is nothing abnormal about panic in an emergency. It would be unusual not to feel panic if you found yourself trapped in a burning room or saw a juggernaut heading towards you at breakneck speed. Panic attacks, however, are extreme attacks of anxiety experienced in circumstances that don't seem overtly threatening but which, for some reason, make the body behave physically as if under serious threat.

Usually the panic attack occurs out of the blue, at least the first time. Someone might be standing in a supermarket queue, driving down a familiar road or sitting in a restaurant when the symptoms occur. The symptoms, which can be quite terrifying, may only last a few minutes although those minutes probably seem like hours. More rarely, the symptoms may come back intermittently over a period of an hour or two.

• Symptoms •

The symptoms associated with panic attacks include:

- breathing difficulties
- dizziness
- disorientation and feelings of unreality
- palpitations
- sweating
- shaking
- tight chest
- tingling in the fingers or feet
- a feeling of choking
- hyper-sensitivity to light, sound and movement
- ringing in the ears
- intense sense of fear
- strong negative feelings, for example sadness or short-temper.

These sorts of feelings and sensations, not all of which occur, are caused by the surge of adrenalin the body produces when it feels intense fear. Some people experience only one panic attack in their lives or only occasional ones, others have them repeatedly. Not surprisingly, after a particularly nasty and frightening first panic attack, people may become very anxious whether, and when, they are likely to experience another.

• Agoraphobia: caused by panic •

The panic attack may itself lead to a phobia about the place the person was in at the time. If you have a panic attack while standing in a busy shopping centre, you may quite reasonably imagine that being in the shopping centre somehow caused it and therefore fear another attack when you next return to the centre. The extreme anticipatory fear may well cause another attack, confirming the belief that the shopping centre, or, gradually, perhaps any crowded place, is the cause and must be avoided. This is agoraphobia (see page 154).

• Who is most at risk? •

Why do panic attacks happen at all and who do they happen to? Anyone can suffer a panic attack, although you are more likely to have them if you are an anxious sort of person. Some people even know that they are likely to have a panic attack at times of general high anxiety and that the attacks will stop when the particular period of anxiety has subsided. Cumulative stresses, however, are often unidentifiable because they are forgotten or long-buried; they may build up and up and eventually something happens which is the final straw. Very commonly, the actual triggering event for the first panic attack is a severely traumatic loss – usually of a person through death or divorce, etc – but the trigger can also be a physical or financial loss or a change of circumstances which feels like a loss. However, it could equally be something comparatively trivial.

Often a long period of stress may result in a panic attack after the stressful time is over, when you are no longer having to fight to stay afloat or in control. Because the stress is over, the panic may not be associated with it and therefore is thought to come out of the blue. For some people, however, particularly those who have very frequent panic attacks, all in different circumstances, there may be a constant level of high inexplicable anxiety in their lives.

• Physical causes •

A common physical trigger for panic attacks is hyperventilation, or over-breathing, where you take too many too shallow breaths instead of fewer deeper ones. There are many possible reasons for over-breathing, including pain, fear, indigestion, anxiety, excitement, talking too fast and excitedly, poor posture or muscle tension that makes more normal breathing seem painful, tight clothing or a stuffy nose.

The effects of over-breathing can be dramatic: you may experience severe anxiety (anxiety can be both a cause and a consequence), panic attacks, feelings of spaciness, tingling in limbs, weakness, numbness, inability to pronounce words properly, loss of concentration, palpitations, dry cough and throat, chest pain and even hallucinations.

It seems amazing that breathing shallowly and quickly could do all that but the breath, of course, has profound effects on the body. In shallow breathing, normal carbon dioxide levels are altered and the brain cannot function efficiently, hence the headiness and feelings of unreality.

In a few cases panic attacks may be caused by an underlying physical condition such as thyroid disorder, low blood sugar (usually caused by poor diet or stress), heart and lung irregularities, epilepsy and inner-ear disturbances. You should see a doctor if you are concerned.

• Getting help •

Very many people who suffer panic attacks end up being prescribed tranquillisers. For those who have very severe frequent and frightening attacks, tranquillisers may well be necessary for a while to restore some degree of control to their lives. However, they are never the solution and may, of course, cause further problems (see Tranquillisers, page 60). Some doctors may prescribe an antidepressant for panic attacks and agoraphobia; imipramine may be particularly helpful for some people.

• Self-help •

Far more useful in the long-term are certain well tried and tested self-help approaches which you can learn to master with the support of caring family or friends, or with the aid of a professional. In order to try the techniques described below, you need to learn how to relax (see Relaxation, page 41) and become comfortable and confident about inducing relaxation at any time and in any place. Also, you may wish to see whether stimulants such as nicotine and caffeine and refined sugars contribute to the severity or frequency of attacks by trying to cut them out.

• What to do during a panic attack •

Control your breathing Although the effects of over-breathing can be considerable, there is an effective and easy remedy. If you feel a panic attack coming on, try to do one of these two things:

- Either concentrate on your breath and consciously make your out-going breath longer than your in-coming one, keeping both of them gentle and regular, rather than gulping at air;
- Or keep a paper bag with you always and when a panic attack threatens to come on, cover your nose and mouth with the bag and breathe normally. This will increase your carbon dioxide levels and quickly help you to feel more normal again.

Go with the attack It is common, when in the grip of a panic attack, to try physically to stop it happening by tensing up. Unfortunately, tensing up actually makes symptoms worse. What you need to do as far as possible is let go and allow the feelings to happen but without fearing them too much.

Watch what is happening to your body as if from outside yourself. Don't let yourself become more fearful or anxious because that will exacerbate symptoms instead of allowing them to pass. See yourself as helping to handle the attack by watching it happen, instead of feeling out of control and at the mercy of your symptoms.

If you do not add to your symptoms with fear, the surge of adrenalin causing the panic will pass very quickly. If you do become frightened about what will happen next or what people will think if you collapse, shake, turn white, etc, the panic is going to last considerably longer.

Try to do an 'instant relax': that is, do your best to put as much tension out of your body as is possible at a moment's notice. Sue Breton, clinical psychologist and one-time panic-attack sufferer, suggests in her book, *Don't Panic* (see Further Reading), doing what she calls 'shoppers' relaxation': imagine coming home carrying heavy bags, your feet and arms aching, and collapsing with relief into an armchair. Practise flopping in a chair and letting go. If you can summon the feeling of that wonderful sit-down when you first go into panic, wherever you are, you will be relaxing a lot of your muscles just when you most need to. Or there may be some other instant-relax scenario you can think of that will work more effectively and reliably for you.

De-power the situation   To get through a panic attack without panicking further, you need to control unhelpful thoughts such as 'what will people think of me?', 'I can't handle this', 'I'm going to die', etc.

First, it's useful to know how to handle fears about dying or collapsing, etc. Because it seems so strange that the body can go into a physical state appropriate for fighting off muggers or facing an avalanche when all you are doing is standing in a queue at a bus stop, it is not an unusual response to think you must be ill, or that the symptoms are a first sign of some serious disorder such as a heart attack, stroke or going mad. Make sure you can fully accept that a panic attack cannot cause you to have a heart attack or a stroke, it cannot choke or suffocate you, make you faint or go mad. Once that is accepted, it may be easier not to fear the feelings so much.

When such thoughts or fears about looking a fool or not coping threaten to intrude, quickly think instead of some positive thoughts that will help you to lessen rather than prolong your fear. You might find certain statements that are particularly helpful or comforting to you and choose to repeat just one or two several times during an attack. For example, you might try any of the following or, better still, think up something helpful of your own:

- 'I can get through this'
- 'I don't like this but I know I can manage'
- 'I know that nothing terrible is going to happen'
- 'I am just going to wait quietly for these feelings to pass'
- 'This is going to pass, this is going to pass'
- 'I am going to concentrate on relaxing'

- 'These feelings can't really hurt me'
- 'There's no rush. Take your time, take it calmly'.

It is probably best to concentrate first on calming yourself and breathing more slowly, then to say your positive statements, or to do the two simultaneously if you can.

Distract yourself Resort to anything that will help take your attention off your physical symptoms or anxious thoughts. What you do will obviously depend on where you are. For example, start talking to someone; do something physical, such as walking briskly, cleaning the windows, some exercises; look at flowers, houses, people's clothes, tins of food in the supermarket; and set yourself some task such as counting how many times you see the colour pink; sing; set yourself a memory task such as recalling nursery rhymes or the last six winners of the Wimbledon men's and women's singles tennis championships.

Say 'Stop it!' If you find yourself worrying in advance whether you are going to have a panic attack, whether you are experiencing the first symptoms, whether it is going to happen in a minute, etc, try thought-stopping. Shout out or say silently (whichever is appropriate) to your thoughts: 'stop it!' 'go away', 'enough!'. Keep doing it whenever the negative thoughts creep back in.

Get angry Women, particularly, may experience anger as anxiety. You may have good reason to be angry with someone or have a long-standing unexpressed anger – for example, towards a partner for thoughtless behaviour – but if anger is an alien emotion for you to express, the feelings may come out as panic.

If you think this could be the case for you, try getting angry instead of anxious when the symptoms come on. If you are at home, do something physical that you can put some aggression into, such as vigorous moving of furniture or digging in the garden. Or you could try hitting a pillow or cushion. Or address your panic attack out loud (or silently, if necessary), 'I'm not having this! I'm not having you get in my way!'

Get out of the situation – for a while If the panic feelings are more intense than you can cope with despite all this, get out of the difficult situation until you feel better and ready to re-enter it. Put down your shopping and leave the shop, if driving pull off the road, get out of the lift at the next floor, etc. But don't avoid going back altogether. You are merely giving yourself a breathing space, making time for your relaxing and positive thoughts to give you strength before you tackle the situation again.

If you go home instead and promise to do better next time, you are feeding your fear and your belief that you cannot really cope in certain situations. However, if you feel absolutely forced to, don't compound your fear with guilt. The important thing is not to give up. Accept that you'll just have to start all over again.

It is simple, of course, to enumerate these suggestions, and much harder to put them into practice when you are terrified. But they do work. Try to make the commitment to yourself to make them work for you, but don't expect instant successes or no set-backs. Gradually, if you persevere, the power of your fear in circumstances that used to panic you should diminish and eventually disappear.

• Preventing panic attacks •

Examine the circumstances   Once an attack is over and you are calm again, try to see if there is anything you can learn from the circumstances in which it occurred to help you avoid another one. For example, were you particularly worried about something? Were you extremely anxious about whether you would have an attack? (This is likely if you tend to have one only in particular circumstances, for example, while shopping.) Were you in some extreme emotional state: unhappy, feeling helpless, angry? Had you had any coffee recently or been smoking a lot? Just identifying a few factors which might help explain why an attack happened at a particular time can help you feel more in control.

Work on learning to breath more deeply   To avoid the hazards of over-breathing, you need to aim to breathe from the abdomen rather than the chest. Lie or sit comfortably, take a long relaxed breath and feel your stomach rising. As you let out the breath, your stomach should fall. If you try to let out every last bit of breath before taking another, you should have the feeling of your stomach being sucked in. It may feel strange or uncomfortable breathing in this way at first, but gradually it will become more natural. And as you get more used to it, you will not have to concentrate so hard in order to do it.

Abdominal breathing is not always appropriate. When you are under exertion, exercising or keyed up in a positive way, you will need to breathe more quickly to meet your body's needs for oxygen.

Rehearse whatever is going to happen   If you have to give a speech, drive over a bridge, attend a church wedding, etc, and fear feeling panic, relax and imagine the situation in advance. See yourself giving your speech, sitting through the wedding, driving over the bridge. See anything that might panic you – a sea of faces looking at you while you speak, the church door shut, a lot of cars stationery on the bridge – breathe, and see yourself coping comfortably.

Ensure you have a way out   The last thing you want is to feel trapped with your panic attack. Arrange in advance some get-out that will give you time to compose yourself. For example, check out where the exits are, sit at the end of aisles, know where you can pull over while driving or that if necessary you can use your flashers and just slow down. If giving a speech, plan in advance a way to divert attention away from you if you feel you need to, for example by showing slides, asking a question of the audience, bending to retrieve a paper, asking for a window to be opened or closed, or even by saying to everyone that you feel a little nervous. Commonly, if you know you can 'escape' temporarily, you will feel more confident of your ability to cope and not need to escape at all.

• Read on •

See Handling Thoughts, Feelings and Needs, page 190, and see also Further Reading.

19

PHOBIAS

PHOBIAS are irrational fears of such intensity that you avoid encountering the circumstance or object which is the focus of your fear. Because they are irrational, it is possible to have a phobia about virtually anything. The most common is agoraphobia, fear of open or crowded spaces. Far rarer – but common enough to have a name – is hygrophobia, a fear of dampness, and ponophobia, fear of fatigue, among many others.

Phobias are usually divided into three groups: agoraphobia; social phobias; and simple phobias.

• Agoraphobia •

Agoraphobia, fear of open, crowded or confined places, or sometimes fear of leaving the home, is a common problem which cannot reliably be quantified because so many sufferers never seek help. About 70 per cent of sufferers are women.

Some experts question whether agoraphobia should really be classified as a phobia at all as it is actually terror of having a panic attack. Usually the way it starts is by a person having a panic attack out of the blue and then associating the panic with the place they were in, often enough a public place such as a supermarket or a train station. If a few attacks occur, fear of an attack happening again leads the sufferer to avoid returning to that place or anywhere similar.

• Social phobias •

These stem from a fear of being embarrassed or humiliated in public. Most people feel anxious about having to perform in front of others but the social phobic may be traumatised by having to write anything or even sign their name in the view of others, be unable to eat in a restaurant for fear of choking or dropping food, be disablingly fearful of blushing or be utterly fearful of anyone watching them while working. Someone who suffers a social phobia may have, or fear, a panic attack at the prospect of being humiliated in public and so may avoid any public event, from activities like theatre-going and parties to using a public convenience. You would be considered to have a social phobia if your fear was enough to interfere with normal life. It is easy to see how that could happen.

• Simple phobias •

These are simple by name but obviously not by nature to the person suffering one. In simple phobias there is one circumstance or one object only which causes such intense fear that it must be avoided. Most common are phobias about animals, insects or reptiles, fear of heights, fear of flying, fear of the dentist, fear of needles, illness and death. Many phobias, because they are so situation-specific, do not unduly disrupt the sufferer's life. However some – for example, a fear of seeing broken glass – are a constant cause of anxiety because the object of fear could come into view at any unpredictable time.

• What causes phobias? •

At the simplest level, usually an association is formed between a circumstance or object and the feeling of anxiety. For example, someone who has experienced a panic attack while having to stand in a bus may think, 'Oh no, suppose I have a panic attack if I can't get a seat on the bus!' The thought causes anxiety and may become firmly associated with anxiety, so that getting on to a bus gradually becomes an anxiety-inducing event. If the anxiety is severe enough, the sufferer may decide to avoid the bus altogether, thus making the fear a phobia.

Another common predisposing cause is an event in one's past that caused deep fear or anxiety. For example, getting accidentally locked in a room may lead to claustrophobia (fear of confined spaces); being bitten or chased by a dog may lead to a phobia about dogs. The fear is understandable; it is irrational only in the sense that we know not every dog will bite us or not every door will be impossible to open, yet we still feel the intense fear and, if we have developed a phobia, end up avoiding as far as possible encountering the circumstance or object that causes it.

• Why some, not others? •

The big question, of course, is why only some people who get bitten by a dog or locked in a room, etc, become phobic. There may be personality differences, differences in upbringing, differing levels and thresholds for stress and physiological factors which have a bearing.

Sometimes a phobia may be just the external manifestation of a deep, unidentified inner fear. For example, a fear that cannot be faced, such as not being wanted or feeling inadequate, may be channelled into an imaginary fear that is initially less threatening to cope with. Gradually, however, the phobia may become so powerful that it takes over and interrupts one's whole life.

Another big question is why women more commonly suffer phobias and panic attacks than men. One likely reason is that women are allowed to express fear more freely than men: it may be seen as endearing for a woman to tremble at the sight of a mouse but feeble for a man to do so. Also, women tend to fantasise and daydream more than men, so phobias may be a more natural way for them to express fears and anxieties in life.

• Jealousy •

Severe agoraphobia can be a means of power play within relationships and can be used by both men and women. It has been known, for example, for some women unwittingly to use inability to leave the house as a way of reducing their fear of their partner straying, as the partner may be forced to take over running the home and caring for the children and clearly have no time for any illicit affair. Sometimes a man who is jealous and fearful of his wife's infidelity may encourage agoraphobia in his wife by constantly making accusations and questioning her whereabouts, but being loving and caring and all too willing to take over when the woman becomes severely affected by her phobia and is forced to stay home.

Interestingly, the ratio of women to men sufferers from agoraphobia is dropping slightly, probably because more women are now more used to working full time outside the home. Women who do not venture far afield, whether because of caring for children, a dependent relative or any other reason, are more likely to suffer agoraphobia than women used to asserting themselves in the outside world. There is less out there that is unfamiliar, unknown and threatening to the working woman. Having said that, however, many sufferers have indeed been active working women, so there are no hard and fast rules, only theories and suppositions.

• NDD •

One unusual cause of agoraphobia in some cases is neurodevelopmental delay (NDD, so named by British neurodevelopmentalist Peter Blythe who discovered it). NDD is failure of certain primitive reflexes to be replaced by adult ones. Primitive reflexes help foetuses to develop and survive in the womb and babies to survive their early weeks and months. There are a number of these reflexes, all well documented, the earliest being the automatic panic reaction (Moro reflex) which makes a baby throw out its arms and legs at the least little fright.

Retention of certain primitive reflexes, which may occur for example because of infection during pregnancy or a familial tendency, may affect co-ordination, vision and balance. Such retention is well known in brain-injured children, but was not realised to occur in normally functioning children and adults until Peter Blythe started his research over 20 years ago. Although more accepted now, it is still a contentious area.

The link with agoraphobia or panic attacks is this. If a sufferer has several primitive reflexes remaining and has had to compensate unconsciously for the problem for years they most probably will, at some point, reach their stress threshold and not be able to compensate reliably any more. Resultant distorted vision or poor balance may suddenly make the ground appear to rise up or the walls close in. If this happens a few times, the sufferer may be confused and panic. Having received short shrift from their doctor and been told nothing is organically wrong, they are quite likely to become fearful of repetition of the experience and may gradually limit their activities or stay indoors.

Peter Blythe and his colleagues have established a testing procedure to check for balance, co-ordination and control over hands and feet as well as special signs that primitive reflexes have not been inhibited. If NDD is diagnosed, the problem is reversible with special exercises designed to mimic the actions babies and children usually make to inhibit each primitive reflex before adult reactions take over. But the whole business takes time, practice and commitment and isn't cheap.

If you think NDD may be your problem, write for details and a list of NDD therapists in the UK to The Institute for Neurophysiological Psychology: see Useful Contacts. You should be sent a questionnaire to fill in to establish, before parting with any money, whether this approach might be appropriate for you or not.

• Treatment •

The most successful type of treatment for phobias of any kind is so-called behavioural treatment, usually carried out under the guidance of a clinical psychologist, using a technique called desensitisation. The thinking behind this method is that the causes of the phobia don't matter, it is the behaviour (that is, the phobic avoidance) which needs to be tackled and helped to change. You can use the technique as a self-help method too (see page 158), if you are confident enough to try and have a supportive partner or friend willing to help you.

Psychotherapy may have a place in helping overcome a phobia but is less likely to be suggested first unless the phobia is just one of many concurrent psychological problems.

• Desensitisation •

The aim is to remove the association between the feared object or circumstance and anxiety by teaching a different response: calmness. For desensitisation to work, you have to be able to relax deeply and then, in the first stage, visualise the feared object/event and, in the second, come into contact with it in real life (if practical; but more difficult, if your fear is of snakes or monsoons, perhaps). It is a gradual process, in which you build up slowly from facing the circumstance that cause you least fear to one that causes you the most. You do this by creating a hierarchy.

• Creating a hierarchy •

Try to think of ten events or possible scenarios relating to your phobia, ranking them from 1 (least frightening) to 10 (most frightening). For example, if your fear is of using the underground, you might decide on a hierarchy like this:

1 Looking at a map of the underground in a book at home.
2 Seeing the underground symbol outside an underground station.
3 Entering the station.
4 Buying a ticket.
5 Walking through the entry barrier.
6 Going down the escalator.
7 Waiting on the platform.
8 Getting on the train.
9 Travelling one stop on the train.
10 Travelling two stops on the train.

• Tackling your hierarchy •

When you are ready to start tackling your hierarchy, you first relax yourself very deeply. Create for yourself a scene which you find peaceful and comforting and every aspect of which you can visualise very vividly: for example, the salty smell of waves on a seashore, the sun warming your back, the muted sounds of children's happy voices, etc. This needs to be a scene which you can summon quickly at will.

When you have relaxed and enjoyed your chosen scene, imagine being in the situation which you have put lowest on your hierarchy. Try to see it just as vividly. Don't see yourself in the scene as anxious, see yourself as calm and unperturbed.

Try to stay with this for about a minute but if you feel panicky, try to breathe deeply and concentrate on feeling calm.

If you feel exceedingly anxious, return to your chosen scene and calm yourself down before trying the phobia scenario once more. Keep going, switching between the two as often as you need to, until you feel no or little anxiety about being in the phobia scenario. At this point you are ready to move to the next one on your hierarchy.

Don't try too much in one go. Give yourself time to relax fully at the outset each time and then limit your actual desensitisation practice to about 20 minutes daily. Begin each day with whatever step you succeeded in dealing with comfortably the day before, then move on from there.

When you have reached the top of your hierarchy and can imagine the most frightening event relating to your phobia with only mild anxiety or none at all (however long this takes), the next step is to begin at the bottom again and face your ten scenes in real life.

• Facing your phobia in real life •

This obviously takes a great deal of courage and commitment. If you tackle your phobia with the help of a psychologist, he or she will probably accompany you. If you are tackling it alone, you might find it helpful if someone you trust and feel comfortable with comes with you. Make sure, however, that you know and they know exactly what their role is: that is, to encourage, support and help distract you if you are in difficulties, but not to set the pace, criticise your progress or lack of it, tell you how to do it better or make you feel embarrassed.

You might find that your previous hierarchy leaves out some important steps when it actually comes to putting them into practice. In this case, add them in as additional steps, so that every step of your journey is in small manageable pieces. Make sure that the last step on your hierarchy isn't too daunting: for example, rather than deciding on 'doing the shopping in a supermarket', set the goal of buying a few specific items only.

You will probably need to repeat each step more often than you did in your imagination, which is fine. However, to ensure that you will progress along your list and not avoid advancement, set yourself a loose time limit by which you want to have carried out all the steps on your hierarchy.

• Coping with difficulties •

You must expect to feel uncomfortable as you undertake your real-life desensitisation, otherwise you wouldn't have a problem in the first place. So don't back out of the situation you are trying the minute you feel any discomfort. However, each time you feel more anxiety than you can cope with, withdraw from the situation, calm yourself by breathing deeply, distracting yourself or by visualising your peaceful scene (see also Preventing Panic Attacks, page 152) and then return to where you were.

You have to be prepared for set-backs. Sometimes a situation you managed well one day causes you intense anxiety on another. Sometimes you will not be able to stay in a situation as long as you hoped. Try to see it all as an integral part of the process. And try to focus on your successes, rather than what you see as your failures. Every step taken is an enormous triumph. Even making the commitment to tackle a phobia at all deserves a huge pat from yourself on the back. So don't let your expectations speed up too much once you get going.

• Further help •

The Phobics Society is a self-help group that has groups throughout the country. The Open Door Association also has self-help groups throughout the country for anyone suffering from agoraphobia. For both associations, write with an SAE: see Useful Contacts.

The mental health charity, MIND, may be able to give details of any other self-help groups or particularly useful books: see Useful Contacts.

20

OBSESSIVE-COMPULSIVE DISORDER

OBSESSIVE-COMPULSIVE disorder (OCD) used to be thought rare: in fact it is now known that this is far from the case. Probably at least a million people in the UK suffer from disabling obsessive-compulsive symptoms, an extreme version of common behaviour traits.

Having obsessions is nothing abnormal. According to research, about 80 per cent of people have obsessions of some kind or another but they don't interfere with normal life – or, at least, not much. There is probably a fine line between some obsessions and enthusiasms.

We would probably consider a teenager to be obsessed with a pop star if they have to attend their every concert, read every magazine article about them, buy every record, dress like them, talk like them, etc, but we wouldn't view it as worryingly abnormal. A man might be obsessed with his car, washing, polishing and tuning it at every opportunity, to the annoyance of his family who might rather they were all using the car to go somewhere interesting and fun.

We are often, in effect, obsessed with someone when we have fallen in love with them, thinking about them almost constantly. An obsession like this does tend to get in the way of ordinary life to some extent and certainly couldn't continue at that intensity and degree of absorption, but no one would consider that they needed help to deal with the problem. People who collect things are also, to a degree, obsessed. They just must have a particular item to add to their collection and will go to extraordinary lengths to achieve it, or suffer agonies if they fail.

There are some activities most of us find compulsive too. It is common for many people to check once or twice that they really did lock the back door or put their child's buggy in the car boot. Some women could not possibly do the washing up and not wipe out the oven afterwards.

All of the above are fairly normal. For someone with obsessive-compulsive disorder, however, the whole business is out of their control. Hand-washing and checking are the most common obsessive-compulsive behaviours and they can take up many hours of an affected person's day, continually disrupting routines and making it impossible to live a normal life.

• What exactly is OCD? •

Obsessions are recurrent ideas, thoughts, impulses or images which keep popping unwanted into the mind. They are usually experienced as frightening, intrusive or, at the least, unacceptable. These thoughts cause anxiety and usually the compulsion develops as a means of reducing the anxiety. For example, an intrusive anxiety about being contaminated by germs on a tea-towel may be removed by going and washing.

Sometimes, the compulsive ritual that develops to deal with the unwanted thought has no apparently logical connection: for example, counting from 100 to 1 and then silently saying the words of three nursery rhymes every time the thought comes into mind.

Someone with OCD knows that what they are doing is irrational. Yet they still feel compelled to go through with their ritual, whatever it may be. They may have to turn the car round after journeying several miles just to come back home and check yet again that the front door is really locked. They may have to perform a hand-washing ritual after just touching a newspaper, with the washing needing to be done in a particular order and begun again completely should someone walk into the room during the ritual.

Because they know what they are doing is irrational, time-consuming and may be destructive of normal family relationships, they may feel deep shame and guilt as well as desperation.

• Why does it happen? •

As with most of these things, no one really knows why. Women do not suffer from OCD any more than men but are more likely to have obsessions and compulsions related to cleaning. Sometimes OCD develops for the first time when someone is depressed but, just as often, OCD is present first and causes depression. Significant or overloading life stresses, such as pregnancy, childbirth, marriage and sex problems, exhaustion, work difficulties and the illness or death of someone close are mentioned by many people in connection with the beginning of their symptoms.

Background and personality are likely to play a part. Sometimes a particular event can be traced which seems to account for the onset of symptoms. For example, a child may have wished that something awful would happen to an adult who tells them off and the next day that adult is seriously hurt in an accident. Although the incident is apparently forgotten, years later the child, now an adult, has the fleeting wish that someone who has hurt or annoyed them would die and the next day learns that the wish has indeed been fulfilled. This may lead to a fear of the power of one's own dark thoughts and an obsessive need to neutralise them with mental or physical rituals.

It is thought possible, in fact, that among those most susceptible to OCD are people who castigate themselves for 'bad' fleeting thoughts that are, in fact, commonplace. Most people, research has shown, have momentary disturbing irrational thoughts such as 'I could stab my son', 'I'm going to push that person in front of the train when it comes into the station', 'I'm going to hit you in the face', when none of the people the thoughts are about have done anything to provoke such a reaction.

Of course, such thoughts are alarming and are a lot about fear of loss of control or of doing something unacceptable. Usually, however, they are shrugged off and forgotten or at least realised to have no likelihood of being translated into action.

For the person who will develop OCD, however, the thought may not just go away. Because they are so shocked by it, they dwell on it, fear it, find themselves thinking it or something like it more often. Or they may try to push it from their minds, only to have the thought come back the stronger. They may come to see themselves as bad.

There is also a possibility that OCD has a biological basis: a deficiency or malfunction of a brain chemical called serotonin. For some sufferers, drugs usually used to treated depression and which act on serotonin levels, have helped dramatically.

• Treatment •

For most sufferers a combination of behavioural and cognitive techniques (changing your actions and the way you think about your thoughts and actions) are most helpful. These are commonly the province of clinical psychologists, within hospitals or private practice. However, the main technique, known rather dauntingly as exposure and response prevention, can be applied as a self-help method.

• Exposure and response prevention •

As with self-help techniques for dealing with phobias and panic attacks, the programme involves doing a little at a time of what you find frightening, learning to reduce the anxiety it causes, and gradually working up from situations that don't cause you too much panic to those that do cause intense discomfort and anxiety. The aim is not only liberation from the most crippling forms of OCD but to realise, in the process, that nothing dire does happen if you don't carry out a particular ritual to ward off anxiety, contamination or whatever.

You need to be very strongly motivated to tackle an OCD situation on your own. Clinical psychologist Dr Frank Tallis, an expert in this field (see Further Reading for details of his self-help book), suggests that, at the outset, you think up and write down the benefits you hope for and the beneficial changes in your life that will occur, once you have kicked the problem. For example, if you have to wash all the time to avoid contamination, you might hope to be free of the compulsion so that you can give family members or friends a hug without fearing germs, go out to restaurants (if fear of dirty plates prevented you before), have more time, not have to fear needing to use a toilet when you are out, etc. If, as is likely during your self-help therapy, there are times when you don't want to go on because the struggle to get better is so painful, you will be able to look at your list for encouragement.

• How to start •

Make a list of situations you find anxiety-provoking and grade them on a scale from one (mild anxiety) to eight (very anxiety provoking). Try to find a situation to match every figure. From these, choose six or eight situations which you could arrange to expose yourself to. For example, if you have anxiety about contamination, you might usefully include touching a newspaper but not touching a rhinoceros so that you have a list going up in severity of anxiety from one to six (or eight, if you want to try the lot).

There will, of course, be some things that are not appropriate for inclusion on your list, however much you would fear contamination by them, because no one, even without OCD, would choose to touch them: such as dog pooh or vomit in the street. However, if just seeing dog pooh sends you home to wash you could usefully include on your list walking somewhere where you might see it, such as a park.

Example: a list for compulsive hand-washing   Someone who fears contamination and must wash might make a list like this:

1 Touching a newspaper.
2 Touching the handle of my own toilet.
3 Sitting on a seat on a train or bus.
4 Eating with cutlery that isn't mine.
5 Using someone else's toilet.
6 Being touched by someone I don't know.

After completing the list, the next step is to work out how long you think you could delay going and washing after exposing yourself to the first action on the list and for how long you would need to perform the washing ritual. For example, you might decide that, on the first day, you could make yourself touch a newspaper for one minute, delay washing for four minutes and would need to wash for seven minutes. The second time you try it, you could touch the paper for two minutes, wait five minutes and wash for six, perhaps. Work on up, giving yourself about 12 exposures to get to a point where you could deal with the circumstance for about 30 minutes (if appropriate) and delay washing for at least 30 minutes. At this point, you probably will not need to wash at all.

A list for excessive checking   If excessive checking is your compulsion, make out a list of the things you are compelled to check many times, grading again from one to eight. Decide how many initial checks you will allow yourself – such as that the fridge door really is shut – and how long you can delay before going back for how many more checks (which should be fewer in number than the initial checks). If what you need to check entails returning to the house after leaving, keep your number of checks down as low as you possibly can. Then, in the same way as for washing and cleaning rituals, work up until you can check just once, delay a re-check for 30 to 45 minutes, and then not check again at all.

• Two important skills •

Before you go ahead, you need to learn two important skills: relaxation and positive self-talk.

Relaxation   Choose a method you feel comfortable with (see page 41) and practise until you feel relatively assured that you can apply it quickly when any anxiety threatens to get out of hand.

Positive self-talk   Try to replace unhelpful negative thoughts such as, 'I can't handle this', 'I'm going to die if I don't wash/check at once', etc, with coping statements such as 'I can handle this', 'My anxiety won't get out of control', 'I'm not comfortable but I didn't expect to be', and 'I'm doing well here'.

If you really can't stop panicky thoughts relating to your obsession from coming constantly into your mind, don't push them away but question their validity. For example, 'Am I really going to pick up a virus if I shake this person's hand? What evidence do I have for this?'

Or: 'Why do I think washing is going to help me now? The more I wash, the more my hands become dry and cracked and the more likely I really will get infected with something.'

Or: 'Do I really need to go back one more time to check the front door is locked? When have I ever left the door unlocked after returning to check it? Why should it be different this time?'

• Avoid seeking reassurance •

While you are working through your OCD in the way described, try to avoid seeking reassurance from others that everything will be all right, advises Dr Tallis. Asking a partner or friend if 'It'll be all right even if I did leave the front door open, won't it?' or 'It won't hurt me not to wash immediately I've emptied the dustbin, will it?' is an attempt to reduce anxiety without carrying out the ritual you usually use to reduce it. The aim of the programme is to experience, not avoid, mild anxiety and be able to handle it, or to reach the point where anxiety doesn't arise in that circumstance at all.

• OCD with depression •

If you suffer from OCD and depression together, it can be very difficult indeed to motivate yourself to tackle situations that make you anxious. You might do better to try to deal with the depression first. See Depression, page 168.

21

POST-TRAUMATIC STRESS DISORDER

THIS is a collection of extremely unpleasant and incapacitating symptoms which may develop after a highly traumatic and terrifying event. Such traumas might be individual, such as being raped or assaulted, or arise from a major disaster, such as being in a rail, car or plane crash, a fire, an earthquake or being in a group held hostage by a gunman. The most common cause of post-traumatic symptoms is a serious road accident.

• Symptoms •

There are numerous symptoms which may be associated with post-traumatic stress disorder. People commonly find their minds returning to the traumatic event and reliving the despair and the distress again and again, or they find themselves subject to dramatic unbidden flashbacks which catch them unawares and terrify them. They may, of course, have recurrent nightmares.

Some people try to cope by blocking out thoughts and feelings about the terrifying event. They may start to avoid doing things which are likely to bring back memories or which might possibly place them in danger again. In one study of road accident victims, a quarter of those who suffered post-traumatic stress went on to fear driving or being a passenger. Many may develop an accident phobia and avoid travelling in cars altogether. Women who have been raped may avoid making new relationships with men. Women who were mugged may avoid ever walking alone.

Losing interest in old hobbies or former pastimes is common. The sufferer may become numb to feeling, withdraw from social life and feel totally untrusting about the future. There may be strong guilt feelings if others died but the sufferer survived. Particularly common are anxiety feelings such as jumpiness, inability to concentrate and inability to sleep.

Post-traumatic stress symptoms may occur for the first time immediately after the traumatic event or within a few days but they can often be delayed and not experienced at all until at least six months have passed. Children may suffer the whole range of symptoms, although once it was believed, wrongly, that they were more resilient than adults. (One reason adults have tended to deny that children could suffer severely is because of an understandable reluctance to acknowledge that a child could go through such pain.)

• Effects •

The extent of suffering from post-traumatic stress is impossible to quantify, particularly as many victims of individual traumas such as rape never officially report what happened to them. However, researchers have been able to estimate that at least 30 to 40 per cent of survivors of major disasters develop significant problems that may last for up to five years.

Post-traumatic stress syndrome is not inevitable, however. Some people do manage to get over even very serious traumas without ill effect. It may be the way that the event is experienced and how someone comes to terms with it which is more important in terms of consequences than the event itself; although research has also shown that a person's closeness to the traumatic event and the length of time they are involved in it has as much bearing on degree of distress as personality. Those who feel guilty or blame themselves for the outcome of the event are more likely to suffer serious problems than those who don't.

The degree to which someone suffers from severe stress after a personal or major catastrophe may depend upon their coping abilities in the past, their usual sense of control over their own life, self-esteem, the strength of the support they can depend on from loving family and friends and their religious or cultural beliefs.

• Professional help •

Psychotherapy or counselling can be extremely helpful, as both provide an opportunity for strong feelings about the trauma to be repeatedly expressed and fully explored. (See page 200 for how to find a therapist.)

• Self-help •

Allow yourself your feelings You may feel a whole range of upsetting or frightening feelings that persist for some time, or you may not. The best guide is yourself. You have the right to grieve, to collapse, to seem foolish or weak; and the worst thing is to try to appear strong and resilient if you don't feel that way. If you keep this in mind, you are more likely to allow your real feelings to surface, whenever they occur.

Expect fluctuations Try to accept that you might feel weepy and frightened one day, calm and more accepting the next and then weepy or numb again another day. Changes up and down may go by the week or month too, for some years.

Talk to others who care Research shows that the more people talk about their experience, the less intrusive thoughts about it gradually become. Talk to someone sympathetic who will listen willingly or just hold you when you need to cry. The more often people re-tell what happened to them, the less intense the emotion associated with it becomes.

Re-tell as often as you need to You may feel you can't keep burdening someone with your same old story. But someone who cares may not feel burdened or you may be able to find a few different people to talk to. Many people find it helpful to seek out a self-help group or others who have had similar experiences. Charities such as MIND (see Useful Contacts) may know of relevant organisations.

Re-telling can help someone make sense of what happened to them or view it from a different perspective or even, in some cases, draw some positive conclusions from what initially seemed unremittingly devastating.

Do it your own way Well-meaning people around you may expect you to feel terrible, or to insist that you let out specific feelings such as anger which they are convinced you must be suppressing. Without hurting their feelings, try not to be pushed and certainly not to feel inadequate for not behaving as they imagine you ought to be behaving.

• Further information •

Post-traumatic Stress Disorder by David Kinchin is a practical guide written by an ex-sufferer. *Understanding Post-traumatic Stress Syndrome* is a booklet published by MIND. See Further Reading.

22

DEPRESSION

DEPRESSION in all its gradations, from a mild case of the blues through to extreme debilitating misery, is extremely common. Few people haven't experienced a low mood lasting at least for a few hours or a day or more, where nothing seems quite worthwhile, including yourself, and you are full of self doubts about your abilities and your achievements.

As many as 60 to 70 per cent of adults will, at some time, experience depression of severity sufficient to have an adverse effect on their daily lives. It may not last long and most of us suddenly just come out of it again. In a small number of cases, however, there are more severe and more persistent psychological and physical symptoms and 'snapping out of it' just isn't possible.

· Symptoms of serious depression ·

Depression in its full–blown state is a mental illness, and to be recognised as such by a doctor someone would be suffering at least five of the following symptoms during a two-week period (but see Brief Recurrent Depression, page 178, for an exception to this).

Depressed mood This is usually an essential for a diagnosis of depression. It is a deep feeling of dejection, despair, despondency and emptiness (rather than sadness), which persists for most of the day, almost every day.

Loss of interest and pleasure This is a lack of interest in normal daily activities and in what the future may hold. Without either this or a depressed mood, a clinical diagnosis of depression cannot be reached.

Marked gain or loss of weight A weight fluctuation of more than 5 per cent of normal body weight in a month may occur, even though you aren't trying to change it. People who are really depressed can easily lose 6 to 12kg (1 to 2 stone) in months or weeks, and in very severe cases may refuse to eat at all. Overeating or eating for comfort is more common in milder depression.

Sleep disturbance This means either sleeping too much or too little. Commonly, depressed people wake in the early hours of the morning (for example, about 4am), and are unable to sleep any more, even if they have gone to bed late. They usually feel extremely despondent at this time, particularly after bad dreams. Others may have difficulty falling asleep when they go to bed, however tired they may be.Yet others use sleep as a means of escape and can sleep from early in the evening until late in the morning or for large chunks of the day, if their lives allow.

Being agitated or slow in actions This nerviness and restlessness or, on the other hand, slowing up of thoughts, words and actions, is apparent to others as well as oneself.

Loss of energy and exhaustion This may happen to such a degree that people often think they must be physically ill. It is difficult to get up, to get going, to do chores. The body seems to ache and there is a constant feeling of being drained.

Feelings of worthlessness or guilt These may be strengthened by constant negative thinking about one's past and future. When depressed you feel like a victim or you feel everything around you and about you is jinxed. You are pessimistic, have no hopes, no pride in achievements and feel responsible for an awful lot of ills, past or present, that may have nothing to do with you.

Inability to concentrate This may be accompanied by a consequent failure to remember things you have been told or are meant to do, an inability to make even simple decisions (such as what to wear or what to eat) and no attention to give freely to others. You often just can't carry things through.

Thoughts of death or suicide Such thoughts may come repeatedly to mind. When people are very severely depressed, they may dwell on accounts of tragic deaths they read about or hear on the news, as well as think about ways they could kill themselves. Tragically, many people do make attempts at suicide and probably about 3000 people manage to kill themselves each year, as a result of major depression.

• Making the diagnosis •

Alarmingly, however, GPs may miss the diagnosis of depression in a staggering 44 to 50 per cent of cases, according to research, because very many people go to the doctor ostensibly for some other problem and GPs are so often too rushed to have time to tease out anything else that may be wrong. So, if you know you are severely depressed and want help, you may need to speak out rather than rely on your condition being detected.

Doctors are nowadays likely to judge the severity of depression, and its need or not for medical intervention, by the symptoms described above. However, it used to be common to try to distinguish between different types of depression and many doctors may still do so. Explanations of the terms follow.

• Reactive and endogenous depression •

It isn't easy to make a completely clear-cut division between these two types, which is why the distinction is falling from favour. Broadly, however, reactive depression means a depression which develops for some concrete and understandable reason, such as the loss of someone dear, extreme financial worries and consequent inability to take care of one's family, etc. Such depression is more extreme than the normal grief or worry and despondency that anyone would feel as a result of such events, but usually will pass without need for medical help, once circumstances have been resolved or grief and loss come to terms with.

Endogenous depression means depression 'from within' and is so called because usually the sufferer doesn't know what has brought it on. There are likely to be explanations in the person's life but they may have been unconsciously suppressed. Alternatively, a recognised outside event may have been the trigger but the depression that ensues is deeper and more incapacitating than that usually associated with the reactive type. Endogenous depression is usually characterised by early morning waking, depression reaching its depths in the morning, loss of appetite and extreme but vague guilt feelings.

• Neurotic and psychotic depression •

Neurotic, to the layperson, is a somewhat denigrating term but, in this context, merely describes the particular symptoms that go with a milder depression: a sufferer has some up days and some down days, is very irritable a lot of the time (with family and colleagues bearing the brunt), evenings are their worst times, they may overeat for comfort and put on weight and may have difficulty falling asleep or sleep too much. Psychotic depression is closer to that described for endogenous depression above but there is always some degree of removal from reality, with the person suffering hallucinations, delusions or morbid obsessions.

However these terms may never be used at all as very many people's experience of depression do not fit comfortably into them.

• Anxiety with depression •

We often tend to think of these two states almost as opposites, the one characterised by constant movement, whether mental or physical, the other by slump and lack of motivation. However the two can and often do co-exist.

In mild depression with anxiety, there tends to be excessive worry about things in one's own life one can or can't control, things 'out there' in the world which one definitely can't control, or worries about possible illness or death.

In major depression, anxiety can take the form of constant crying, pacing, hand-wringing, or clutching at others' coat-tails and begging for help. Sufferers may think they are dying or about to collapse or are unable to move their legs or arms, although to the observer this is clearly not the case. As a result, they may be ignored or deliberately side-stepped, through embarrassment. The risk of suicide is greater when severe depression is coupled with this extreme form of anxiety.

• Manic depression •

Some people suffer from bouts of extreme highs and lows, commonly known as manic depression. There is no clear order of events, although a period of mania is usually followed by a period of depression. In a manic phase, everything seems wonderful, exciting, the world full of opportunity. Manic people tend to talk fast and incessantly, stay up until all hours, eat little, and act on mad impulse, which can often mean running up huge telephone bills phoning friends in foreign parts for lengthy (one-sided) conversations, splashing out on expensive items and even acting on extravagant ideas such as hiring a chauffeur-driven car for a week. Unfortunately, there usually isn't the money to back up the lifestyle and severe financial difficulties can result. Family and friends may be castigated for not sharing their enthusiasms or being spoilsports.

The manic phase usually ends with the sufferer suddenly coming down to earth with a bump and then deep depression follows. A lot of manic people do not have alternating bouts of mania and depression but several of one and then one of the other. Their behaviour may be normal for years, with only occasional weeks or maybe months of highs and lows.

• Brief recurrent depression •

This is a type of depression which has only been recognised relatively recently because it doesn't fit the standard criteria for depression that doctors look for. As its name implies, it is a short-lived recurrent depression (see page 178).

• Special risk times •

Women may be more susceptible to depression with irritability before a period, a familiar symptom of premenstrual syndrome for sufferers.

One in four women may suffer from depression ranging from mild to severe after the birth of a baby, regardless of whether the baby is wanted or not (see Post-natal Depression, page 179).

Women may also be susceptible to depression around the time of the menopause, especially if they have already had a tendency towards depression in their lives. But a depressive episode may often occur for the first time ever at this time.

For both men and women, depression may sometimes be brought on when the days shorten and there is less light, during autumn and winter. This is known as Seasonal Affective Disorder or SAD (see page 180).

• What causes depression? •

There are many factors that may affect the development of depression.

Childhood experiences Loss of one's mother during childhood is known to increase risk of depression later. A child who is continually hit, told off, criticised or treated without warmth may learn to repress feelings of hurt and pain, which in later life may surface as depression.

Children also copy the way their parents behave so, if a parent is depressed a lot, a child may learn this way of responding to events too. This is different from inheriting a tendency to depression, although heredity does play some part, particularly in manic depression and sometimes in severe depression.

There is also a theory that babies can be frightened by their own angry feelings, when, for example, they don't instantly get what they want, and especially if their anger is not accepted by their carer or is met with anxiety. They may unconsciously turn their anger inward, into depression.

Painful feelings   Anger turned inward as an adult can be an explanation for depression, as can other painful feelings, such as grief or fear, which are not fully expressed. People who feel helpless a lot of the time in life and that their efforts don't amount to much are particularly susceptible to depression; 'learned helplessness', as it is called, can often start in childhood if independence is thwarted at crucial moments of development.

Personality   This has a bearing on whether we tend towards depression or not. People who are naturally more optimistic, flexible and adaptable are less likely than pessimists and perfectionists to suffer. The way we think about ourselves and our lives can contribute considerably too. If we tend to be negative about our abilities, our potential and about how we feel others see us, we are more likely to succumb to depressive feelings.

Life events   What happens to us during our lives naturally makes a major contribution to the experience of depression. Crises or catastrophes in our personal lives, an over-demanding or unsatisfying job, chronic pain or disability are understandable precursors. So too are feelings of loneliness, boredom or uselessness.

Physical causes   These may include the effects of certain viral infections, particularly influenza and glandular fever, hormonal changes during the menstrual cycle, pregnancy, the menopause and fluctuations in the functioning of some brain chemicals.

• Women and depression •

Women are twice as likely as men to suffer from depression but this is probably not the inevitable nature of things. Women are more likely to admit to feeling depressed whereas men traditionally are more likely to demonstrate bravado or drown their sorrows in drink. Married women are more likely to be depressed than either married men or single women, probably because they play most of the supporting role: for example, mothers who work full time are still more likely than fathers to organise running the home and caring for children. Part of the extra depression in women is accounted for by the effects of the female sex hormones, oestrogen and progesterone.

• Drugs and physical treatments •

It is fashionable to think that there should be no need for drug treatment for depression, and that dealing with life difficulties or working to alter undesirable aspects of one's personality should be able to do the job. This is not always the case, although life problems which are responsible for triggering or maintaining depression obviously need addressing in any treatment. However, in a small minority of cases, depression has purely biochemical causes which only the appropriate medication can help and, in some others, deep depression may be so debilitating and disabling that it is only after that state has been lifted with drugs that a sufferer can even look to make life changes.

Antidepressants, as their name indicates, are drugs designed to combat depression. They are only useful for severe depression, need to be taken for some months for full effect and are not addictive. There are various different types but all work to increase the availability of neurotransmitters, chemical messengers that belong to a class of compounds called monoamines, and which are thought to be deficient in severe depression.

• Tricyclics •

Tricyclics belong to a class of drug known as MARIS (monoamine re-uptake inhibitors) which have the effect of stopping nerve cells from reabsorbing their own monoamines once they have carried out their messenger work. There are various tricyclics and they work mainly on two neurotransmitters, noradrenaline and serotonin.

Those which have been in longest use and have the most side-effects, to varying degrees, include imipramine, amitriptyline, clomipramine and dothiepin. Common likely side-effects are blurred vision, dry mouth, constipation, sweating, and weight gain. Some have the effect of making a person more energised, others have sedative qualities. So-called newer tricyclics such as lofepramine, trazodone and viloxazine, may have fewer side-effects. Mianserin is a tricyclic-related drug that works as an antidepressant but sometimes has been found to have an adverse effect on bone marrow.

• Selective serotonin re-uptake inhibitors • (SSRIs or 5-HT inhibitors)

These relatively new drugs work by increasing availability of serotonin, a major neurotransmitter, deficiency of which increasingly appears to be linked with depression. They are more expensive than tricyclics, so are less likely to be tried first. There are currently four, called fluvoxamine, sertraline, fluoxetine and paroxetine. The main side-effect is nausea and also indigestion if taken on an empty stomach.

The brand name version of fluoxetine is Prozac, about which a lot of fuss has been made in America. It seems to enhance mood and became something of a fashionable drug to take for all sorts of anxiety conditions as well as depression and bulimia – or even for no problem at all.

Prior to its popularity it was associated with scare stories about its leading to violence and suicide attempts, but these are largely considered unfounded. However, some experts do think that it may increase agitation or aggressiveness in some people. British psychiatrists mainly see it as just another SSRI without any special life-enhancing properties but a useful drug for the right people if cheaper ones don't work.

Hair loss may be an infrequent side-effect of fluoxetine, according to the US equivalent of the UK drugs datasheet compendium.

• RIMAs •

This stands for reversible inhibitors of monoamine oxidase subtype A. RIMAs, of which only one is so far available – moclobmide – are a new version of the oldest drug treatment for depression, the MAOIs, monoamine oxidase inhibitors. However, these were problematic because of a side-effect on the metabolism of an amino acid called tyramine, found in many foods and drink but particularly cheese and wine. If these were consumed while taking the drug, a very unpleasant reaction including a banging headache would result.

The new RIMAs do not have this effect so are far safer and far less life-disrupting to take. Both they and the old MAOIs (still sometimes prescribed) may be very useful when anxiety is present with depression.

• Lithium •

This drug is commonly used to treat severe manic depression. The dosage has to be exactly right both for it to work and to avoid adverse effects on the kidney, so periodic monitoring is essential. It is often taken for years if necessary. In about half of users, relapse may occur if the drug is stopped.

• Oestrogens •

Oestrogen implants or oestrogen patches seem to be effective in treating depression related to premenstrual syndrome, post-natal depression and depression around the time of the menopause or up to two or three years earlier. In one study of women with severe premenstrual depression, it lifted when they wore patches twice a week for three months. In another study, a daily oestrogen patch used for one month helped women who developed severe post-natal depression within three months of giving birth. However, research in this area has been carried out by gynaecologists and is only slowly being recognised by psychiatrists, and antidepressants may still be given as first line treatment, perhaps inappropriately.

• ECT •

Electroconvulsive therapy (ECT) is a means of producing fits via electrodes placed on either side of the head. The patient is anaesthetised and also given a muscle relaxant beforehand. It sounds barbaric and probably is. However, it can be remarkably effective in very severe cases of depression where antidepressants don't work or the depression is too life-threatening for antidepressants to be given the time to work. There can be nasty side-effects, such as loss of memory and quick thinking which many claim is permanent. Headache and confusion are temporary.

• Psychotherapy and counselling •

These are so-called 'talking' treatments. They are not direct treatments for depression but ways of looking at circumstances in one's life which may be causing depression, or events in the past which may predispose to it, and seeing how to make some helpful changes.

Although psychotherapy and counselling are supposedly different techniques, the distinction is becoming somewhat blurred. Traditionally, counselling is more about crisis management. You go to see a counsellor about a particular problem and work on what you can do to change your situation or alter your approach to it, or on how you can explore and come to terms with something emotionally painful. You might go to counselling for marriage problems or for help in coming to terms with bereavement or infertility. However, many counsellors are trained to work with clients in a more open-ended way too and on problems which are less specific.

Psychotherapy and psychoanalysis go into more depth than traditional counselling. Usually you explore your emotional make-up and emotional past in a more all-encompassing and detailed way. It is less relevant as a solution to a particular problem but may throw light on lots of important aspects of your life and why you are as you are.

It is crucial, whichever you choose, that the practitioner is properly qualified. (See Where to Go for Help, page 200.)

• How to help yourself •

There are many ways that you may be able to challenge your depression or, once the worst is handled by drugs or other means, take some steps to minimise chances of a repeat experience. It can be hard to get yourself going or to believe you can really do anything much to help but the evidence says that you can.

Express your feelings Make a point of letting things go somehow, whether it is by talking to a sympathetic friend, bashing a pillow or crying into it or writing all your feelings down, if there is no one you can or want to tell them to. Don't just think about things that bother you today. Was there something that happened recently or long past that you haven't fully expressed your feelings about? If so, do it, if you can, by one of the means suggested.

Think about what you think   Negative thinking exacerbates depression and keeps it going. Try to catch all those negative thoughts that fly into your head and challenge them (see The Power of Self-talk, page 190). It is very hard to do this when you are depressed and very easy to put it off until tomorrow or next week. But if you really want to help yourself, try to do it now. Aim to write down 40 or 50 negative thoughts. That sounds a lot but it is amazing how quickly you will get there if you are depressed. Look at them and consider whether you would have thought those particular thoughts if you weren't depressed. That might help to give you a different perspective.

Get started   Getting motivated to do anything is very hard when you are depressed. Do something, anything, to go against those negative thoughts which are saying, 'I can't do anything', 'I'm useless'. The littlest things will show you are not: fetching the children from school, getting to work, cleaning the house or whatever. If you get involved and absorbed, your mood will lift at least a little, enough to take another step upward.

Take some exercise   Do something physical, whether it is a brisk walk or cleaning out some cupboards. (Californian research has shown that a ten-minute brisk walk had a more lasting effect on mood than comfort-eating of a chocolate bar.) If you can do something physical, you will have more energy not less and the mental benefits will be more space to think of other ways out of depression.

Forget sleep – or rather, forget to worry about sleep. The more you worry about being awake when others are asleep, the less you are likely to drop off. Read a book, listen to the radio, do a jigsaw, watch television. You are still relaxing, even if not sleeping, and may fall asleep sooner because you are relaxed.

Help someone else   It might seem unthinkable when you are in the throes of depression but doing something, however small, for the benefit of someone other than yourself can be an enormous step forward. Depression is about self-absorption, however involuntary. Helping an elderly person by getting their shopping, helping a harassed mum by minding one child while she fetches another after school or babysitting one evening to enable parents to go out will help them and help you too, research shows. Doing something helpful for others distracts from depression and is good for self-esteem.

Don't get things out of proportion   Be aware that you are suffering depression. That means that you can accept black thoughts with more equanimity because you know they are a symptom of depression, not a permanent accompaniment to your life nor, necessarily, a true representation of things as they are.

Go for sensation   All too often, during depression, nothing feels real or strong. Try to give yourself sensation, just to remember what it is like to feel normally. Have a hot perfumed bath, a cold shower, get someone to give you a massage, exercise until you feel it in every bone, dance to music that used to make you happy, rent a funny video and really let yourself laugh.

Don't block out the good times   It is so easy, when you are depressed, to experience everything as all bad. For example, you may remember easily that you stumbled and scuffed your shoe, but you may block out the fact that you went to the library and found the very gardening book that you had been trying to buy for weeks. Write down the good things that happen every day and look back at them a few days later. It can be a shock to realise that not all is negative when you seem to be experiencing life that way; and it can be a pleasant shock which may be the lift you need to move on.

Don't set unrealistic expectations   Catch yourself when you think negatively, 'I always do this (sort of thing) wrong' or 'I never do that (sort of thing) right'. It isn't helpful or true, most of the time: no one always or never does anything. The more you criticise yourself inappropriately, the more you blame yourself unnecessarily. When you catch yourself feeling guilty or self-critical, examine the facts and don't take the responsibility if, on reflection, you see that it isn't really yours.

Brush aside as many of your 'shoulds' and 'oughts' as you can; that is, the ones that you carry with you because you learned them from parents or peers but you don't really believe them yourself and which you aren't harming anyone by not acting on.

And don't have unrealistically high expectations of others either. You may be feeling insecure but that is no reason why your partner should realise – without an explanation – that you didn't really mean it when you told him to go away and that really you wanted him to give you a big bear hug. We are all responsible for the messages we give out and can't expect others to see through them when we are not being honest about what we feel, for whatever reason.

Do the opposite   Whatever it is, do the opposite of how your depression is pushing you to feel. If you can't sleep, get up. If you feel lethargic, set yourself some physical tasks. If you feel compelled to do everything slowly, compel yourself to run. Running or brisk walking on a regular basis can benefit depression as much as psychotherapy, some studies have found. If you don't care how you look, make yourself get dressed up or buy yourself new flattering clothes.

Make lists   Try listing all sorts of helpful positive things: all the good qualities that you like about yourself; all the achievements you are proud of, dating from however far back; all the most important, memorable and flattering things people have said to you over the years, all the things or activities you have enjoyed, etc. It will help to improve the perspective and to boost the spirit.

Above all, remember that depression can be strengthening. If you have been down and can get yourself back up, that is positive indeed.

• Recurrent brief depression (RBD) •

This is a form of depression very different from that so far described. It was only recognised by the World Health Organisation as recently as 1992. And although it is believed to affect up to 6,000,000 adults in the UK, or 7 per cent of the population, very many doctors are likely to miss it or to mistakenly diagnose it in women as premenstrual syndrome, even though the symptoms are not related to specific times in the menstrual cycle. Also making diagnosis more difficult is the fact that still not all psychiatrists accept its existence.

RBD is a devastating condition which can easily wreck lives. It is depression which lasts only for a few days at a time but during that time the symptoms are as severe as those of conventional deep depression. Normally, doctors are unlikely to diagnose depression unless there have been symptoms for at least two weeks. In RBD the problem for doctors is that by the time patients have made an appointment to see them, the symptoms have usually gone away again.

Sufferers from RBD descend very suddenly into the depths of depression, stay down for about three days at a time and then their depression lifts just as suddenly as it came upon them. They may have over 20 of these short attacks in a year, often two a month, and there are unlikely to be any life-event triggers, such as divorce or redundancy.

Dr Stuart Montgomery, a consultant psychiatrist at St Mary's Hospital in London, who has researched the condition for nearly 20 years and who gave it its name, claims that RBD is classic depression but in small doses. Sufferers become despairing, pessimistic and often aggressive verbally or physically. Alarmingly, the risk of suicidal feelings and actions is even higher among RBD sufferers than those with the usual recognised forms of depression. Carrying on a job may be almost impossible and relationships with family and friends may be severely, if not terminally, strained especially as sufferers usually don't realise that anything is physically the matter with them. It is thought that there is a biological cause.

Unfortunately, none of the existing drugs used to treat depression work in the case of RBD and there may not be a treatment until a new drug is developed especially to prevent or lessen attacks. In the meantime, all that doctors can do is give the condition a name – it does help people to know that there is a reason for why they are behaving so unpredictably so often – and to advise sufferers to try to make whatever lifestyle changes they can, such as to try not to work during attacks or to arrange to do aspects of their jobs least likely to bring them into confrontation with others.

· Postnatal depression ·

There are three forms of postnatal depression. These are:

Baby blues   This is so common that it is hardly even thought of as a depression. It tends to come on a few days after the birth of the baby and is a tendency to become extremely emotional and tearful over nothing very much. It is thought to be the effect of the very sudden and large changes in hormone levels that occur after birth. The condition passes quickly and most mothers accept it as just a brief phase. Knowing it is likely to happen makes it easier not to imbue the tearfulness with any greater significance than it warrants.

Puerperal psychosis   At the other extreme is puerperal psychosis, the most severe form of postnatal depression which probably affects about one in every 500 new mothers. It usually begins a few weeks or a month after the birth and the first symptom is an inability to settle or to sleep. Behaviour may become very strange. The mother may have extreme highs and lows in mood, be manic in her behaviour, suffer delusions of grandeur or have hallucinations. It is very frightening for those close to her, and requires medical help.

The one without a special name   The most common form of postnatal depression is the one which is most often missed. Yet it may affect more than one in six new mothers, and not necessarily always after a first baby. It can come on suddenly or gradually in mild or severe form, usually within four to six months after the birth but at any time in the first year.

There are many possible symptoms, familiar in depression, but no one is likely to suffer them all. They include: difficulty falling asleep or getting back to sleep, even when not disturbed by the baby; feelings of inadequacy as a mother; fear of not loving the baby enough; loss of appetite; excessive anxiety about the baby's health; frightening thoughts about the baby dying or your own death; severe anxiety about everyday things which don't usually bother you; loss of appetite; loss of desire for sex; a change of feelings towards a partner; irritability; tearfulness; hopelessness.

· Causes of postnatal depression ·

Hormonal changes may precipitate postnatal depression and treatment with oestrogens has been found helpful for many who suffer from it severely (see Drugs and Physical Treatments, page 173). More controversial, although some success is claimed by its main proponent Dr Katherina Dalton, is treatment with progesterone, the other main female hormone.

In one in every 100 women with serious postnatal depression, the cause is a disorder in which the body makes antibodies against its own thyroid gland. About 11 per cent of women produce thyroid antibodies and are at especial risk of postnatal depression as well as thyroid-gland damage. Treatment of antibody-positive women with the thyroid hormone thyroxine after they have given birth may prevent development of depression.

There are many psychological factors which may help explain why new mothers so often experience depression. Becoming a mother can be an enormous shock, however much wanted and anticipated the baby is. Suddenly you are responsible for another life. You have to learn how to look after the baby, how to read its signals, you worry about it, think about it, are often consumed by its needs. You may worry that you are not loving enough or expect that you should be able to give fully and freely all that is demanded of you, without getting frustrated, upset and exhausted – a human impossibility.

Commonly, you do not have much time for yourself any more, or at least at the beginning. You may feel trapped at home. Some women physically feel trapped, if they are isolated or have other young children and cannot get out easily. Many women feel they have lost their identity, particularly if they were used to working full time in stimulating careers . They may feel society views them differently and definitely doesn't accord them the same status as before.

Our past experiences may also be a deciding factor in who does or who doesn't develop postnatal depression. As in any other kind of depression, personality and our own experiences of childhood may play a role but having a baby can bring up unresolved feelings connected with parents particularly strongly.

• Getting help •

Research shows that the chance to talk through feelings with, for example, a health visitor trained in counselling techniques, can make all the difference. Quite a lot of GP surgeries now employ counsellors to give sessions to any patients who might benefit. It also helps to be in touch with other mothers.

You may find a group locally or you can get in touch with MAMA (Meet-a-Mum Association) to be put in contact with a local group. If possible, MAMA will try to put a mother who is depressed in touch with another mother who has herself been through postnatal depression, and who has successfully come out the other side. Another useful organisation that can offer advice is the Association for Postnatal Illness. See Useful Contacts, and please send an SAE when writing to either.

• Seasonal affective disorder (SAD) •

This is a depression which occurs in autumn and winter, when there is less natural light around. It is thought that over 10 per cent of the population is affected to some extent by the darker wintry days, and in 5 per cent the depression is severe enough to warrant treatment. Women are three times more likely to suffer than men and symptoms usually first start in the twenties or thirties, although it is not unknown for SAD to occur in some children, teenagers and older people.

• Symptoms •

Classic symptoms are depression, sleep problems (usually a desire to sleep excessively), lethargy, loss of interest in social life or sex, extreme mood swings, irritability and a tendency to overeat, usually with a strong craving for carbohydrates. Symptoms come on any time between the middle of September and the middle of November and tend to disappear some time between February and mid-April.

• Possible causes •

Doctors now know that SAD isn't just a case of feeling blue once the sunny days of summer have gone. In true SAD, the body's natural balance is disturbed and many systems are affected. It is thought to have a biochemical basis, although the exact cause is as yet uncertain.

The first school of thought was that excessive production of the hormone melatonin, which in animals notably occurs in the hours of darkness and promotes sleepiness amongst other things, was to blame. Bright light entering the eye brings melatonin production to a stop. But there is no evidence of such an effect in humans: there don't appear to be any abnormalities in melatonin secretion in SAD sufferers and drugs to prevent melatonin from being produced do not help in SAD.

Another possibility is faulty circadian rhythms or body clock. Receiving most attention currently, however, is a theory that the hormone serotonin is affected by the seasons, more markedly in some than others.

• Treatments •

SSRIs, antidepressants which work to increase availability of serotonin (see Drugs and Physical Treatments, page 173), can often be effective.

The most favoured treatment is with natural light from special light boxes. Four out of five people who receive this treatment are helped. You have to sit a few feet in front of a lightbox for a few hours each day, during which time you can carry out sedentary activities such as writing, reading or watching television. Very many users claim they start to feel better in a couple of days if they follow the procedure fully. Some people suffer a headache or eyestrain, but this might be expected if walking or sitting for a long time in bright sunlight too.

Experiments are still going on to find the best equipment to use and the best methods. Both full spectrum and standard fluorescent bulbs appear to be effective, the latter being stronger and therefore enabling treatment sessions to be shorter. The equipment must be custom-designed, however. Standard sunlamps used for skin conditions and sunbeds are not effective and could be dangerous to the eyes.

Several hospitals in the UK now provide treatment for SAD on the NHS. The SAD Association, a support group which keeps up to date on all the research, can provide information on how to get help, where to buy lightboxes (likely to cost over £100) and will also hire out lightboxes for a small weekly fee for people to try at home. Send an SAE to SADA: see Useful Contacts, and also Further Reading

As SAD is a form of depression, self-help methods recommended for helping in general depression are often also advised, in conjunction with light treatment.

23

EATING DISORDERS

THE EATING disorders anorexia nervosa and bulimia nervosa (more commonly referred to as anorexia and bulimia) are not only suffered by women. However, there are 10 women sufferers for every one man, which is not surprising when women suffer so much pressure to be slim. Images in the media so heavily promote slim women as beautiful that women themselves have come to value slimness and to imagine that slimness in women is also highly valued by men. But of course this isn't the whole story. Both anorexia and bulimia are complicated conditions with no easy explanations nor, unfortunately, any easy solutions.

• Anorexia nervosa •

The symptoms of this tragic and often fatal illness are an extreme fear of getting fat, eating very little and losing excessive amounts of weight. Commonly, sufferers exercise obsessively too, as a means to keep weight down. As weight falls below a healthy level, monthly periods cease.

• Who gets it? •

Usually anorexia starts half-way through the teens, with one in every 150 15-year-old girls likely to be affected. Sometimes, however, it begins in childhood or doesn't develop until the twenties or thirties. Usually it is girls from middle-class backgrounds who suffer and it is very common for someone else in the family to have had similar problems.

Anorexia usually stems from a desire to diet; a third of sufferers are overweight before they begin trying to lose weight. However, once weight loss starts to be achieved, the anorexic becomes obsessed with the desire to lose more and more, until she is well below a healthy weight for her body. However, she does not see herself that way: she sees herself as still fat, even when she is clearly emaciated.

It may not always be obvious at the start that someone is developing anorexia nervosa. A girl or young woman may just seem keen to eat healthily and eat a lot of fruits and vegetables or salads. Also, she is not necessarily repelled by food and may delight in buying food or cooking it for other people.

Although the word anorexia means loss of appetite, sufferers do not lose their appetite at all: they deliberately curb their eating for the sense of control this gives them. Often, when they can control themselves no more, they may have a binge on many foods and then desperately try to vomit or use laxatives in a bid to undo the (calorific) damage. Many anorexics may also use slimming pills as a regular aid to weight loss.

• Physical consequences of anorexia •

As a young woman loses more weight than is right for her body, the functioning of her body systems starts to suffer. Periods stop. Her metabolism reacts as if she were starving (which of course she is) and slows down. She feels extremely cold, particularly in her hands and feet as her circulation becomes sluggish; but, if she suddenly has a binge, she may feel briefly hot and feverish because of the sharp surge in her metabolism. Usually she is constipated.

If she is repeatedly making herself vomit, the chemistry of the body is also affected (see Consequences of Bulimia, page 186). If she continues to starve herself, her muscles will weaken, she will be unable to sleep or to concentrate properly when awake and will probably be depressed.

Another serious consequence is brittle bones. One study has found that women who had been anorexic four years previously for just nine months had the backbones expected of a 70-year-old. Anorexics can lose up to 15 per cent of their bone in a year, ten times the speed at which bone is lost from post-menopausal women who lose 1 to 2 per cent of bone per year and who are the ones most usually considered at risk of osteoporosis.

The study, which was carried out at the Royal Edinburgh Hospital by consultant psychiatrist Dr Chris Freeman and colleagues, found that even when the women had gained weight and resumed periods, their bones stayed fragile or even continued to thin. Their bone density rose only by 1 to 2 per cent a year.

Anorexia is notoriously difficult to treat. The condition may become chronic, lasting ten years or more, or end in death through metabolic disorder or suicide.

• Causes •

Anorexia is a very complex condition and it is unhelpful to be simplistic about its causes. It probably arises from an intermeshing of many factors rather than any single one. Those which may be involved include:

A desire to be slim To fit the perceived ideals of our culture.

A way to feel control Weight loss may be the only thing teenage girls can feel full control over during a turbulent time in their lives.

Mixed feelings about sexuality Anorexia leads to a lack of curved female form as well as loss of periods, or failure to start them. It may therefore serve as a way of pushing away the frightening prospect of womanhood. It may be a way of dealing with confusion about sexuality perhaps learned from within the family, either where any talk of sex and relationships is avoided or where it is too overt. Sometimes, but only sometimes, sexual abuse is at the root of anorexia.

Mixed messages about food   These are also often learned through the family. Every child quickly learns that eating or not eating has an impact upon the giver of food and brings attention. In a family where something is awry, not eating may be the only way an unhappy adolescent feels she can have any influence over her family and express her unhappiness or need for feelings to be taken into account.

Difficult life events   One recent study found that in 80 per cent of cases some severely troubling event or difficulty had occurred in the year before onset. Certainly it is known in a number of cases that anorexia has related back to unexpressed grief over the loss of a parent or another close person. However, it is also not uncommon for the trigger event to have been an apparently positive one (such as marriage) or a milestone (such as leaving home), about which the sufferer had confused feelings.

• Finding help •

Usually it is family or friends who have to persuade a sufferer from anorexia to seek help, as commonly the sufferer doesn't perceive she has a problem. Even if she does accept something is the matter and would welcome help, the power of the illness is very strong: she may find herself sabotaging efforts to help her.

There are, however, many psychiatrists and psychologists who are very experienced in dealing with anorexia nervosa and very sympathetic to anyone who suffers from the condition. There are, also, a number of hospitals which have a specialist eating disorders unit, some of which will take referrals from outside their area, but all are likely to have waiting lists and are not an option in emergencies. If possible, anorexia is treated on an out-patient or day-care basis. In-patient care is restricted to an emergency when someone refuses food to such a degree that their life is in danger.

The usual, more enlightened, approach to this condition is to try to come to an understanding, as far as possible, of what lies behind it and what circumstances or feelings perpetuate the 'need' for it. Counselling or psychotherapy, either as part of hospital treatment or separately and more long term, are very important. Also, of course, a sufferer needs help to accept the amount of food he or she needs to eat in order to return to a normal weight and maintain it, and to prevent excessive fear of weight gain. All this is very difficult and needs to be extremely sensitively handled.

A very helpful organisation is the Eating Disorders Association which offers advice to sufferers and families about the condition and how to find help. It also recommends reading materials and runs a network of self-help groups. See Useful Contacts, and enclose an SAE if writing.

• Bulimia nervosa •

It is enormously difficult to quantify the prevalence of bulimia because so many women who suffer never reveal the fact and, as they are not emaciated or even underweight, no one else may recognise what is happening. One estimate is that three out of every 100 women will suffer it at some time. It is generally accepted, however, that bulimia is far far more common than any experts have ever realised, or had evidence for, however familiar the problem may long have been to women.

• Symptoms •

Women with bulimia are terrified of being fat but choose to try and maintain a normal weight by bingeing and then vomiting. For a diagnosis of bulimia, this will occur at least twice a week for months. In extreme cases women may consume more than 15,000 calories in an hour and may binge and vomit up to 30 times in a day. They commonly use laxatives, often to marked excess, in the mistaken belief that using laxatives after a binge will prevent food absorption. (Laxative use removes fluid from the colon but does little to prevent absorption.) There is often some small fluctuating weight gain of about 3 to 4.5kg (8 to 10lb).

The binges are usually secret, pre-planned and are commonly followed by guilt, depression and even suicidal behaviour. There is an enormous disruption of leisure activities and relationships, as the need to eat and then vomit is constantly on sufferers' minds, taking precedence over any normal social life.

• Who gets it? •

Women who develop bulimia tend to be older than those who develop anorexia. Most usually they are in their twenties, have commonly been overweight as children and are very concerned about their weight as adults. Very often they are extremely successful women and appear to be happy and confident but beneath this competent exterior lies low self-esteem and distress about being so controlled by food. Unlike anorexics, sufferers from bulimia know they have a problem but often feel too guilty or ashamed to tell anyone, let alone seek help. They are likely to be very concerned about their appearance and also to be perfectionist about their performance in other areas of their life, such as work.

Often they start out just trying to diet, using the extreme method of trying not to eat in the day and then just having a few hundred calories in the evening. But by evening they succumb to a binge. Eighty per cent of women with bulimia are on a diet when symptoms begin. For some not well understood reason, bulimia (and anorexia) is more common than expected amongst diabetic women. Bulimia may be preceded by anorexia nervosa or by alcohol problems in some cases.

• Causes •

As with anorexia, social pressure, conflicting messages about food and a need to experience control over some aspect of one's life may be precipitating factors. Commonly, women have marked depressive symptoms, which it is thought may be an underlying cause, and depression may run in their families. When depressed, eating is very often used as a form of comfort and, for many sufferers, binges may develop as a result of episodes of eating to cope with unhappiness.

It has also been suggested that premenstrual cravings for carbohydrate may be a trigger for periodic excessive eating which then starts to occur at other times throughout the month.

In bulimia, there is a particularly high likelihood of the sufferer experiencing stressful life events concerning relationships with family or friends before symptoms started and there is also a strong connection with a traumatic childhood, according to recent research.

• Consequences of bulimia •

Apart from the depression, guilt and inability to have a normal lifestyle, there are many physical consequences. The woman who vomits repeatedly risks stomach acid dissolving the enamel on her teeth. Salivary glands swell, giving the face a puffy appearance. There may be calluses on the back of the hand caused by continual abrasion of the skin against the teeth during induced vomiting (although many experienced bulimics can induce vomiting just by thinking about it or pressing a hand lightly on their stomachs). Other signs may include swollen ankles and fingers, breast tenderness, and menstrual disorders.

It now appears that three out of four sufferers from bulimia have polycystic ovarian syndrome (see page 249), though it is unclear whether the syndrome predisposes to the bulimia, or bulimia followed by starving results in the polycystic ovaries.

The most severe effects include muscle weakness, damage to the kidneys, stomach ulceration and even epileptic fits. Over-use of laxatives can lead to severe bowel problems as well as stomach pain and sometimes removal of part of the bowel becomes necessary.

Women who carry on episodes of bulimia while pregnant seem to be at higher risk of giving birth to babies with abnormalities such as cleft palate and cleft lip. They are also more likely to have multiple births and obstetric complications. Diabetics who are bulimic are at higher risk of complications from the diabetes.

• Finding help •

Psychiatrists and psychologists who specialise in eating disorders are interested in bulimia as well as anorexia. The main emphasis of treatment is both to help a woman understand what leads her to binge and vomit and to deal with these issues in some more direct way; and to help her re-establish a more normal eating pattern by keeping an eating diary and changing the way she thinks about food.

Most bulimics who have binged for a long time have forgotten what normal body signals of hunger feel like. The aim is for three balanced meals a day and to learn self-control instead of bingeing. Very often, for example, a woman who eats one chocolate when she is supposed to be on a diet takes this as a sign of failure and decides she might as well binge. Changed thinking patterns, such as recognition that one chocolate is really neither here nor there, can help develop self control.

Antidepressants are also sometimes of value, the most effective being fluoxetine, from the group of antidepressants called SSRIs (see page 173). However, effects are only short term and so their use is viewed as less valuable than intensive psychological treatments but worth trying if these have failed and a woman does have symptoms of depression.

Useful self-help measures include deliberately planning activities so as to be busy at times when at highest risk of bingeing (such as evenings), avoiding excessive food shopping and having too much food at home, planning and sticking to three meals a day, enlisting support from a friend, no weighing and no laxatives.

These kinds of measures are more likely to work if a woman is receiving some other sort of help or support at the same time. A ten-year follow-up study at the Royal Free Hospital in London of 49 women with bulimia found that those who had a supportive partner were the most likely to make a full recovery.

Reassurance that eating normally does not lead to overweight may be helpful in preventing lapses into dieting, which in turn may lead to lapses into bulimia.

The Eating Disorders Association can offer advice and support: see Useful Contacts.

24

PSYCHOSOMATIC ILLNESS AND HYSTERIA

PSYCHOMATIC disorders are illnesses in which the physical symptoms are thought to have psychological origins, either in total or in part. This doesn't mean that psychosomatic illnesses are any less genuine than any others, although many people are under the mistaken impression that psychosomatic means that they are imagining it. Far from it. In fact, it has been estimated that 90 to 100 per cent of illnesses are psychosomatic.

Most of the serious diseases of the modern day can be included in this category: for example heart disease, cancer, stomach ulcers, asthma, high blood pressure and many skin diseases. The psychological factor might be stress (which adversely affects much normal body functioning), withholding of emotions (which then break out physically, such as in skin eruptions) or a mental disorder such as depression which not only depresses the person but appears to depress the immune system as well.

Most illnesses with a psychosomatic component also have clear physical risk factors. For example, it appears that people who are habitually hostile and self-centred are more prone to heart attacks than others, but eating a fatty diet, smoking and not doing exercise will play a fair part in deciding which self-centred people are more likely to succumb.

While psychosomatic disorders are indeed physical illnesses requiring, usually, physical treatments of the appropriate kind, an understanding of the psychological factors behind the illness and a resultant change of lifestyle are also essential, in order to reduce the likelihood of recurrence.

• Hysteria •

This is included not because it is common but because it is commonly a wrongly used term, levelled at women. Many women may have had the unpleasant experience of being dismissed by a doctor as 'just an hysterical woman' and wish to know what, in fact, this expression means.

The word hysteria comes from *hystera*, the ancient Greek word for womb, because the condition was once thought to be associated with the womb, though goodness knows why. Used colloquially, it tends to mean over-the-top histrionic behaviour such as screaming, waving the arms about, fainting and generally causing a commotion for trivial causes.

However, this isn't what psychiatrists mean if they use the term, and in fact many avoid it, as there is some controversy even among themselves as to what it means.

Someone may be diagnosed as suffering from hysteria if they have physical symptoms for which no organic cause can be found. The most usual hysterical symptoms are paralysis of an arm or leg, loss of memory and even temporary blindness. The development of a multiple personality is also an hysterical symptom.

Whatever the symptom, though, it is caused by a (perhaps unconscious) psychological conflict over a certain circumstance. Although the symptom is not produced knowingly, it obviously must have some advantage to it, in order to have been produced as a 'solution' to the conflict at all. Perhaps the internal conflict is so great that the symptom, however unpleasant, is preferable to the stress caused by the conflict. It may reverse of its own accord if the circumstance precipitating it passes. If not, psychotherapy is the treatment most likely to help.

However, hysterical symptoms in isolation are rare and are more likely to be associated with another mental illness. Also, psychiatrists would be reluctant to settle too quickly on hysteria as a diagnosis, in case there really was some underlying physical disorder which has so far gone undetected.

Some doctors believe that there is no such thing as hysteria, but just malingering: that is, deliberate manifestation of such symptoms for certain gains, such as avoidance of work. Although malingering does of course occur, this isn't a terribly helpful approach.

25

HANDLING THOUGHTS FEELINGS AND NEEDS

WE CAN do a lot to safeguard our own happiness and mental health by making simple changes to many of the unconscious ways we behave in our daily lives. The way we handle our feelings, think about ourselves and our lives and take care of our needs, for example, are all very bound up with the experience of anxiety and depression. Learning to think more positively, to experience our emotions more fully, to stand up for our needs and rights and to value ourselves for the good that is in us can dramatically improve our own quality of life, and that of those who share it with us.

• The power of self-talk •

We all have silent commentaries running through our heads the whole time we are awake, and most of the time we aren't really conscious of their content. People who tend to be anxious, worry a lot or to suffer from depression undoubtedly have many negative, although usually unconscious, statements in their self-talk. This could include things like,

- 'What if I don't get done in time?'
- 'I'm sure to be the only one who isn't dressed right for the occasion'
- 'It's all my fault'
- 'They'll blame me even if it isn't my fault'
- 'What if they don't ask me back to dinner again?'
- 'I'm no good at small talk'
- 'Everyone will see how nervous I am'
- 'I can't do it'
- 'I'll never get through'
- 'I shouldn't have said I'd give that talk',
- 'She's so much better dressed/looking/qualified/ than me', etc.

Thoughts are powerful. They affect not only the way we feel about ourselves and our mental health but our physical health as well, as they appear to alter the chemical signals the brain sends to various parts of the body, including the immune system. Positive thoughts benefit us, negative ones bring us down. Fortunately, there are some well-tested techniques for exchanging a predominantly negative attitude for a positive one so, if you think excessive negative self-talk could be a problem, you might like to try the suggestions below.

Identify negative thoughts The first step towards disempowering negative thoughts is to identify what they are. For a week, try to make a point of tuning in, when you can, to the stuff that runs through your mind. Carry a pen and pad and note down every negative thought you have. (Be aware of abbreviated negative thinking too. For example, you might think 'here we go' when what you mean is 'I can feel myself getting panicky and I'm terrified that, the minute it is my turn to answer, I'm going to blush terribly or shake and someone is going to notice.') When you add the negative thoughts up at the end of the day, you might be quite surprised by how many there are – and that's only the ones you managed to catch yourself thinking.

Try making it positive To start with, it is hard to even catch the negative thoughts but once you have got them, you can start to get them under control. As soon as one of them slips into mind, make the conscious effort to rephrase it in a positive but believable way.

For example, instead of 'I'll never be good enough,' say silently, 'I'm doing my best'. 'I can't cope'; 'I am coping. I'll just take it step by step.' 'They'll say it's my fault, I suppose'; 'It isn't my fault and I don't see why anyone should think it is. If they do, I shall explain quite clearly what actually happened.'

Question unrealistic assumptions A lot of negative commentary isn't founded on fact at all. The power and frequency of it can be quite significantly reduced if we call particular statements into question. For example, 'I daren't go out to the theatre with them because the pain in my injured leg will probably be bad and it will be embarrassing and miserable,' could be questioned with 'Why should it be bad? It will actually probably be worse if I stay at home thinking about it. Seeing the play will take my mind off things.'

Shy away from 'shoulds' Should isn't a negative word but it might as well be. Should is largely about critical self-judgments; it's about events or qualities which aren't but ought to be – or so we think: 'I should be cleverer.' 'I should be quicker.' 'I should be thinner.' 'I should be able to run my family and my job.' 'I shouldn't lose my temper.' 'I should listen to my mother more often.'

Not all shoulds are bad, of course. We should take care when we cross the road, we should respect other people's rights. But many smack more of rules laid down for us by others – parents, partners, the media – and they don't fit with what we really feel we want to do.

Take a look at your shoulds. Where did they come from? Are they beliefs you genuinely hold or are they beliefs passed on to you by parents or held by peers?

If you think you should have a job befitting your qualifications as a solicitor, for example, is that because you genuinely don't want to settle for anything less (fine) or because really you would like to move to the country and learn to be a potter but assume that wouldn't be right? If you are only hurting yourself with your shoulds and are genuinely not hurting anyone else without them (don't count upsetting mother's ideas of what is best for you: count whether the children will suffer); try to allow yourself to make a few choices instead of settling for what you imagine to be your duty or what others expect of you.

Don't jump to conclusions   It is very easy, when you are in a negative or victimised frame of mind, to jump to conclusions from a single event. 'He didn't ring back. I'll never be attractive to men.' 'I can't do this essay. I'll never get my degree.' 'The boss criticised me. Everyone is going to think I am a fool.' If you catch yourself doing this, try the 'challenging yourself for evidence' technique.

Don't make events into catastrophes   Try to avoid making things worse than they are. If, for example, you lose your job don't instantly go into the frame of mind of thinking you will never find another one. Often, however, people make catastrophes out of events that may not even be negative at all. 'The boss didn't smile at me when he passed me. He is going to fire me today.' 'My husband didn't ring me when he said he would. He's found another woman.' Again, challenge the evidence.

Sometimes people catastrophise about future events. 'It will be absolutely unbearable if I go to the wedding and have a panic attack in front of everyone.' One way to deal with this sort of thinking is to give it credence and examine it. Would it be so unbearable to have a panic attack? Wouldn't there be somewhere you could slip away to?

By avoiding using words or expressions such as 'the worst possible thing', 'insupportable', 'terrible', etc, you can think about things in a much better perspective.

Accept compliments   How do you respond if someone says they like your dress? Do you say, 'What, this old thing?' or 'I don't really think it's my colour, actually' or 'Oh, it only came from that bargain shop down the road'? Or do you say, 'Thank you, I enjoy wearing it' or 'Thank you, I like it too'?

Don't be self-absorbed   Being anxious to make a good impression or not feeling confident can lead someone to dwell on herself in an unconstructive way. For example, in any new situation where others are present, she is likely to be thinking 'Does he think I'm intelligent enough? I hope my jacket isn't dirty. Is she noticing that the muscle in my eye is twitching? Will they laugh if I tell my joke? Will they think I'm rude if I go over to the buffet and get a plate? Will they think better of me if I just nod appreciatively or if I make comments?' Usually the worry is about not coming up to scratch. Unfortunately, this kind of self-absorption prevents you from being present in the moment, whatever it is, and really giving it your attention and interest.

Go for greys   Black and white thinking tends to be uncreative and cuts off opportunities. For example, 'If I can't get this right this time, I might as well pack the whole thing in'. Better to think, 'If I still can't do it after this go, I'd better give myself a break and then come back to it/ask for help/ see if there is another way of tackling it altogether.' Labelling is another form of black and white thinking. If you think of yourself as always a failure or clumsy or unattractive or irresponsible, it is difficult to get out of that set. Don't consider yourself as 'always' anything negative: judge each circumstance by its merits or demerits and be realistic in your reasoning about your own role in it.

Don't take the blame   We very often volunteer for the blame for things when they are not our fault. Or we unconsciously blame ourselves without voicing it. 'It didn't work because I'm stupid.' 'I'm so sorry. If I hadn't called hello and waved, you wouldn't have looked across the street and then you wouldn't have walked into that lamp post.'

• Expressing feelings •

Feelings are not always what they appear to be. Unconscious suppression of feelings we might not be comfortable with, for example anger or intense grief, may lead them to emerge in a more familiar form, such as anxiety and depression, which we then assume to be what we are feeling. We imagine that we are prone to free-floating anxiety or depression that comes out of the blue, when in fact there might be a very specific but masked cause.

It can be frightening to let go of intense feelings, whether excitement, anger or pain, and often we hold the feeling in unconsciously by tensing some part of our bodies such as the neck, shoulders or stomach. Another possible way that uncomfortable feelings emerge indirectly is through bodily symptoms such as an irritable bowel or a migraine.

It is never healthy, emotionally or physically, to push down and suppress feelings. The important thing is to find a safe way to express them. So when you feel particularly tense, anxious or depressed, for no clear reason, try to think about what is going on in your life and whether there is anything that you could unconsciously be trying to damp down. It may be that you are angry with a partner, or you could be angry with yourself for not taking a good opportunity to do something.

Of course, the problem may not be that you don't know what you are feeling but that you don't know how to deal with it. If your partner is threatening to leave you and you are frightened about how you will cope, he may not be the best person to express such feelings to. Better to talk over your strong feelings of fear with a trusted friend or a supportive third party, and then you can clear some space in your mind for tackling the actual issues with your partner. Does he really plan to leave? Is he prepared to make another go of it? What could you each do to improve things?

• Feel what you are saying •

Expressing feelings, whether to a friend or to the person you have the feelings about, needs to be done from the heart. Just saying you feel angry or sad in a neutral or dead voice doesn't communicate the real feeling and doesn't fully express it in the literal sense of getting it out of yourself. You need to feel safe because you will have to experience your anger or your grief as you talk, and that will cause discomfort or pain. Try to stick with feelings. Don't analyse what you are saying or blame yourself or make any kind of judgments. Feelings are irrational. Get them out of the way first and then look at facts or practicalities.

Use feeling words. Saying 'You are mean and horrid to me,' is an accusation. Saying 'I feel really hurt that you didn't phone me when you promised you would' expresses a feeling.

• Be positive •

Anger is often experienced as a dangerous emotion. It can be expressed destructively, in a way that hurts yourself and others, or constructively. If you have had a difficult day at work and it was all topped off by waiting an hour for a bus and then having to get off it in the pouring rain, you could vent your feelings safely by getting stuck into something physical, such as scrubbing walls, doing some energetic exercise or beating your fists into a pillow. If you are angry with someone about something you consider they have done to you, you need to find a way to express your view that doesn't mean things degenerate into a shouting match. (See Being Assertive, below.)

• Write it down •

If it is impractical to talk to someone else about whatever you are feeling – your best friend is away, or it is 3am and it seems unreasonable to phone – try writing down what you are feeling, for your eyes only. Use feeling words. Relive and express the feelings through the power of the words you choose.

If you think of yourself as someone who tends to get stuck with feelings, you might try keeping a feeling diary, which you write in whenever you feel the urge. It can be very useful to delve back into the past to any trauma that you know you didn't really talk about or experience fully at the time – perhaps the death of someone close or the loss of an important relationship – and get those feelings down on paper. Releasing the words and feelings can release you from them too and free you to move on.

• Being assertive •

If you tend to

- always put others before yourself
- say yes when you would like to say no
- be nervous about offending anyone at any time
- be anxious that no one should ever think critically of you

assertiveness training could benefit you greatly. There are many courses available through evening institutes as well as self-help books: see Further Reading.

The word assertiveness is often misunderstood to mean aggressiveness. In fact it is far from it. Assertiveness means respecting yourself enough to say what you want and feel while respecting others enough not to do it at their expense. An assertive request or response does not leave anyone feeling bad or that their dignity has been taken from them. Being assertive means being able to accept that everyone has rights and responsibilities.

Women traditionally have been less forward about expressing their needs than men. We are less likely to refuse requests because we are taught to put others' needs before our own. But that doesn't mean that we give in gladly. When we agree to do a favour that will inconvenience us enormously, we probably experience resentment and bad feeling. Sometimes this stays below the surface; sometimes not.

Imagine agreeing that two friends of relatives of yours in Australia can stay at your home for a week while travelling through London. In fact you haven't the space, you work from home and are trying to meet a deadline, so could do without extra demands, let alone the noise and distraction in the day-time. You find you don't even like these people very much, when they do turn up, and they seem to take you for granted; of course you are smiling as you offer to cook them breakfast, lunch and tea and tell them it is no problem. Maybe you will get through the week without losing your cool. But just as likely you will go over your tolerance threshold and have a screaming row with your guests, accusing them of all sorts of ingratitude and requiring they pack their bags and leave at once. And they are genuinely startled and hurt, because you had given no indication whatsoever that you were not happy with their behaviour. This is an example where saying no at the outset, for good reason, would be fairer than saying yes.

Being assertive is not easy, of course. And there may well be occasions when following your own feelings would not be appropriate: for example, when being taken out for a special meal by a friend and finding your meal

---

AN EXAMPLE OF ASSERTIVENESS

Suppose someone was in the process of parking their car across your driveway so that you could not drive your own car out. The aggressive response would be to run outside and yell abuse at the driver, demanding he or she move at once. The passive response would be to stay inside and seethe in silence.

The assertive response would be to go outside and say, 'I realise it is difficult to find parking around here. However, you have parked across my drive and I need to go out very shortly. Please would you park elsewhere?' Whereas being aggressive hurts other people and being passive makes you feel bad, assertive behaviour leaves everyone able to feel OK. Should your assertiveness be met with an abusive response, you can at least feel respect for yourself because you said what you wanted to say in a manner you felt good about.

unsatisfactory, but thinking the occasion would be spoilt for your friend if you called the waiter and complained, however politely. Once you are able to be assertive you also have the choice about whether you want to be assertive in a particular situation or not. There are probably times when you are only too happy to leave all the decisions to someone else or when you just need to blow your top, but you have to be prepared to accept the consequences and not agonise over it all for ages afterwards.

• Assertiveness techniques •

When you are assertive you don't make excuses for other people or yourself. You are clear about your position and take responsibility for communicating your needs but you also acknowledge the other person's. It is helpful to think in terms of three basic points.

Acknowledge the other person's position or point of view This is not the same as agreeing with it, just confirmation that you have understood where they stand or why they have acted in some way. For example, if your child minder is consistently late arriving, delaying your departure for work: 'I know you have a difficult journey to get here.'

Say how you think or feel Make a clear statement without apologies or preamble. 'However, it is crucial for me to leave here at 8am so that I can fulfil my own obligations.' Using the word 'however' is preferable to 'but' because it gives the impression of taking you on from your previous statement whereas 'but' just seems to negate the previous statement.

Say what you would like to happen next or in the future Always use the word 'I' to start this statement, whether it is 'I would like', 'I would appreciate', 'I want'. For example: 'I would like to be able to rely on you to be here on time.'

This kind of three-part statement makes your own position clear but doesn't have to put the other person on the defensive. There is room for negotiation or discussion of preferable arrangements without bad feeling.

There are many other specific techniques for specific situations. Here are a few which may be of most use.

• The broken record technique •

This means repeating a key part of the message you are trying to convey so that the person you are talking to realises there is no room for negotiation or argument. For example, a friend who is rather disorganised rings you yet again at the last minute, begging you to babysit tonight so that she can attend an evening meeting she has forgotten with a prospective client. You have tickets to see a play. Using the broken record technique would mean saying something like: 'I realise you are really in a spot and I would like to be able to help you. However, I have made arrangements for tonight that I cannot break. I'll try and think of someone else who could help, as I cannot break my arrangements. Or, if you could re-schedule your meeting and give me notice, I'll be happy to help out another time, as I cannot help you tonight.'

• Say no •

Saying no assertively is not about being unco-operative or selfish, it is about standing up for your own rights not to be used or taken advantage of. No one has to feel guilty about saying no to a request if they have a good reason for declining. Once you can accept you have the right to say no, you don't have to invent elaborate excuses for turning someone down. You can be straightforward and honest. For example, suppose you have just started working for yourself from home. Friends who are free in the day now seem to assume that they can drop in on you at any time, as you will be glad of a visit. Sometimes you are glad and sometimes you aren't, depending on how much work you have to do. If the doorbell rings at the wrong time, rather than invite the caller in with a false welcoming smile (while gritting your teeth and worrying about your workload) or appearing at the door wearing your coat pretending you were on your way out, the assertive response would be: 'I think it is really nice that you have called by and I would love to be able to say come in for a chat. However, at the minute I am up to my eyes in work and I just can't stop for anything. Another time, it would be lovely to see you.'

• Fogging •

This is a useful little ploy for preventing a criticism made of you from escalating into an argument. It involves agreeing to part of the criticism so that there is nothing further to say. Imagine, for example, your partner wants you to grow your hair long like it used to be when you met, while you don't want that image any more, 15 years on. It is a constant battle. When your partner says, 'Why don't you grow your hair long? Your friend Marilyn has long hair and it really suits her,' the fogging response could be, 'Yes, it does really suit her'.

• Don't say sorry •

This is different from not apologising when apologies are really due. We tend to say sorry when we aren't or when we needn't be, such as if someone treads on our foot. Because it is such an over-used and abused word, it has something of the feel of a victim about it. If you really are sorry, say 'I apologise for. . .', 'I hope you can excuse me for. . ', etc.

• Self-esteem •

Self-esteem is self-value. It, or its lack, underpins the whole way we live our lives. If we can accept ourselves and our talents, trust and respect ourselves, believe our opinions are worth listening to and our company worth having, the result is self confidence and, probably, inner happiness.

If we don't trust our judgment, don't like our own company, don't value our abilities, thoughts and feelings and are constantly looking for reassurance or approval from others, we probably experience a considerable degree of anxiety and depression in our lives. Usually it is hard to make close friendships or form satisfying, intimate relationships when self-esteem is low because how can you believe someone likes or loves you if you don't think you are likeable or lovable yourself. Groucho Marx's famous quip, that he wouldn't want to belong to any club that would have him as a member, is a classic example of low self-esteem talking.

People aren't born with low self-esteem. It can develop as a result of our upbringing. Having parents who were never quite satisfied with what you achieved as a child can contribute to low self-esteem and excessive self-criticism. But it isn't just negative attitudes from parents, such as neglect or abuse, that can have detrimental effects. Parental over-protectiveness and over-indulgence, done with the best of intentions, can significantly affect the way a child feels about him or herself while growing up. The over-protected child may not learn independence, not dare to take risks or trust her judgment. The over-indulged child may expect too much and not learn a sense of responsibility for himself which can result in lack of effort, failure and broken dreams. By contrast, those lucky enough to come from a home where there was much love, encouragement and acceptance of who they were as emerging people are likely to have a high self-esteem and sense of security.

Parents, of course, are usually trying to do their best but don't realise how sometimes their best efforts may work against the best interests of their child's developing sense of self. Sometimes, it is just the nature of families that someone's sense of self suffers. For example, very many eldest children never quite recover from what they experienced as catastrophic displacement by a new baby, however much harassed parents may have tried to compensate.

Fortunately poor self-esteem isn't set in stone. Just because someone has had difficulty valuing themselves fully in the past does not mean things cannot dramatically be changed in the present.

• Ways to improve poor self esteem •

1 Actively start to accept yourself. Write down all the things you do like about yourself. This might seem hard at first but there are probably plenty. Maybe you are nice to animals and old ladies, you like the colour of your eyes, you are good at listening to children, you always keep your word, etc. Try to make this list as long as possible and give yourself a few surprises.

2 Stop criticising what you are. Instead, look specifically at what it is you do that you don't like. First, write down the things you think you don't like about yourself. Easy! Now try to challenge them. Are they things you could do something about? Are they sweeping generalisations? Are they someone else's opinion rather than your own? For example, if you think

your clothes don't look good, instead of dismissing yourself as a hopeless wreck, say to yourself, 'I'm not very good at putting accessories together,' or whatever, and give yourself something specific to aim to change. Or if you have written down, 'my legs are too short', who told you that? Perhaps a former and now unloved lover?

3 Please yourself. Other people's opinions shouldn't be crucial to what you do or think about yourself. Self-esteem comes from within, not from others' acceptance of you. Try to start making up your own mind about how you want to be, what you think about certain issues, what pleases and annoys you, what decisions you would like to take: and trust your own judgment. Of course, it is good to have the good opinion of those we trust and respect but even the minds of friends don't always have to be in accord. Never mind what others think if you truly feel good about something yourself.

4 Nurture yourself. Pamper your body with exotic bath oils, buy yourself a bunch of flowers whose colours attract you, have a manicure, pedicure or massage if this is something you would never normally do, treat yourself to a fine wine, invite a new friend for a lovely country walk, abandon the ironing and go for a swim etc. Love yourself in little ways as often as you can. The more you feel good about yourself, the more you will have to give to others.

5 Work more deeply on change, if it would help. Although it isn't essential to understand why we are as we are before we can make changes, it may be liberating for some. Think about trying therapy or counselling where you can explore vague or specific concerns about yourself. (See Where to Go for Help, page 200.)

26

WHERE TO GO FOR HELP

THERE are very many different kinds of help available for people who want to try to sort out some crisis in their lives, or to explore aspects of themselves with which either they are unhappy or which are making them ill.

As a nation, we have a considerable resistance to seeking any sort of therapy, feeling somehow that it is weak not to be able to solve our own emotional problems; although we don't feel in the least bit weak not being able to solve any physical ones. Disadvantages are that the process can be expensive (some kinds of help are free on the NHS, but most aren't) and painful. But no therapy is all just pain. When therapy works, people commonly start to feel more positive about themselves, feel more self-respect and more enthusiastic about the furture. For women, particularly, who often spend a large part of their time being carers and nurturers, therapy is a chance to nurture oneself. For an hour you need think about no one else's needs. The attention is all yours.

Nevertheless, undertaking therapy requires motivation, commitment and courage. It is far from being a support for the weak. The following is a brief guide to different helping professionals, and what they can offer.

• Psychiatrist •

A psychiatrist is a medically trained doctor who has specialised in dealing with disorders of the mind. You can be referred to a psychiatrist at a local hospital, by your GP, or you could ask to be referred to one privately. Psychiatrists can prescribe drugs or may recommend psychotherapy or counselling – so-called talking treatments – according to individual problems and needs. Some psychiatrists also have skills as psychotherapists.

• Psychologist •

A psychologist is not a medical doctor, although a psychologist with a PhD will have Dr as a title. Psychology is the study of how the mind works and clinical psychologists use this knowledge, through behaviour therapy or cognitive therapy, to help people handle mental health problems in which a change in behaviour or way of thinking is the most useful approach. There are psychologists in very many NHS hospitals and they are the people most likely to help with problems such as phobias, obsessive-compulsive disorders and panic attacks.

You are not usually referred directly to a psychologist in a hospital, but to a psychiatrist who will then refer you on to a psychologist if deemed appropriate. However, you can also consult psychologists privately, in which case it is important to ensure that the person you see is properly qualified. Those who call themselves chartered psychologists have undergone a lengthy specific training and abide by the code of conduct laid down by the British Psychological Society. You can find the names of individual chartered psychologists in all areas of the UK, and the specific services they offer, by consulting *The Directory of Chartered Psychologists*, which should be available in every public reference library.

• Psychotherapist •

A (reputable) psychotherapist is someone who has trained with a recognised body to help people explore their own mental state and come to a greater understanding of themselves and their problems. A skilled therapist will listen intently, direct, suggest or guide gently where appropriate and always be supportive and understanding, so that the patient (or client, if this is the term the therapist uses) can reach important insights into herself and see the way towards change or self-development.

Psychotherapy is available on the NHS but services are thinly spread and there will probably be waiting lists. Private practitioners abound. As anyone can call themselves a psychotherapist, it is important to try to find someone who is properly qualified. The United Kingdom Council of Psychotherapy has a register which represents organisations in the UK whose practitioners are qualified and accredited, and abide by a specific code of practice and ethics. See Useful Contacts.

• Psychotherapy •

This is an umbrella term for all therapies for mental or emotional disorders that do not involve the use of physical treatments such as drugs or ECT. In actual practice, the word psychotherapist usually denotes someone quite specific, with a particular range of skills. Other non-physical treatments which may broadly be classified under psychotherapy – such as behaviour therapy or cognitive therapy – tend to be referred to by name.

There are very many different kinds of psychotherapies, all with different orientations. These can loosely be divided into two categories: the psychodynamic tradition associated with Sigmund Freud, Carl Jung and their followers (in which it is held that a person's mental state and behaviour can be explained through unconscious early childhood experiences); and the humanistic therapies, devised more recently and particularly concerned with enhancing normal life experience rather than confining themselves to definite problems.

The aim of psychotherapy is to reach a greater self-understanding by look-ing at yourself in a new way and getting in touch with unconscious, sup-pressed feelings and past experiences that may be leading you to act or react as you do in certain circumstances of your life. It can be both an intensely painful and exhilarating process and takes courage to embark on.

In standard psychodynamic psychotherapy, the session usually lasts 50 min-utes, during which the client sits and talks. According to the orientation of the therapist, you may be encouraged to free associate (say whatever comes into your mind) or more emphasis may be placed on dreams. Transference, in which the patient or client transfers on to the therapist feelings which she had or has for some key person in her life (usually a parent) is an important medium for exploration and interpretation of feelings which come up.

As psychotherapy is more to do with self-exploration than crisis manage-ment, you need to make a commitment to it and expect to go to sessions for a couple of years or more, perhaps twice a week. (However, there is now a variant which is shorter and called, appropriately enough, brief psychotherapy – see below).

Several useful books on psychotherapy are listed in Further Reading.

• Psychoanalysis •

This is the grand-daddy of psychotherapy. It was devised by Sigmund Freud as a very in-depth exploration of the unconscious self, using tools such as free association and transference. It is not designed for problem-solving. Usually you attend 50-minute sessions four or five times a week for several years, so it takes much commitment and dedication. It is also expensive, as it is not available on the NHS.

Not all psychoanalysts work in the same way. Specific methods and aims developed by other pioneering analysts, such as Carl Jung and Alfred Adler, differ from those devised by Freud, so you need to know the orientation of your analyst. To find out whether psychoanalysis or psychotherapy would suit you, and to understand the difference between a Freudian and a Jungian therapist/analyst see Further Reading. To find an analyst contact the British Psychoanalytic Society for Freudian/Kleinian analysts or the Society of Analytic Psychology for Jungian analysts.

• Behaviour therapy •

Behaviour therapy starts from the premise that bad or unhelpful behaviour, reactions or habits are learned and can therefore be unlearned by special training. It is most often one of the techniques practised by clinical psycholo-gists and particularly useful for overcoming phobias, panic attacks and obsessive-compulsive disorders. Psychiatrists and nurses may use these methods too.

• Cognitive therapy •

This is a type of psychotherapy which is concerned with changing the way people think about themselves. It may be used in conjunction with behaviour therapy, when it is called cognitive behavioural therapy, or with more conventional psychotherapeutic methods, when it is called cognitive analytical therapy. The aim is to help people with poor self-esteem or little self-confidence gain conscious control of the negative inner commentary that is probably running constantly through their minds, challenge such negative thinking and replace it with more positive attitudes. Many of the techniques described in the sections of this book on phobias, panic attacks, obsessive-compulsive disorders and handling thoughts and emotions are cognitive therapy techniques. Psychologists, psychiatrists and some psychotherapists may use them.

Many health professionals are now choosing to be trained in cognitive therapy, including doctors, nurses and psychologists, so it is gradually becoming more available. It also, to some extent, can work as a self-help method.

The particularly good news about cognitive therapy is that studies have found it to be the most effective way of dealing with moderate depression: as effective as drugs and longer-lasting. Where appropriate, treatment with both antidepressants and cognitive therapy may be most useful.

• Counselling •

Counselling tends to be more concerned with helping clients explore or come to terms with a particular problem or crisis in their lives than with exploring feelings and motivations more generally and in depth. You might attend an agreed, fixed number of counselling sessions, such as six or twelve. Often, counselling is subject specific. Many counsellors are connected with charities and are concerned only with bereavement, stepfamily problems, marriage guidance etc.

Just to complicate matters, however, very many counsellors have been trained quite extensively and have skills more akin to those of a psychotherapist. They would be able to offer more in-depth and general help. Others, such as nurses, health visitors and GPs may have taken counselling courses so as to use counselling as an adjunct in their day-to-day work. Some GP surgeries have counsellors who provide sessions as part of their service. If you wish to see a private counsellor, check that they have trained with a body recognised by the British Association for Counselling (BAC). The BAC can also help you find a suitable counsellor.

• Brief psychotherapy •

This, as its name implies, is a shorter version of psychotherapy, with a different emphasis. The aim is to help a person in maybe half a dozen sessions and the stress is on looking at specific issues or problems and how they have developed, rather than why. Used in depression, for example, the therapist will concentrate on helping a person explore how they think, react, behave, make decisions, etc, in such a way as to exacerbate depression, and then help the person to find a more positive way forward. It has similarities to cognitive therapy, using some of its techniques. Brief therapy is only just starting to become more available in the UK and may particularly be used in hospitals or family therapy settings, where relationships between different members of a family are seen as important in understanding whatever problem has brought one of them for treatment.

• Hypnotherapy •

This is a form of psychotherapy in which the therapist induces a state of deep relaxation .(hypnosis) which relaxes the patient/client sufficiently perhaps to recall experiences and feelings that are buried and which it might have taken a conventional psychotherapist a long time to help tease out. In this sense it can be an adjunct to psychotherapy. Also, however, it can be used to help a patient gain control over certain mental or bodily processes. It is often successful, for example, in helping with problems in which stress or anxiety may play a part, such as migraine, skin problems, irritable bowel and phobias. Often, it is used to try to bolster self-confidence and thus increase an individual's ability to overcome a problem such as smoking or overeating. The outcome is successful for some.

Alas, anyone can set up as a hypnotherapist. To find someone bona fide, send a large SAE to the Institute for Complementary Medicine: see Useful Contacts. Then make it quite clear when you contact the practitioner what exactly you are looking for, to ascertain whether they are equipped to help you adequately.

• Humanistic psychotherapies •

Humanistic therapies concentrate on what is happening now in people's lives, rather than delving into their pasts for explanations and insights. The aim is to help people come to understand themselves better, value themselves more, express themselves, communicate more fully and generally feel more alive and positive about life. It can suit people who just want to get more out of their lives, without being conscious of any specific problem, or those who feel that life has more greys than yellows or who feel they have difficulties, for example, in relationships or personality, that they would like to tackle.

There are many different types of humanistic therapies and many different techniques which may be used in different combinations by individual therapists. Below are some of the better known but, for a useful fuller guide, read *Innovative Therapy in Britain*: see Further Reading.

The Association for Humanistic Psychology Practitioners (AHPP) is a professional organisation which aims to promote high standards among humanistic therapists. It gives accreditation, based on peer assessment and 'reasonably strict criteria of training and professional competence'. For a list of therapists in the UK, using various different humanistic approaches and accredited to AHPP, send an SAE for their membership directory: see Useful Contacts. The Association advises contacting several practitioners to discuss your needs and to find out what is offered. This may be done by phone or by an initial meeting which many offer free of charge.

• Gestalt therapy •

Gestalt techniques were very often used in the encounter groups of the 1960s and '70s. Its philosophy is that we are all a whole that is greater than the sum of our parts and the techniques aim to put us in touch with it. Body and mind are seen as inextricably linked and both must work together. Words, thinking, ideas and bodily defences are all explored as a way of integrating a whole personality.

Gestalt concentrates on the 'here and now' and doesn't separate out the past, believing that we are in fact carrying much of the past with us in the form of 'unfinished business'. Techniques for breaking down mental and physical defences include asking someone to role-play two aspects of her own personality, having a duologue between the two parts (for example, one's aggressive side arguing with one's timid side) or to have a duologue with a part of one's own body. Emotions which surface are discharged in a safe way, such as anger by thumping a pillow. Gestalt can be a group or individual therapy. To find a therapist, contact the Gestalt Centre London: see Useful Contacts.

• Bioenergetics •

This therapy, which may be group or individual, starts from the view that emotions such as anger and grief that are unreleased, instead express themselves in muscle tension, reducing energy and vivacity. It may use special bioenergetic exercises designed to reveal where tension is held and then work on these tensions, in the process of which the suppressed emotions and anxieties start to be released. Because of the approach, this starts to happen quite quickly but should be handled safely and supportively by a skilled therapist. It is difficult to find a therapist in the UK but some members of the Association of Humanistic Psychology Practitioners (see Useful Contacts) may use its methods.

• Psychosynthesis •

As its name suggests, this is a blending of all things, a method that sees man and woman as an integral part of the whole universe. It emphasises will and choice and aims not only to sort out one's personal needs but to inculcate a more spiritual awareness and a sense of being part of the whole of nature. For a suitably qualified practitioner and more details, contact the Institute of Psychosynthesis: see Useful Contacts.

• Psychodrama •

This is a group method of acting out real-life concerns, with the chance to express feelings which might never otherwise be expressed. For example, someone who has a distressing relationship with her mother might play herself while another acts the part of her mother. Also, roles may be reversed, so that the person with the problem mother gets to play her mother and perhaps comes to understand more of her mother's point of view. Some members of the Association of Humanistic Psychology Practitioners may use this method.

• Transactional analysis •

A combination of humanistic psychotherapies and behaviour therapy, which explains development, thinking, feelings and relationships in simple terms. TA has it that everyone has three aspects to their personality: the parent (nurturing but also perhaps judgmental and authoritarian), the adult (reasonable, grown-up, objective) and child (the needy and spontaneous part of ourselves made up of all that has happened to us and still affects us). The child is further divided into two: the natural child is the creative loving part of ourselves which we don't tend to value and express enough; the adapted child is the part that may act inappropriately, be aggressive or selfish, etc, because this behaviour was learned as a defence against hurt in our past.

The aim of TA is to integrate all three parts of the personality effectively. It is a useful method if you want help with a particular problem or set of attitudes but it is not one intended to bring deep understanding. For a list of qualified therapists, write to the Institute of Transactional Analysis: see Useful Contacts.

• Handling specific life crises •

Life inevitably makes many demands, particularly on women who generally take on the major caring role in families. We may have serious difficulties in our relationships with our partners, our children or other close members of the family. We may have to learn to cope with serious illness in someone we love, with the exhausting demands of caring for an elderly or seriously sick dependent (or the decision not to), and trying to spread ourselves somehow so that the healthy members of the family still also feel sufficiently cared for.

Many of us may suffer the trauma of divorce and separation and then the very different challenges of becoming a stepfamily if a new relationship is formed and becomes permanent.

There may be financial insecurities, job insecurities, career advances, career set-backs. There may be loneliness, bereavement or a struggle to come to terms with disability, chronic pain and perhaps impending untimely death. Or we may have difficulty just coming to terms with growing older.

At any of the difficult times in life, we may want someone to talk to, or we may just want to contact someone who can give us practical advice. There are many organisations that can offer help for different needs, which may not be mentioned in specific sections elsewhere in this book: see Useful Contacts.

Part III

....

OUR
SEXUAL SELVES

A WOMAN'S sexual self is a very important part of her life, regardless or not of whether she has a sex life.

All the workings that make us women are usually deeply connected with our sense of selves, even if we never want children, or even a partner. For men, there is nothing equivalent to the menstrual cycle and the delicate interplay of the many hormones required every month to make it all work correctly. That interplay of hormones also affects our feelings and how we are as individuals. And although there is often talk of the male menopause, there is nothing truly equivalent to the female menopause, with its clear message that fertility is finished and the emotional and physical experiences that may accompany it.

The complicated way our reproductive organs work means that most of us, at some time, experience some minor or major disorder connected with them. By dint of anatomy, our reproductive organs are more at risk of infection and disease than those of men, so there is much we need to know to ensure we can keep healthy or act early on signs of trouble. As these organs are such an intimate and important part of us, it is wise for women to be well-informed about the least drastic options for treatment, if required.

This section looks in depth at the whole range of gynaecological conditions, investigations, treatments and feelings about them, in our reproductive years and after. It also looks at everything to do with those other important organs in the reproductive system, the breasts. Love it or hate it, breasts are a sexual signal. They are also for very many women a deeply important aspect of their sense of femininity. Concerns about breast appearance and breast health are fully covered here.

So too are sexual health and sexual problems, both physical and emotional. A major cause of serious gynaecological ill-health is undetected sexually transmitted disease, so the full range is explained, with plenty of advice about treatment and self-help.

If you have an active sex life, you should also find all you need to know to decide which contraceptive method is best suited to you, at which stage of your life; and how best to approach getting pregnant if and when you do want to. The practical and emotional aspects of an unplanned, unwanted pregnancy, and of inability to become pregnant, are sympathetically treated.

27

....

THE FEMALE SEX ORGANS AND THE MENSTRUAL CYCLE

THE VULVA is the name given to the area of the female genitalia which you can see outside the vagina. The entrances to both the vagina, and the urethra, along which passes urine from the bladder, open from here.

The urethra is a very short tube, just 4cm (1½in) long, and the opening is very narrow. The opening to the vagina beside it is larger and the length of the vagina is longer, all of 10 to 12.5cm (4 to 5in). Behind, close to the vagina, is the opening to the anus. Because the entrances to the vagina, urethra and anus are all so close, it is easy for bacteria that live in the anus without causing problems there to enter either the vagina or the urethra and cause infections.

The bone you can feel between your legs is the pubic bone and on top of this lies the mons, an area of soft fatty tissue from which pubic hair grows at its most profuse. (Pubic hair extends between the legs, often some way down the thighs and around to the anus.)

Underneath the pubic bone, on either side of the opening to the vagina, lie two sets of fleshy skin folds like lips: the labia majora (outer lips) are

────────── **GYNAE GUIDE** ──────────

The resource and information centre Women's Health is a charity which answers enquiries and provides information about all aspects of women's health, particularly gynaecological health. The staff keep details of women's health groups, support groups and relevant voluntary organisations on computer as well as publishing leaflets and booklets on many gynaecological conditions. They also sell items such as speculums for self-examination and fertility awareness posters. Their office in London has a library of books, articles and pamphlets that women are welcome to browse through if you ring to arrange when to come. Send a SAE for full details: see Useful Contacts.

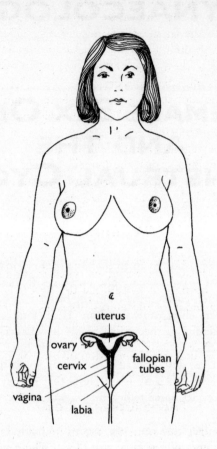

covered with hair and, just inside these, are the sensitive and hairless labia minora (inner lips).

The labia minora join at the end nearest to the pubic bone to form a soft hood of skin underneath which lies the clitoris, the most sensitive spot in the genital region. Under the hood of the clitoris lies the glans, which contains erectile tissue (like the penis) and swells during sexual arousal.

On either side of the vaginal opening are small round raised areas called the Bartholin's glands, which produce a little lubrication during sex and which sometimes get infected and swell.

• The vagina •

The vagina is often thought of as a tunnel but in fact its muscular walls are collapsed and only open to accommodate something that is inserted such as a penis, speculum or tampon. They open most spectacularly, of course, to enable a baby to be born.

The vagina is kept naturally moist by secretions from the cervix (the neck of the womb) and the vagina itself. The moistness will vary from woman to woman and according to the time of the month or the time of life, as the vagina is responsive to the female sex hormones oestrogen and progesterone and their differing levels during the menstrual cycle (see page 212) and after the menopause. When these hormones cease to be produced after the menopause, the vagina often becomes dry.

The moistness lubricates the vagina, helps keep it healthy and prevents painful friction during sex. Bacteria called lactobacilli which live in the vagina keep it slightly acid, which helps keep it infection-free.

The entrance to the vagina is partly blocked before sex has first taken place by a thin stretchy membrane called the hymen. Usually it is stretched before first intercourse by the use of tampons or during masturbation. If not, there can be initial pain and a little bleeding at the first penetration.

• The uterus •

The uterus or womb is about the size of a pear in a woman who is not pregnant. The bottom third is the cervix, which opens into the top of the vagina and can be felt with the fingers; it feels like the tip of the nose. The other two thirds is the main body of the uterus. Its walls are thick and muscular and the cavity in which a foetus develops stretches to the fallopian tubes that lie on either sides. The uterus usually tilts forward against the bladder and is described as anteverted. In a small proportion of women, it tilts back towards the rectum and is described as retroverted.

• The fallopian tubes •

The fallopian tubes curve out from the uterus and downward towards the ovaries. They have fringe-like tissue at the ends, called fimbriae, that stretch

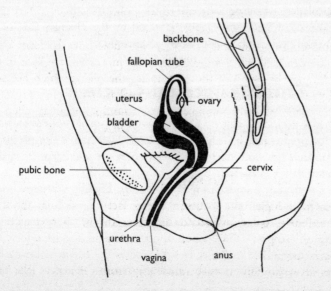

towards the ovaries and 'catch' the eggs as the ovaries release them. The fallopian tubes are muscular organs lined with tiny hair-like structures called cilia which help waft an egg towards the uterus. Sometimes a fertilised egg gets stuck in the tube, most commonly because of a previous undiagnosed infection, and begins to develop here.

This is termed an ectopic pregnancy (ectopic means 'in an unnatural location') and results in a medical emergency because after a couple of months, if undetected, the tube may burst. An ectopic pregnancy may also occasionally occur in the abdomen if the egg released by the ovary is not caught by one of the fallopian tubes and is fertilised outside them.

• The ovaries •

The ovaries are the organs which produce a female's eggs and the female sex hormones. They are about 3 to 4cm (1¼ to 1½in) long in an adult woman and half that in width; about the size of a walnut, although actual size varies from woman to woman and they shrink considerably after the menopause. Each ovary contains fluid-filled sacs or glands called follicles which each contain an immature egg. When we are born, we have about 2,000,000 eggs in our ovaries. This number has dropped to the still awesome figure of 200,000 to 500,000 by puberty. Every month a number are stimulated by hormones to start to mature but each month only one fully develops and is released.

• The pelvic organs •

The uterus, fallopian tubes and ovaries are together termed the pelvic organs. They lie in the abdominal cavity, partly covered by the peritoneum, the lining of the abdomen. The pelvic floor muscles – those you use if you try to stop a flow of urine – help to hold them in place. Weakness in these muscles can result in a prolapse, or falling forward, of the pelvic organs.

The breasts are also female sex organs, affected by the changes that occur during the menstrual cycle and, of course, by pregnancy.

• The Menstrual Cycle •

Menstruation, or a period, is the end of the monthly process in which the body prepares for pregnancy. It only occurs when a woman is not pregnant. Part of the tissue that lines the uterus in preparation for a pregnancy is shed because pregnancy hasn't occurred.

The average age to start menstruating is 12½ years. Usually women continue to have periods until their late forties, although there is nothing abnormal about starting periods as young as nine or as late as 18 and their not ceasing until the mid-fifties.

The time from one period to the next is known as the menstrual cycle and on average lasts 28 days. This is very much an average, because individual women vary widely in the length and frequency of their cycles. Some might menstruate every 26 days, others every 33 days; still others may have a few periods at relatively short intervals, then a few months before they have another.

The first day of bleeding is called day one of the cycle because this is when the whole cycle of preparing for pregnancy begins again. The process is very complex, depending upon a finely orchestrated triggering of hormones. The following is as simple a description as possible.

• First hormonal cues •

On day one, levels of the hormones oestrogen and progesterone, produced by the ovaries, are very low. This is the cue for the hypothalamus, a control centre in the brain, to produce GNRH (hormones called gonadotrophins) which in turn signal to the pituitary gland at the base of the brain, just below the hypothalamus, to make the hormones FSH (follicle-stimulating hormone) and LH (luteinising hormone). These two hormones gear up the ovaries to start developing its egg follicles and producing the female sex hormone, oestrogen. Each month, all the egg follicles in the ovaries are exposed to the effects of FSH but only about 20 start to develop and only one will mature. This leading follicle appears to control the development of the others, preventing the egg inside them from maturing. Gradually, the others shrink and the egg inside dies. The egg that matures usually comes from alternate ovaries each month.

As the leading follicle grows, more and more oestrogen is produced. The glands of the cervix start to secrete more and more mucus which is very hospitable to sperm and the lining of the uterus (the endometrium) starts to thicken and grow, ready to support a pregnancy.

• Ovulation •

By about day 12 or 13 of the cycle there is a sufficient surge of oestrogen to signal the hypothalamus via the pituitary to produce a sharp surge of LH. This is the hormone that triggers the rupturing of the follicle and the emergence of the egg. Within 36 hours of the LH surge the follicle opens and the egg is released. This is ovulation. Cervical mucus is often so thick and sticky now that it may appear like an excessive vaginal discharge.

At ovulation there is such a plentiful increase in cervical mucus in some women that it can even be enough to drench underwear. This is called, rather poetically, the 'ovulatory cascade' and is nothing abnormal. Some women feel a cramping in their lower abdomen or back at ovulation and there might even be a little blood in the vaginal discharge. Some experience headache, feel very lethargic or have very strong gastric pains which then disappear. One possible reason for the pain is that the follicle from which the egg emerges fills quickly with blood which then clots.

Once the egg has emerged, it is propelled towards the entrance of the

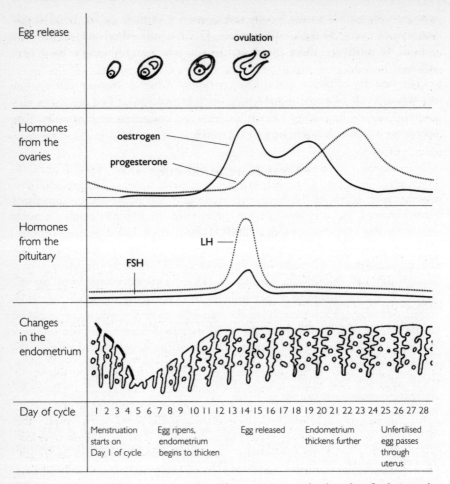

fallopian tube on that ovary's side. The egg is caught by the fimbriae, the fringe-like projections at the end of the tubes and the hair-like cilia, which line each tube, assist its passage down towards the uterus. If there are viable sperm in the fallopian tube at this time, fertilisation may take place. The egg is only capable of being fertilised by sperm for 24 hours after ovulation but healthy sperm can live in the hospitable pre-ovulation mucus of the vagina for up to five days, so sex well before ovulation can still lead to pregnancy.

If the tubes are blocked through infection, the egg, which is absolutely minute at this stage, is lost in surrounding tissue and soon disintegrates.

• Preparing the uterus •

The egg follicle, once ruptured and collapsed, becomes stained with a vivid yellow pigment and is then known as the corpus luteum, Latin for yellow body. The corpus luteum starts to produce, as well as oestrogen, the other female sex hormone, progesterone, a process triggered by the surge in LH that precipitated ovulation. Progesterone is needed to help the uterus prepare its lining, the endometrium, ready to receive a fertilised egg. It thickens the endometrium and helps its glands secrete substances that will nourish an embryo. In this second half of the menstrual cycle, progesterone is dominant and has the effect of making the cervical mucus thick and unfriendly to sperm.

Oestrogen and progesterone both carry on being produced for about the next ten days. At about day 22 of the cycle, progesterone is at its peak. The endometrial lining of the uterus is now thick and ready to provide sustenance for an embryo.

If, however, no fertilised egg materialises, the corpus luteum starts to degenerate and levels of both oestrogen and progesterone fall, progesterone particularly dramatically.

• Menstruation •

When all the hormones are back to their lowest levels again, around day 27 and day 28, the thickened endometrium can no longer be supported and starts to loosen. When it begins to be shed, this is menstruation and we are back to day 1 of the cycle.

About two-thirds of the new enlarged endometrium is lost in the menstrual flow, which may last for only two or three days or for up to eight and be either heavy or light. As well as blood in the menstrual fluid, there are cells, bits of membrane from the lining, mucus and other fluids. Blood makes up over half of the flow but only amounts on average to about half a wineglass-full, over the whole period, although it seems like more to most women.

In a menstrual cycle of 28 days, ovulation is likely to occur around the 14th day. In shorter or longer cycles, ovulation time is more difficult to calculate. It is the part of the cycle before ovulation which may vary in length. After ovulation has occurred, and if there is no pregnancy, it is usually 14 days until a period starts.

• Anovulatory cycles •

Ovulation does not occur in every menstrual cycle. Before the age of 20 and after the age of 38 failure to ovulate may occur as often as one cycle in four. Between the ages of 20 and 38 a woman may not ovulate perhaps in one in ten cycles. Consistent failure to ovulate is the most common cause of female infertility.

In an anovulatory cycle, the follicle ripens but no LH surge occurs, either because there is not enough FSH stimulation to increase oestrogen production sufficiently, or because the hypothalamus, for some reason, doesn't respond in the correct way when oestrogen reaches its peak. The follicle carries on secreting oestrogen until it dies, which may take longer than normal, making a period late that month. Women who never ovulate may regularly have long cycles. However, failure to ovulate does not always affect cycle length and menstruation may equally often occur at the same time as usual.

28

INVESTIGATIVE PROCEDURES

THERE are a number of procedures that may be carried out in order to investigate possible gynaecological problems.

• Pelvic examination •

This is a routine check which may be carried out periodically at a well-woman clinic or GP surgery (and should be done regularly, to some degree, after the age of 35). You may receive one if you are being prescribed any form of contraception, if you are having a cervical smear or if you think you are pregnant. It is also the first investigation you will receive if you complain of gynaecological symptoms.

The pelvic examination can be carried out with the woman lying either on her back with legs wide apart and knees bent or while she is lying on her left side (for a right-handed examiner) with the upper leg bent. The latter position is experienced by many women as more comfortable and less exposing than lying on one's back. However a GP, or even a specialist, may demur if they are not used to using that position for examination.

A full pelvic examination will consist of a manual investigation and a look

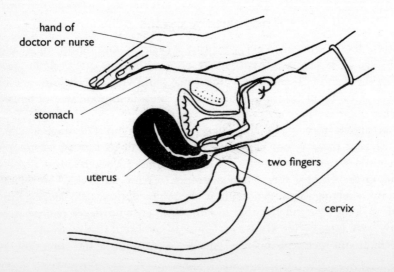

at the cervix via a speculum. In the manual examination, the doctor inserts two fingers of a gloved hand into the vagina to palpate the cervix. The other hand is placed on top of the abdomen to palpate the uterus and ovaries at the same time. The examination can reveal the position, size and shape of the uterus and whether it is mobile (normal). It is usually tender when squeezed between two hands. The fallopian tubes can never be felt when normal; the ovaries sometimes can be felt and sometimes can't when all is well. If they can be felt, they are usually extremely tender. Ovarian cysts may be revealed and their size gauged by manual examination.

The speculum is used to inspect the vagina and the cervix. This is a metal or plastic instrument with two 'arms' which are inserted into the vagina in the closed position. Then the handles of the speculum are pulled so that the arms open inside the vagina, stretching out its walls and making the cervix visible. It should be warmed and lubricated before insertion. Insertion of a speculum doesn't hurt if a woman is relaxed but it is hard not to stiffen when you know something relatively cold and inflexible is about to be pushed inside you. Making a deliberate effort to relax all your muscles really helps.

While the speculum is in place, swabs will be taken from the cervix or top of the vagina if an infection is suspected and a cervical smear may be carried out. Swabs, in which cotton-tipped sticks are introduced into the vagina to take a sample of any discharge, is painless; a cervical smear feels like a little nick as a few cervical cells are scraped off with a special spatula or brush for analysis in a laboratory.

Some women find the whole procedure embarrassing and therefore quite stressful. In the end, the experience will largely depend upon the attitude of the doctor performing the examination and the feelings a woman brings to it. It can be very hard, for example, for a woman who has been sexually abused to tolerate internal examinations.

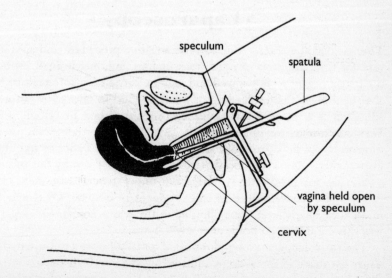

speculum

spatula

vagina held open
by speculum

cervix

• Pelvic ultrasound •

Ultrasound works by sending sound waves either through the skin via a special instrument held on the abdomen, or through the vagina. A computer that is part of the ultrasound machine converts the sound waves – which reflect differently according to whether they are bouncing back off bone, blood, soft tissue or whatever – into a hazy picture of the pelvic organs which you see on a screen.

For an abdominal ultrasound scan, you have to drink a lot of water beforehand so that you have a full bladder. This is because in abdominal ultrasound the operator is having to look through bowel and bladder to see the pelvis, and a full bladder serves to push the bowel out of the way and to lift the uterus up. Vaginal ultrasound, which is becoming more available, allows a slightly clearer view because there are no such obstacles.

Ultrasound scanning can be used to see ovarian cysts, both benign and malignant, polycystic ovarian syndrome (multiple cysts on the ovaries, a condition which is confirmed by biochemical tests), fibroids in the uterus and polyps. When a trans-vaginal probe is used, the thickness of the endometrium can even be measured.

Ultrasound is most commonly used in pregnancy, of course. It can also be a helpful aid in assessing whether a woman with severe pelvic pain is suffering an ectopic pregnancy by showing whether there is a foetus in the uterus (in which case an additional ectopic is unlikely) or that the uterus is empty, leaving the likelihood of an ectopic pregnancy very high if a pregnancy test has been positive.

Another use for ultrasound is to locate whether an IUD is still in the uterus if the threads cannot be felt in the vagina or were cut too short.

• Laparoscopy •

This has become a very common investigative procedure and almost obligatory for firm diagnosis of conditions such as endometriosis. It enables all of the pelvic organs to be viewed and may be carried out to establish causes for abnormal pelvic pain, bleeding or infertility and to check for fibroids, cysts, adhesions (scar tissue causing organs to stick together) or ectopic pregnancy. Very commonly, treatment may be carried out laparoscopically too, with a surgeon using the laparoscope to see by while using a laser or minute cutting instruments. Quite commonly, sterilisation is carried out by this means.

Usually, the procedure is carried out under general anaesthetic, in which case you are likely to need to stay the night in hospital. Or it may be done under local anaesthetic, depending upon the reason for the investigation, and you may be able to go home after a few hours.

The laparoscope is a long illuminated metal tube which is inserted through a tiny cut made in the abdomen just below the navel. At one end is a lens, at the other a telescope. Before the laparoscope is inserted, carbon dioxide gas is pumped into the abdominal cavity via a needle so that the pelvis and its contents can be seen more clearly. If treatment is being carried out in conjunction with the laparoscope, other instruments are inserted through a second incision.

Laparoscopy is often described as a painless procedure with little discomfort experienced afterwards. That doesn't fit very many women's experience of the after effects, which is more akin to being being beaten in the stomach by a gang of thugs. The soreness only lasts a few days but it is helpful to know it may occur. Plans to go direct from the hospital to work, for example, may be somewhat ambitious.

The other common after effect is a seemingly inexplicable pain in the shoulders. This is known as a referred pain: that is, experienced in the shoulders although not the site of the problem, and is caused by the residual carbon dioxide gas. It is actually possible for surgeons to prevent it happening by taking steps to help the residual gas find its escape route when instruments are being removed, but whether this is actually done, or the method known to most surgeons, is another matter.

• Hysteroscopy •

The hysteroscope is a similar instrument to the laparoscope but it is passed through the vagina into the womb where it may be used to find out the cause of abnormal periods, take endometrial tissue for biopsy, to see suspected polyps or fibroids and to locate and remove lost IUDs. It is a far less invasive diagnostic method than dilatation and curettage (D&C, see below) and far more sensitive. Surgery to remove fibroids and polyps can, where suitable, also be carried out hysteroscopically, using tiny cutting instruments requiring just tiny incisions and eliminating the need for a large cut in the abdomen.

A little gas or fluid is pumped into the uterus to open it slightly and make viewing via the hysteroscope easier. Discomfort afterwards is mild: maybe period-type cramps for a day or two. Usually, hysteroscopy is carried out under local anaesthetic and women can go home within an hour.

• Dilatation and curettage (D&C) •

This is a surgical procedure in which the cervix is stretched open under anaesthetic (general or local) and a spoon-shaped instrument called a curette is inserted to scrape out the endometrium, the lining of the uterus. Traditionally, it has been used to investigate heavy bleeding, treat painful periods or uterine adhesions, take tissue samples from the endometrium for investigation and remove lost IUDs as well as being a means of performing abortion or clearing the uterus after miscarriage.

It can be an effective treatment for menorrhagia if problematic polyps are removed along with the endometrium or if the endometrium was inflamed (endometritis). However, it is never a good treatment for dysmenorrhoea and it is gradually falling out of favour altogether because it is often diagnostically inaccurate and may easily fail to effectively treat the real problem. For example, a tiny fibroid is easily seen and removed via a hysteroscope but may be missed by a sweep with the curette, leaving the woman with the symptoms she first complained of and well down the road towards an unnecessary hysterectomy.

Alarmingly, it is, or was, over-used in this country, with six times as many women undergoing D&C here as in the United States, according to an Oxford study. It should never be used before conservative treatments have been tried for menorrhagia and it shouldn't be used in women under 35 unless hormonal treatments have failed. Its investigative and treatment benefits have now been completely overshadowed by hysteroscopy, which is becoming increasingly available.

If you undergo a D&C you may experience cramps and some bleeding for a couple of days afterwards.

• Colposcopy •

A colposcope is an instrument which provides a magnified view of the vagina and cervix and is the procedure which is carried out if a cervical smear has indicated some possibly suspicious cells. A speculum holds the walls of the vagina apart when the colposcope is used. (See page 217.)

·······································

29

MENSTRUAL DISORDERS

A VERY high proportion of women suffer from problem periods of one kind or another. The most common problems are severe menstrual pain and premenstrual syndrome. Others are failure to have periods at all, having too few, having too many and having periods that are too heavy. Sometimes there is an underlying disease causing these complaints so they always warrant investigation.

· Amenorrhoea · (absence of periods)

This is a failure to have periods and may be described as either primary or secondary. Primary amenorrhoea is the non-appearance of menstrual cycles by the time a girl reaches 16. Commonly puberty is just late, but sometimes there may be a physiological or hormonal problem which should be investigated.

Secondary amenorrhoea is the diagnosis when a woman who has established her periods suddenly or gradually stops having them. There are numerous possible causes and the most common, of course, are pregnancy and the menopause. Women who breast feed usually take longer to restart periods after a pregnancy; often, but not always, several months.

Some women who have been on the contraceptive pill and then stop using it may find their periods do not return after several months. Although a short delay of a month or two is quite common, as natural hormones get back in balance, several months or more than a year without resumption of periods probably means an underlying cause for the amenorrhoea which the use of the pill, with its false bleeds, only masked. In other words, using the pill does not cause amenorrhoea when you stop: there is likely to be some other cause which warrants investigation.

Excessive dieting or losing more body weight than is naturally healthy for you, and also excessive exercise, can play havoc with oestrogen levels and lead to loss of periods. Anorexia is not only dangerous in itself but loss of oestrogen increases risk of thinning, easily broken bones (osteoporosis) at a very early age.

Cysts, polycystic ovarian syndrome and tumours may all cause amenorrhoea. So may stress, severe depression, certain drugs such as some tranquillisers and antidepressants, and certain illnesses such as thyroid disease and anaemia.

Hormone imbalance may commonly be responsible for amenorrhoea. In about 20 per cent of women with secondary amenorrhoea, the cause is over-production of prolactin (hyperprolactinaemia) by the pituitary gland. Prolactin, which stimulates milk production, suppresses oestrogen production. Only in one in three women with this condition, however, is there any watery or milky discharge from the nipple (galactorrhoea).

The drug bromocryptine can be given at a dose just sufficient to reduce prolactin to normal levels. In some cases a pituitary tumour known as a microadenoma may be the cause of high prolactin. This also responds to bromocryptine.

In about five per cent of women who have amenorrhoea, the ovaries fail early causing a premature menopause (before the age of 40). Sometimes, however, the ovaries fail only temporarily because the body inexplicably decides to produce antibodies that prevent the process which stimulates ovulation from being triggered: in women to whom this happens, one in three may find that ovulation and menstruation suddenly start again out of the blue some years later.

Unfortunately, as the blood test of hormone levels which reveals ovarian failure cannot distinguish between ovaries which have packed up and ovarian function blocked by antibodies, it is impossible to know in advance whose cycles may restart.

Loss of periods should always be investigated, if the natural causes mentioned above do not explain it.

• Oligomenorrhoea •
(infrequent periods)

Periods, although infrequent, may be regular. Technically, any cycle length at least two weeks longer than that which a woman was experiencing before – that is, if a woman used to menstruate every 28 days but starts to menstruate every 42 days – is termed oligomenorrhoea. Alternatively they may be irregular. You might only have a few scant periods a year. Oligomenorrhoea isn't usually a problem (although it can be a nuisance if you are trying to get pregnant), as ovulation is likely to occur as normal but just less frequently. It becomes more common in most women towards the menopause. It may sometimes occur as a result of thyroid or adrenal disease but there would be other symptoms as well.

• Polymenorrhoea •
(too frequent periods)

This is the name given to normal periods with normal (for the woman concerned) blood loss but occurring regularly in cycles of less than 22 days.

Usually, a hormone disturbance or ovaries less than normally responsive to hormone triggers are the cause. The cycle can be regulated by the oral contraceptive pill or by a progestogen given from day ten of the cycle for 15 days. If the bleeding is excessive as well as too frequent, this may be a symptom of an illness, such as pelvic inflammatory disease.

• Breakthrough bleeding •

This is bleeding which occurs between periods. One in ten women has slight spotting at ovulation and women sometimes experience breakthrough bleeding on the contraceptive pill. In all other instances, however, it is not normal. It may signal the beginning of a miscarriage or the fact that an IUD, if fitted, is becoming dislodged. It may also be a sign of cancer of the cervix or uterus. Bleeding that occurs after sex may be explained by a cervical erosion or cervical polyp (both harmless).

• Menorrhagia •
(heavy periods)

Suffering excessively heavy periods is the most common reason for a woman to be referred to an out-patient gynaecology clinic. Far from being a problem mostly in the imagination, 40 per cent of women seen in these clinics have menorrhagia severe enough to cause anaemia.

There may often be a gynaecological disorder which is causing the problem, such as endometriosis, pelvic inflammatory disease, fibroids or endometrial cancer. Thyroid problems can also cause very heavy periods.

Where there is no disease, heavy bleeds may have been caused by the fitting of an IUD, which can make periods heavier initially; the progestogen-only pill, which can sometimes play havoc with periods; or a thickening of the lining of the uterus, which particularly starts to happen as a woman approaches menopause. In these cases, the main concern is anaemia and the effect on your lifestyle of having to suffer such heavy and perhaps prolonged bleeds.

• Investigations due to heavy periods •

If you see your doctor because of heavy periods, you should receive a manual pelvic examination and then, according to findings, you may be referred on for a pelvic ultrasound or hysteroscopy, the best method of checking the uterus for causes of heavy bleeding. A hysteroscope is a kind of telescope which is inserted via the vagina to view the uterus. It is powerful enough to see even the tiniest fibroid which can also be removed via hysteroscope with tiny cutting instruments.

If hysteroscopy is not locally available, you may be referred instead for a D&C (dilatation and curettage), a procedure in which a spoon-like instrument called a curette is used to scoop out the endometrium. This may be suggested as especially suitable if a fibroid is suspected, because the fibroid should then be removed along with endometrium.

However, with a D&C it is quite possible for a small fibroid to be missed. So if your menstrual problems do not resolve after a D&C and you are told a hysterectomy is the only course left, insist on being referred first to a hospital that does hysteroscopy, so that you can be sure there isn't a little fibroid still lurking inside.

• Self-help for heavy periods •

If no disease is found on investigation of menorrhagia, many women are reassured sufficiently to be prepared to carry on coping with heavy bleeds. If your blood loss is very heavy, however, and blood tests have shown you to be anaemic, it is important to take iron supplements which your doctor should prescribe. As well, make sure your diet is rich in iron by upping your intake of foods such as liver, dark green leafy vegetables and eggs. Have some fruit or vegetables containing vitamin C (or drink a glass of vitamin C-rich fruit juice) at the same time as eating iron-rich foods because vitamin C increases iron absorption. You could also try using cast-iron cooking pots, so that iron leaches out into food during cooking.

• Drug treatments for menorrhagia •

When menorrhagia causes intense discomfort and inconvenience, there are a number of treatments which can be tried, both medical and surgical. For many women, non-steroidal anti-inflammatory drugs (NSAIDs) may be effective in reducing excessive blood loss. The drugs, such as mefenamic acid, ibuprofen or naproxen, need to be taken through the duration of each period and from a short while before, particularly if a woman has premenstrual pain.

Sometimes the contraceptive pill is prescribed to prevent the build-up of endometrial tissue before menstruation; and sometimes both NSAIDs and the pill may be useful.

Very encouraging for sufferers from menorrhagia is the development of new IUDs which release the progestogen levonorgestrel. They are becoming known as intrauterine systems rather than IUDs because they are so different from ordinary ones. (See page 412.) They give contraceptive protection for five years and may reduce menstrual flow by up to 90 per cent within three months. It is the most effective drug treatment so far and should become widely available as manufacturers receive their licences. There could be side-effects, however, which may include irregular bleeding, breast pain, nausea, fluid retention, the development of ovarian cysts and depression, but the risk of them is low because such a small amount of progestogen is used.

Therapies which have more traditionally been used to suppress hormones involved in the menstrual cycle include the synthetic steroid danazol. This drug is effective in reducing blood flow and making periods more regular but has significant possible side-effects such as weight gain, acne, hirsutism, deepened voice, loss of libido, reduction in breast size, hot flushes and vaginal dryness. For this reason, it is not usually prescribed for more than six months initially, and blood loss is likely to return to pre-treatment levels some months after stopping treatment. Gestrinone, a similar drug, may be slightly better tolerated.

Other drugs called LHRH analogues which suppress pituitary function and cause amenorrhoea are effective but also have the side-effects of menopausal symptoms such as hot flushes, vaginal dryness, loss of libido and reduction in breast size. As well, importantly, they cause a decrease in bone density (with the increased risk of osteoporosis) because of suppression of oestrogen.

• Surgical treatments for menorrhagia •

Hysterectomy used to be the surgical treatment for menorrhagia but now there are other options. Transcervical resection of the endometrium (TCRE) involves removing the lining of the uterus vaginally but leaving the uterus itself intact. Using the hysteroscope to provide a view of the womb and an electric current passed through a cutting loop, almost all of the womb lining can be cut away in 20 minutes. Either local or general anaesthetic may be used for the procedure but the patient is usually able to return home within a few hours whichever is used.

About a third of women find that their periods stop completely after this procedure and the rest have periods which are very light. The technique is not simple technically, however, and a proportion (at best estimate 5 per cent, at worst 30 per cent) may need repeat surgery or a hysterectomy afterwards.

The endometrium can also be removed by laser (endometrial laser ablation). A very fine fibre is used to introduce the laser energy into the uterus which, by its very size, increases safety over the larger cutting loop used in TCRE. However, the downside of the laser method is that the laser beam destroys the endometrium, whereas in TCRE it is removed and can be checked for any malignancy. One or other of these procedures is available in most hospitals, most commonly TCRE. Both can affect fertility, however, so will not suit those who want to try for a child.

It is usually recommended that for two months before removal of the endometrium women should be given a GNRH analogue (a drug which prevents the ovaries from functioning), such as goserelin, which prevents stimulation of the pituitary gland, thus stopping oestrogen production and 'thinning' the endometrium. This makes it easier for the surgeon to see what he or she is doing and increases safety. Goserelin may have unpleasant side-effects, however: mainly those that mimic menopausal problems.

If you do opt to have a hysterectomy or are recommended to have one, bear in mind you may undergo an earlier menopause even though your ovaries are not removed. In uncomplicated hysterectomies, the operation can be done vaginally, without any need for an abdominal incision at all. Often for menorrhagia, however, an abdominal hysterectomy, where a large cut is made in the abdomen through which to remove the uterus, has been necessary and recovery can take months.

Increasingly, however, there is another less traumatic option: laparoscopically-assisted vaginal hysterectomy, which women can recover from within a week. The laparoscope, a kind of telescope inserted into the abdomen close to the navel, enables a surgeon to see to use tiny cutting instruments to extract the uterus and remove it through the vagina. The whole procedure requires just three tiny cuts around the bikini line and the one around the navel, so scarring is minimal.

• Dysmenorrhoea • (painful periods)

Painful periods probably affect about a third of menstruating women. There are two types: primary and secondary dysmenorrhoea.

Primary dysmenorrhoea is severe, often incapacitating, cramps during menstruation that come on for the first time within three years of starting to menstruate. Other accompanying symptoms may include soreness in the groin, back and thighs, bloated stomach, feeling or being sick, diarrhoea and sweats. Primary dysmenorrhoea is most common in younger women but may continue into a woman's thirties, and not necessarily be resolved by pregnancy and childbirth.

Secondary dysmenorrhoea is menstrual pain that is caused by some underlying condition such as endometriosis, pelvic inflammatory disease or fibroids. It is not likely to be experienced at such an early stage as primary dysmenorrhoea, although endometriosis can cause pain in teenage girls sometimes and may not be investigated because it is not expected. If you are aware of persistent and particularly increasing pain, seek investigation and treatment, whatever your age.

Primary dysmenorrhoea is most probably caused by an excess production of the hormone prostaglandin, which, among other things, causes the uterus to contract; helping the uterus contract during labour is one of its important roles. It is not known why some women but not others should be affected.

• Self-help for painful periods •

Tried-and-tested self-help methods include taking to bed with a hot water bottle; practising relaxation exercises (to relax the uterus and reduce the extra tension caused by expectation of pain); lying in a warm bath perfumed with three drops each of the essential oils chamomile and sweet marjoram; ginger tea (a cup of hot water added to one teaspoon of grated fresh root and infused for 10 minutes before drinking); homoeopathic remedies available from pharmacies (check correct remedy for your specific symptoms); massage of painful areas. Many women find professional acupuncture helpful.

• Drug treatments •

Doctors can prescribe an anti-prostaglandin drug such as mefenamic acid, which is usually very effective, and good old aspirin also works against prostaglandins. Some doctors may recommend the contraceptive pill as a means of dealing with dysmenorrhoea. Fine if you want to be on the pill anyway, otherwise not really an ideal solution. A contraceptive approach that is looking good is the new, soon-to-be-marketed progestogen-releasing IUD (see page 412). In research studies, it has been found to put a halt to period cramps within a couple of months.

• Premenstrual syndrome (PMS) •

Premenstrual syndrome (PMS) is characterised by a variety of possible physical and mental symptoms which regularly occur from some point in the second half of the menstrual cycle, worsening or intensifying until a period starts but not necessarily continuing during a period and definitely not present for at least seven days after menstruation finishes.

Between 20 and 40 per cent of women of reproductive age suffer emotional, behavioural and physical symptoms severe enough to lead them to seek help from their doctors. Five to 10 per cent of women find their symptoms incapacitating, badly disrupting their family and working lives.

• Symptoms of PMS •

Physical The range of possible symptoms is dauntingly large (150 have been cited) but the most common physical ones are headache; breast tenderness; swollen breasts; weight gain; backache; abdominal bloating; swollen fingers and ankles; acne; and irritable bowel symptoms.

Emotional The most common emotional and behavioural symptoms are depression; irritability; anxiety or panic attacks; crying for no known reason; forgetfulness or loss of concentration; loss of sex drive; aggressiveness; fatigue; and food cravings.

PMS is thus very different from the milder mainly physiological symptoms which at least 95 per cent of women suffer before a period. It is also different from what doctors may term 'menstrual distress' where existing physical or emotional problems are made worse premenstrually but continue in some form throughout the cycle (that is, with no symptom-free stretch of a week to ten days).

• Possible causes of PMS •

What causes PMS is still not known for certain, although particular theories have been put forward with force by particular parties. Progesterone deficiency, progesterone excess, excess of oestrogen, prostaglandins or prolactin, vitamin deficiencies, defects in the metabolism of fatty acids, low blood sugar (hypoglycaemia), fluid retention, abnormalities in brain opiates (endorphins) and psychiatric problems have all been suggested as possible causes.

Although hormonal activity during the second half of the cycle was believed to be a major contributor to the problem even this has been challenged. No consistent hormonal abnormalities have been found in women with PMS and, also, in a trial in which cycles were artificially manipulated in a group of PMS sufferers, symptoms were the same regardless of the balance of oestrogen and progesterone levels.

So, as there is no firm consensus about causes, it is necessary to experiment with measures to help overcome it, in order to find out what suits you. Certainly, self-help measures should be the first to try.

• Self-help: diet •

Carbohydrate and sugar   It is claimed by some that women with PMS are over-sensitive to lowered blood sugar. Low blood sugar triggers a rush of adrenalin to correct it, with effects such as panic attacks, migraine and outbursts of temper. Therefore, it is worth trying to keep your blood-sugar levels steady by eating a starchy food (a piece of bread, rice cake or crispbread) at three-hourly intervals.

Initially, the cause of the problem is a sudden blood-sugar boost caused by eating simple sugar: the pancreas is forced to produce insulin to bring it down and the over-sensitive adrenal glands then produce adrenalin to bring it back up again. Some self-help advocates suggest cutting down on sugar altogether. (However, detractors of this theory say there is actual evidence that premenstrual symptoms are not related to low blood sugar.)

Caffeine   There is plenty of anecdotal evidence of the benefits of cutting down on caffeine, so it may be worth giving this a try. However, there is no actual scientific evidence that drinking less tea, coffee and cola drinks reduces symptoms.

Salt   There is no evidence that cutting down on salt improves anything.

Vitamin B_6 (pyridoxine)   A supplement of this vitamin has been popular treatment for PMS in recent years. The thinking is that high levels of oestrogen could cause a deficiency which would have an adverse effect on certain brain chemicals. Some trials have shown benefit, but most have not and the trials which did show benefit have been accused of flaws. It is known, however, that taking too much can be dangerous and problems with the nervous system may occur with long-term treatment of more than 200mg per day. (The usual recommended dose is 50mg per day.)

Other vitamins and minerals   Many nutrition and PMS experts still think there is a place for vitamin B_6, however, together with other vitamins and minerals. There are several studies that support the use of magnesium supplements (such as Magnesium-OK, containing magnesium, B vitamins and zinc) or magnesium combined with multivitamins (Optivite). Magnesium, vitamin B_6, niacin, zinc, vitamin C and other nutrients are known to be co-factors in the metabolism of essential fatty acids. Defects in essential fatty acid metabolism have been found in some PMS sufferers and so have low levels of magnesium. One study has found that magnesium supplements are more effective than drug therapies but there are also studies that find no benefit.

Evening primrose oil This may help women with breast symptoms but is not so likely to help other symptoms.

• Other self-help measures •

Taking regular exercise can help, as it improves mood and also relaxes the muscles which improves blood flow. Relaxation techniques and stress management techniques may be helpful too, not necessarily as a way of eliminating symptoms but as a way of enhancing ability to cope and thus reducing their impact. Many women try yoga, acupuncture and hypnosis, with varying degrees of success.

• Drug treatments •

The National Association for Pre-Menstrual Syndrome (NAPS) has found that most women with PMS can be helped with diet, exercise and relaxation and that only one in three needs drug therapy.

There are quite a number of drugs in use, but they don't necessarily work well for everyone or else have drawbacks such as unpleasant side-effects. Diuretics to treat fluid retention are only likely to be of any help if you gain a significant amount of weight in the second half of the menstrual cycle. If you don't gain weight, no matter how much bloating you feel in your abdomen you are not retaining fluid.

Progesterone treatment with vaginal or rectal suppositories or injections has been the treatment recommended by PMS expert Dr Katherina Dalton for many years, and she has certainly claimed many successes. However, the theory that PMS may largely be due to a deficiency of progesterone in the second half of the cycle has not been borne out by most other investigators, and several trials have not shown that progesterone treatment is a benefit. Large doses given rectally can cause diarrhoea, wind and soreness.

Some drug treatments are aimed at suppressing the ovarian cycle altogether. The contraceptive pill may help some and be an acceptable treatment if you want contraception and are happy about the pill. However, some women have found the pill made their symptoms worse.

The synthetic steroid, danazol, works but alas has many unacceptable side-effects such as weight gain, hirsutism and acne which limits how long it can be used. When lower doses (200mg a day rather than the traditional 400mg) are given, however, the side-effects are likely to be less and the treatment still appears to be effective. Drugs called GNRH analogues, which prevent the ovaries from functioning, have been shown to work but they too have side-effects such as menopausal symptoms and they increase the risk of osteoporosis, so can't be prescribed long-term either.

Oestrogen patches may be helpful, particularly when depression is experienced as part of PMS. One study has found that in women with severe premenstrual depression, oestrogen patches worn twice a week not only lift depression but reduce other mood swings and relieve pain and water retention. However, a progestogen must be taken during the second half of the cycle and this can cause PMS symptoms in women who are particularly sensitive to progesterone or its artificial versions. Oestrogen can also be implanted. The pellets take about six weeks to work and the treatment needs repeating every six months. While very effective, it works for two years after the last implant, so a progestogen has to be taken for the following two years as well.

Minor tranquillisers have sometimes been given for PMS. The benzodiazepine alprazolam has been shown have some effect, but taking tranquillisers for PMS is not a good idea at all, particularly with their known risks of causing dependence. The antidepressant fluoxetine may be helpful where depression is a major symptom of PMS.

The most drastic treatment for PMS is surgical: hysterectomy with removal of both ovaries. Obviously, this must be kept as a very last resort.

• Psychological factors in PMS •

There is still a view that PMS is largely in the mind and it is held not only by old-fashioned doctors but by some modern psychologists. At a special symposium held at the British Psychological Society conference in 1993, one psychologist claimed that women are more likely to blame periods for irritability and depression when they are premenstrual but put their moods down to stress at other times. Even she, however, didn't claim that PMS does not exist; just that more may think they experience PMS than really do.

• Abnormal vaginal bleeding •

The only normal bleeding from the uterus is the bleeding that occurs during a period, and after childbirth. Only about half a wineglassful of blood is lost during an average period but this is difficult to use as a gauge for whether periods are heavy, as other fluids are lost as well, making it seem more.

The term abnormal uterine bleeding may include menstrual periods that are unusually heavy (menorrhagia) or unusually light or very irregular (oligomenorrhoea) or absent altogether (amenorrhoea). Other causes of heavier-than-usual bleeding or bleeding or spotting at odd times during the cycle include:

- Use of the IUD or the contraceptive pill.
- The approach of the menopause, which may make your periods different from normal; but irregular heavy bleeding is never a feature of the menopause and needs investigation.
- Vaginal dryness, particularly in women who have passed the menopause and are not on hormone replacement therapy, because inflammation caused by soreness and chafing may cause some bleeding.
- Gynaecological conditions such as fibroids, endometriosis, pelvic inflammatory disease, polyps or ovarian cysts.
- Miscarriage or ectopic pregnancy (if pregnant).
- Cervical erosion (if bleeding occurs after sex).
- Cervical cancer or endometrial cancer.

For further information, see separate entries or sections on all the above.

30

COMMON GYNAECOLOGICAL PROBLEMS

THIS chapter looks at the main internal problems for which a woman may find herself referred to a gynaecologist for investigation.

• Pelvic pain •

Pelvic pain is a symptom, not a condition. It is experienced as a pain in the lower abdomen but, because it can have a variety of causes, the actual type of pain varies. It may be constant, intermittent, sharp, dull, colicky; occur mainly before and around period times, etc, and will probably be accompanied by other symptoms, depending upon the condition which is causing it, such as bowel disturbance if the problem is irritable bowel, or heavy periods if the problem is fibroids.

• Causes •

Possible gynaecological explanations for this extremely common female complaint include pelvic inflammatory disease (PID), endometriosis, ovarian cysts, fibroids, pelvic congestion and, in rare cases, advanced malignancies of the cervix or ovaries.

However, it may also be caused by problems that have nothing directly to do with the pelvic organs at all, although they may be affected, such as irritable bowel syndrome and back problems.

Very severe persistent pain could be a sign of ectopic pregnancy or appendicitis. Sometimes, but not as often as some doctors like to suggest, pelvic pain may be a manifestation of a non–physical problem, such as psychological discomfort with sex or unhappiness in a relationship.

• Difficulties with diagnosis •

Because pelvic pain is likely to have other seemingly unrelated symptoms (and because other seemingly unrelated complaints may cause pelvic pain) it can often be hard to get the correct diagnosis. For example, pain during sex may be the only symptom of lower back pain but by doctors is more usually associated with PID, endometriosis and pelvic congestion.

Some conditions, such as endometriosis and sometimes PID, can only be confirmed by laparoscopy, so a clinical examination which reveals nothing wrong should not be taken as adequate reassurance if your pain still persists. Also, sometimes swabs taken to test for pelvic infections are taken incorrectly or the wrong organisms are tested for, so a negative result may not in fact be firm proof that infection is not the cause of the pain.

If you suffer from pelvic pain it is very important that you do all you can to help a doctor come to the correct diagnosis. Gynaecologists are only human and when they are running busy clinics may omit to ask one vital question when taking your history that would have set them on the right track. Volunteer as much information about your pain and any related symptoms as you can. Sometimes women are embarrassed to mention bowel problems such as diarrhoea or constipation or think they are not relevant, but this could be crucial in reaching a correct diagnosis.

Inevitably, there will be an element of trial and error if symptoms or tests do not clearly point to one condition. However, a full account of all related symptoms could save a woman undergoing unnecessarily invasive investigative procedures such as laparoscopy if not initially warranted.

• Be persistent •

Sadly, many doctors still aren't particularly interested in pelvic pain, preferring to dismiss it as related to periods or as psychological in origin. Many may not even have heard of severe pelvic congestion, for example, let alone know how to treat it. So you may not be referred to a specialist or given any real help. In these circumstances, it is important to insist on being referred if you know you have a problem that needs investigation.

It is also important to keep an eye on your own symptoms and carry on taking them seriously, even if you are given a diagnosis for your pain and you undergo treatment. A woman can have two conditions simultaneously, such as endometriosis and fibroids. It may even be that only one of these conditions is causing the pain but because the other is discovered by laparoscopy, naturally that is the condition which is treated, despite its being asymptomatic (causing no symptoms). Endometriosis, for example, can be asymptomatic even in seemingly severe cases.

The simple rule of thumb has to be that if your pain doesn't get better after treatment and you are not given a good reason why (the consequences of very severe PID, for example, may sometimes only be controllable by pain killers), go back and ask for further investigation.

• Pelvic congestion •

This is congestion in the pelvis created by enlarged pelvic veins. It can cause severe pelvic pain but is not very commonly recognised. It is, however, the most common cause of pain in the 70 per cent of women who, on investigation by laparoscopy for pelvic pain, are found to have perfectly normal pelvic organs.

Research into pelvic congestion has been pioneered by Professor Richard Beard of St Mary's Hospital in London who runs a clinic for women with unexplained pelvic pain. Women are referred from all over the UK, having already had investigations locally, and Professor Beard has found the majority of them to be suffering from pelvic congestion.

• Symptoms •

The pain is usually one-sided, depending upon the side on which ovulation occurs, but some women experience it as a general ache in the lower abdomen. You may find you have a background dull ache with acute flare-ups of great intensity, such as before a period or after having sex.

Standing for any length of time or walking usually make it worse. Or it may be triggered only when pressure is put on the affected side, for example when crossing your legs or when pressure is put on the ovaries during an internal examination. Once triggered, the pain may be excruciating.

Pain may, for some women, start during sex and be particularly strong at orgasm. Stressful times during your life may be the times when the pain is worse, although it is not always easy to make this association when pain is chronic.

• Causes •

If the veins are enlarged, they become slack, slowing down the circulation of blood in the pelvis and creating congestion and pain. Congestion is common before and around the start of a period but it is when the pain continues throughout the cycle that a diagnosis of pelvic congestion for chronic pelvic pain may be made.

Emotional stress appears to be involved in the problem as well. It is known and accepted that stress can affect the circulation, making the heart beat faster, for example, and pelvic circulation may sometimes be affected too. Women suffering from this condition are usually also found to have tiny cysts on their ovaries.

Simple activities such as standing, exercise or having sex may induce the congestion and bring on pain.

• Diagnosis •

Tests used to see whether the pelvic veins are enlarged are either a pelvic venogram (in which, under local anaesthetic, dye is injected into the veins in the pelvis which makes the veins show up clearly on X-rays) or, more usually now, an ultrasound scan. A laparoscopy is also usually required, for a good view of the uterus, ovaries and veins.

• Treatment •

Treatment with the progestogen Provera has so far been the most successful. In Professor Beard's studies, Provera taken every day for an initial four months improves symptoms in three-quarters of women. Usually during this time periods stop altogether but sometimes bleeding just becomes irregular. If the treatment is successful, women commonly continue taking the drug for several months and when they stop, find the pain does not necessarily return, or does not come back immediately and by no means as strongly as before.

Counselling is an important element of treatment to help women recognise the particular stresses that may be affecting them and worsening their pain (for example, exhaustion, money worries, relationship difficulties, etc), and to find effective ways to reduce the experience of pain when it occurs, such as by relaxing, doing something distracting and using mental strategies to prevent the pain from taking over.

Stronger hormone-suppressing drugs and also local surgical treatment of the ovary are currently under research to see if they might help the minority of women with pelvic congestion who are not helped by Provera and counselling. For those in severe pain for whom nothing is found to help, hysterectomy with removal of both ovaries may be the only remaining but drastic solution. It is, however, always a cure, but brings its own problems of premature menopause.

•Pelvic inflammatory disease (PID)•

Pelvic inflammatory disease (PID) is an overall term for a group of infections that may infect the uterus, the fallopian tubes and the ovaries and related pelvic structures. When it is the uterus which is affected, the specific diagnosis is endometritis; fallopian tube infection is salpingitis; ovarian infection is oophoritis; and combined tubal and ovarian infection is salpingoophoritis. The most common pelvic organs to be affected are the fallopian tubes. In very severe, undiagnosed cases, the infection can spread beyond the pelvis to tissues around the abdomen, appendix and liver.

PID is alarmingly common. It has been estimated, for example, that 15 per cent of all women born between 1945 and 1954 would have had symptomatic PID by the age of 30 and, as the incidence of this illness continues to rise, this figure is likely to rise too.

• Causes •

PID is almost always caused by micro-organisms ascending from the vagina and cervix and a number of infections have been implicated. Well over half of all cases of PID are caused by chlamydia or gonorrhoea, two sexually transmitted infections (see pages 373 and 377). Chlamydia, the most common sexually transmitted disease in the Western world, is more likely to account for PID in more affluent countries or areas; gonorrhoea in poorer parts.

Other micro-organisms can also be responsible, some of which, such as bacterial anaerobes and *Escherichia coli* (*E coli*), quite commonly live in the vagina or the gut without causing a problem. Sometimes, however, they may proliferate and cause problems in certain circumstances, or may be carried up to higher organs (where they can do harm) during surgical procedures such as IUD insertion, D&C, complicated childbirth or abortion. Very occasionally, PID can be caused by the organisms responsible for pneumonia or tuberculosis.

Although PID has not been treated with the seriousness it deserves by many gynaecologists and only now is the true extent of it becoming apparent, it is a potentially serious disease, causing infertility in a quarter of cases and increasing sevenfold the risk of ectopic pregnancy, a dangerous and even potentially fatal condition.

• Symptoms •

Symptoms vary from woman to woman and according to the level of infection. Any of the following might or might not occur:

- fever
- nausea
- vomiting
- aching back and legs
- abnormal vaginal discharge
- abnormal menstrual bleeding
- spotting between periods
- a need to urinate more often and a burning pain when doing so
- pain or bleeding during or after sex
- swollen abdomen
- dizziness
- depression
- fatigue
- weight gain or weight loss.

While some women have symptoms so sudden and severe that they end up in hospital, others may just feel slightly unwell in a way that is difficult to pin down. They may be aware of a dull ache in the pelvis which might be there all the time or just during sex or any physical activity.

There is clearly enormous variation in the experience of PID but one piece of research has shown that, after one attack of PID, about 80 per cent of women experience painfully heavy periods or irregular bleeding, 40 per cent suffer deep pain during sex – often severe enough to make sex an impossibility – and 20 per cent continue to have chronic pelvic pain.

• Acute and chronic infection •

Symptoms vary so much because infection may be acute or chronic. If there is an acute infection, a woman is likely to have a great deal of abdominal pain and a fever. When the infection is less than acute (sub-acute), there is a lower level of infection giving rise to less pain and perhaps no raised temperature at all.

However sub-acute PID may become acute at any time. Alternatively, it may become chronic, where the infection continues for years at a low level but sufficient to cause pain and damage to organs. Acute PID can also become chronic if not treated properly. Commonly too, women may appear to get over an episode of PID and feel well for a time only to find the problem occurring again and again.

• Who is at risk? •

You are particularly at risk if you have a number of sexual partners and don't use a barrier method of contraception. Even if you don't have more than one partner but your partner does, you are at increased risk, of course. There is always the possibility, too, that a partner may have had an infection, without symptoms, for years which is then passed on to you, however monogamous your relationship.

IUDs have been implicated in increasing the likelihood of PID, with most of this increased risk occurring within a few months of insertion, when any active and potentially problematic organisms present may be carried upwards to do damage. Infections can also ascend the threads of IUDs. There is less risk of this when threads are smooth rather than rough.

Surgical procedures or events such as miscarriage or childbirth are unlikely to be the direct cause of PID, but they increase the risk of any infection that is present in the vagina ascending. It isn't impossible that infection might be introduced at this stage, but it is unlikely because of the emphasis on creating sterile conditions for surgery.

• Diagnosis •

You are far more likely to get an accurate diagnosis, and it is likely to be quicker, if you go to a genito-urinary clinic rather than via your GP to a gynaecologist. Because there are no absolutely specific PID symptoms, apart from tenderness in the abdominal area, pelvic pain caused by PID may be confused with a number of other possible causes (see Pelvic Pain, page 231). A GP may not think of PID first and even some gynaecologists may not order further investigations.

There are genito-urinary clinics at most large hospitals and they have walk-in or appointment systems which do not require you to go through your GP. At genito-urinary clinics, swabs are taken to test for all sorts of possible agents, whereas a gynaecologist might possibly not take a swab at all, or take only a high vaginal swab that can show up a number of micro-organisms but not chlamydia, commonly responsible for PID. If chlamydia is to be detected, cells must be taken from the endocervical canal (the endocervix is the mucous membrane lining the neck of the womb).

The doctor will also do a manual examination: palpation of the abdomen is likely to cause pain if infection is present. Usually there is rebound tenderness: no pain when pressure is put on the abdomen but tenderness when it is removed. The doctor will look into the vagina via a speculum to see if pus cells show on the cervix, indicating active infection.

Negative results to tests are not, however, definite confirmation that you do not have PID. Sometimes organisms that are affecting the tubes or the uterus do not show up in cervical tests. If you are still having pain and any treatment you are given doesn't work, insist on being referred for a laparoscopy, so that your internal organs can be looked at. Certainly, any inflammation of the fallopian tubes will show up quite clearly during this procedure and specimens of any micro-organisms found in the tubes can be taken and tested, so that the specific causes of the infection can be identified. It may even become apparent that PID is not the correct diagnosis for you and that you have some other pelvic problem.

Laparoscopy is not always a complete answer, however, because PID in the form of endometritis (infection of the uterus) can be missed and so can very subtle fallopian-tube disease. There is even the risk that doing a laparoscopy could itself aggravate any existing and active infection. It may be suggested that antibiotics are given a try first.

• Treatment •

Antibiotics are used to treat PID infection. Amoxicillin, tetracycline and either metronidazole or clindamycin should take care of the various bacteria that may cause PID. If the offending micro-organisms haven't been tested for or haven't revealed themselves, it is a good idea to ask to take all of these drugs, and on-the-ball GPs do indeed prescribe them all at once. (You must finish all courses to gain the benefit.) However, a GP or gynaecologist not highly experienced with these infections might just prescribe one type of antibiotic and if this drug is the wrong one or insufficient, it could have the undesirable effect of damping down the infection but not curing it, opening the way to recurrent infections and more internal damage.

Unfortunately, if the infection has long been rife, even the correct antibiotics when finally given may not be able to reach the responsible micro-organisms because they are holed up too far away in the damaged tubes to be touched.

It is absolutely vital too that a partner is seen, tested and treated, otherwise any infection that he is passing on to you will be passed back yet again once your treatment stops.

Treatment of PID is almost always dealt with on an out-patient basis. However, if a woman has a very severe attack, particularly where there is the possibility of a surgical emergency, such as ectopic pregnancy or appendicitis or the suspicion of a pelvic abscess, treatment must be carried out in hospital. Sometimes a short hospital stay may be beneficial when PID is chronic, as there is sometimes a chance that antibiotics given intravenously can better fight a more resistant infection.

• Treating the consequences •

As well as treating any infection, any consequences of having had the infection for some time must be treated as well. In chronic PID there is likely to be damage to one or more organs for which the only treatment may be surgery. Sometimes removing one tube or one ovary is sufficient to deal with the infection. However, a big part of the problem may be adhesions, scar tissue which develops as the body's defence against infection. Adhesions are not painful in themselves but cause other organs to stick together. This is what causes the pain in chronic cases, even after infection is cleared.

A hysterectomy, with or without removal of both ovaries, may be suggested if a woman has had her family or is clearly going to be unable to have one; but this is drastic and may not even deal with all pain, although it will certainly lessen it.

To preserve fertility where possible, adhesions can be removed by laparoscopic surgery and, in suitable cases, tubes can be opened during laparoscopic surgery too.

What can be done depends upon where adhesions are and the extent of the damage. If adhesions are close to the bowel, a surgeon cannot take the risk of cutting the bowel. If adhesions are so severe that a lot of organs are stuck, surgery cannot be tried at all and the best help conventional medicine can offer is long-term pain killers. Pain clinics, which a number of hospitals have and to which a hospital doctor or GP can refer you, may be able to teach psychological techniques for coming to terms with pain, if the clinic is large enough to have a psychologist on the team.

• Self-help and prevention •

Go regularly for checks at a genito-urinary clinic if you have a number of sexual partners or if you or your partner have sex with anyone else. Do not use the IUD as your means of contraception if you or your partner are likely to have sex with others.

Be wary of any pelvic pains you might experience after having a surgical procedure such as D&C, insertion of an IUD or abortion, having a baby or experiencing a miscarriage. Even if you experience nagging pelvic symptoms that you consider only minor or intermittent and you can put up with them, this is the time to go to the genito-urinary clinic for testing. Take your partner with you for treatment too, if anything does show up.

If you suspect you may have PID but with symptoms not severe enough to warrant hospital, take care of yourself straight away. For any flare up, the PID Support Group (see Useful Contacts) emphasises the importance of rest, preferably bed rest, until you feel better, and not doing anything that might encourage the infection to spread further. Avoid penetrative sex, but masturbation to orgasm may be helpful because it increases blood flow to the pelvis and may help the body fight the infection. If that feels out of the question, a hot water bottle against your stomach will also increase pelvic blood flow and the body's ability to fight any localised infection. Eat as nutritiously as you can to keep your defences up. When you feel better, go for tests.

Try not to be ground down by any resistance you may meet from anyone in the medical profession who is less than helpful. Don't be fobbed off with course after course of antibiotics. If they are not working, they are the wrong ones or the diagnosis is wrong. After two or three courses at the most, demand further investigation such as laparoscopy. Keep on until someone takes you seriously. Negative findings, either in tests or by laparoscopy, don't necessarily rule out PID. Fortunately, thanks to the efforts of the PID support group and more enlightened thinking among doctors, PID is treated with more sympathy and understanding now.

If you have chronic PID that treatment, even the correct type, doesn't seem to help, try to keep your natural body defences up by ensuring you regularly get enough sleep, eat well and try to avoid more stress than you can comfortably cope with. Taking vitamin and mineral supplements may be beneficial and many women have found complementary therapies of different types useful.

• Support •

For the chance to talk to, share experiences with and/or seek advice from others who have suffered from PID but learned to cope, you might like to get in touch with the PID Support Group, a self-help network. It can be contacted through the charity Women's Health: see Useful Contacts.

• Endometriosis •

This is a very miserable condition which may in some form affect as many as one in ten women. When symptoms are severe, it can seriously disrupt a woman's working life and relationships and destroy her self-esteem and confidence. It can also impair fertility.

It is because endometriosis so often goes undiagnosed for years that the problems may become so serious. It is therefore important to insist on proper investigations if you think your symptoms may signal the presence of this condition.

• What is it? •

Endometriosis occurs when bits of the tissue that normally line the uterus (the endometrium) stray to other parts of the body and implant themselves there. Usually the stray tissue stays within the pelvic area, most commonly attaching itself to the outside of the uterus, the fallopian tubes and the ovaries. But it may also be found on the bladder or bowel and it is not unknown for the tissue to migrate much further. Endometriosis has been found in the lungs, the kidneys, the pancreas and even the eyes, amongst other places.

Although far from their normal home, these patches of tissue react to the hormones that govern the menstrual cycle in just the same way as normal endometrial tissue. They swell as oestrogen starts being produced in increasing quantities early on in the cycle, fill with blood and then may bleed a little at menstruation.

Inflammation commonly occurs around the patches and then scar tissue forms, a process which may be repeated every month until the build-up of scar tissue is so great that adhesions may form. This is when scar tissue sticks together organs that normally lie freely side by side. Sometimes large cysts form, particularly when endometriosis is on the ovaries, and these can disturb hormone balance and affect ovulation.

• Who is at risk? •

Endometriosis can affect any woman of any race at any time from the onset of menstruation until the menopause. There may be a hereditary element, as between 7 and 8 per cent of sufferers have a relative with the condition. Many gynaecologists don't expect to come across it until a woman is in her thirties, which means that the diagnosis may not even be considered in some teenagers and they certainly aren't usually offered the surgical investigation necessary for diagnosis. Understandably, no one wants to inflict what might be unnecessary surgery on someone so young but years of misery might, on the other hand, ensue as a result.

• Symptoms •

The most common symptoms are:

- pelvic pain, particularly a few days before a period
- pain during sex.

  Other common symptoms include:

- painful urination
- painful bowel movements
- back pain
- swollen abdomen
- pain at mid-cycle
- pain at any time during the menstrual cycle.

A major survey of sufferers carried out for the Endometriosis Society and published in 1994 found that 83 per cent of women were in pain during periods, nearly half of them very severely. Two-thirds had severe pain mid-cycle and up to 15 per cent experienced severe pain at other times during the cycle. Six out of ten suffered pain irregularly throughout the month. Nearly half suffered moderate to severe pain during sex (one in five women under 29 reported very severe pain during sex) and one-third experienced some pain at least some time during every single day.

Another highly important symptom, but one unlikely to be discovered until trying for pregnancy, is infertility. Fertility may be compromised in about 40 per cent of women with this condition.

The degree of pain can vary dramatically because endometriosis can be present in so many places in the body and because adhesions, once formed, will themselves cause pain, with or without the endometriosis. Where the endometriosis is, rather than how much there is, will tend to dictate the degree of pain. Huge cysts on the ovary may actually be painless whereas small patches of endometriosis, in places where pressure is put on them during sex, are likely to be excruciating. Some women, when being investigated for another condition are found to have extensive endometriosis that causes no symptoms at all. Others have fewer patches and more pain.

It was once thought that endometriosis, if found, should be treated anyway but now it is only defined as a disease if it causes symptoms, increases in amount or affects fertility in those who wish to become pregnant.

• Causes •

There are no certainties about the causes of endometriosis, only theories. The one which has probably been around longest is 'retrograde menstruation', which is actually something that happens to all women every month. The term refers to muscle spasms during a period which force a tiny amount of the menstrual flow containing the womb lining back up the fallopian tubes instead of downward and out. As the fallopian tubes are open at their other end, to catch eggs emerging from the ovaries, the bits of tissue may be routed towards the ovary or out and around the pelvic cavity to other organs where the tissue may become implanted.

It is suggested that, whereas normally this tissue disintegrates and is reabsorbed, in 10 per cent of women the implants are larger and remain in place, becoming endometriosis. Retrograde menstruation may be compounded by the fact that women now commonly have periods consistently every month for years, as we have the option to control our fertility and often don't choose to have a first pregnancy until later in reproductive life. However, this does not explain endometriosis in young women.

Another theory is that the stray endometrial tissue reaches other organs because it is carried there by lymph, a fluid present in all our tissues and which acts as a rubbish truck, collecting waste products and running them back to the depot (the lymph nodes) for disposal. Most recent interest has been directed towards the possibility of an immune deficiency in women with endometriosis, which might explain why only some women are susceptible to endometriosis from retrograde menstruation or endometrial cells circulating in the lymph.

It is even possible that endometriosis is an auto-immune disease, in which the body attacks some part of itself as if it were a foreign body.

• Effects •

The effects in terms of symptoms and possible infertility have already been described. However, the psychological and social effects can be pretty devastating too, if the illness is not satisfactorily treated. The Endometriosis Society survey found that three-quarters of sufferers felt the illness had severely disrupted their lives and that their ability to do everyday things such as drive, shop or complete ordinary household chores was affected.

One in five had had to stop work or had lost a job and a sixth of women were unable to work for more than 24 days in the previous year because of severe pain. Many felt forced to work part time because of pain and a third felt their work was adversely affected when they were in pain.

The illness commonly takes a huge toll on relationships, too. About 15 per cent of women surveyed felt it had ruined their relationship with a partner and nearly eight out of ten had had to stop having sex because of the pain (over eight out of ten young women found this). But a quarter, fortunately, found that having to cope with their illness had actually strengthened their relationship.

More than half of all women with severe endometriosis, according to the survey, are likely to avoid socialising or doing sports because of fear of pain, which can be as powerful a deterrent as pain itself.

• Diagnosis •

It is clearly vital to get a diagnosis for endometriosis as quickly as possible after symptoms start, so that much of the long term physical and psychological damage can be prevented. Sadly, a large number of women may be too embarrassed to tell their GPs that they are experiencing pain during sex, a symptom which should alert an aware doctor to the possibility of endometriosis, and a busy GP may not think to ask.

Even if a woman does mention her symptoms, there are still some GPs unsympathetic to gynaecological complaints who dismiss pelvic pain, particularly if related to the menstrual cycle, as normal period pain that a woman should be prepared to put up with.

The Endometriosis Society survey found, most alarmingly, that a quarter of women had suffered from endometriosis for more than ten years before they received a correct diagnosis. The average time between onset of symptoms and diagnosis was seven years. Fortunately, with more awareness on the part of both doctors and women, this should definitely be changing for the better.

However, it is important to be as comprehensive as possible when describing your symptoms so that you are sent for the right investigations. A GP whose questioning focuses on whether you have a bowel problem as well as pelvic pain rather than on whether you have pain during sex may well refer you to a gastroenterologist instead of a gynaecologist.

Your GP should give you a manual pelvic examination to check for anything out of the ordinary, such as enlarged ovaries or whether the uterus is in the right place (it may have been pushed backwards if it has become stuck to the bowel) but will not be able to say for sure, at that stage, whether you have endometriosis or not. So if your doctor gives you an internal examination or no examination at all and reassures you that nothing is abnormal, do not be reassured.

Endometriosis can, at present, only be diagnosed by laparoscopy (see page 218). It isn't, alas, a sure-fire way of coming to the correct diagnosis because endometriosis is not always easy to detect. It can be missed if patches are very small, if the surgeon is looking in the wrong place, if adhesions are obstructing vision or if a surgeon is looking for the wrong thing: endometriosis may look different at different stages of the disease, ranging from transparent blisters to red, brown or black areas with scarring.

Research into less-invasive methods of diagnosis has been going on for some years. Effort is mainly directed towards finding antibodies reliably produced by all women with endometriosis with the aim of then developing tests for them; or using known antibodies to locate the sites of endometriosis by injecting them into the bloodstream with radioactive markers that show up on special pictures.

• Drug treatments •

The aim of drug treatment is to stop a woman ovulating and menstruating for at least six months to give the patches of endometriosis a chance to shrink. Research has shown that pregnancy has a beneficial effect and often there is no recurrence of the disease after childbirth. However, as 40 per cent of women with endometriosis develop infertility problems, they have difficulty becoming pregnant even when they want to. Drug treatments are an artificial means of suppressing the menstrual cycle. Some women find they are able to become pregnant, if they want to, after a course of drug treatment.

The combined contraceptive pill Taking this pill, without stopping for a week's break that allows an artificial period, can help women with mild endometriosis (as long as they are not smokers, for whom the pill is not advised). A brand with a high level of progestogen (synthetic progesterone) is usually recommended because progestogen will oppose oestrogen's usual (and in this case unwanted) effect of starting to make the endometriotic tissue thicken. Breakthrough bleeding may be a problem, however, and many women find they still have their symptoms, which is why this method is only likely to help in mild cases.

Danazol This is, or has been, the most widely used drug in the treatment of endometriosis. It is an androgenic steroid, which has the effect of suppressing much of the pituitary gland's output of FSH (follicle-stimulating hormone) and LH (luteinising hormone), hormones which trigger the ovaries to start producing oestrogen. Danazol therefore stops ovulation and usually menstruation, although this depends on the dose.

An androgen is a male sex hormone. All women have some androgens but danazol contributes rather more than usual causing, as some of its most troublesome side-effects, the possibility of weight gain, acne, deepened voice (which may, very rarely, be permanent), and hirsutism. Because oestrogen levels are low when danazol is taken, the same side-effects that often accompany the menopause may occur, such as vaginal dryness, hot flushes and reduction in breast size, as well as an altered sex drive. A lower dose of danazol may reduce side-effects but will probably allow some breakthrough bleeding.

Very many women find the side-effects of danazol too unpleasant or depressing to tolerate. Others are so relieved to be freed from pain that they will more willingly put up with its consequences. Usually danazol is only given for six to nine months at a time, because of its side-effects, and it puts an end to pain in probably nine out of ten women who take it. The endometriosis may or may not recur after treatment.

Gestrinone   Another drug which has the same action as danazol is Gestrinone, which is taken twice a week instead of daily and may not have as many side-effects. It may not be as effective for many women, but could help some who do not find danazol helpful or who cannot tolerate it.

GNRH analogues   These are newer drugs which are as effective as danazol and which most women find easier to tolerate. They stop the pituitary gland from stimulating the ovaries at all, meaning that no oestrogen is produced. This effect, while good for endometriosis, is however the main drawback of these drugs, as lack of oestrogen may reduce bone density and increase risk of osteoporosis. They also may bring on all the other undesirable side-effects of the menopause: vaginal dryness, hot flushes, reduction in breast size, unpredictable emotions and loss of sex drive.

The main GNRH drugs are Goserelin and Leuprorelin, given as monthly injections of an implant under the skin, and Buserelin and Nafarelin, given in the form of nasal sprays. Women who take them may experience more menopausal side-effects than women who are taking danazol. Because of the osteoporosis risk these drugs should not be taken for more than six months. As with danazol, symptoms may or may not recur after stopping treatment.

Progestogens   These are usually only prescribed if danazol doesn't work or can't be tolerated. However, according to the few small studies which have been done on them, progestogens can be as effective as danazol. Progestogens may be given as pills, implants or in the form of the progestogen-releasing IUD (see page 412). The possible side-effects are fewer but include weight gain, breakthrough bleeding and breast discomfort.

• Surgical treatments •

Surgery is usually a second-line approach, for women whom drug treatments do not help. Minimally invasive surgery has now made it possible for patches of endometriosis to be cut or lasered away via a laparoscope. The method can also be used to divide the ligaments to the uterus, which helps reduce pain, and remove small cysts and simple adhesions. Surgery may often have to be repeated, however, because patches of endometriosis are easily missed or more develop.

In cases where laparoscopy is not possible (for example when cysts are large), a laparotomy may have to be done. This is a major operation in which the abdomen is opened and from which recovery may take several weeks. Sometimes, however, surgery is not possible at all because adhesions are too extensive or because the uterus is stuck to the bowel in such a way that removal of the adhesion risks damage to the bowel itself.

Many women are offered hysterectomies and, after years of agony, may gratefully accept in the belief that the surgery will cure them. However if the ovaries are not removed as well, oestrogen may continue to be produced and the problem will not be over at all. The Endometriosis Society survey found that 39 per cent of women who had hysterectomies for endometriosis still had some pain every day.

If hysterectomy is to be done, removal of the ovaries as well as the uterus is now thought by experts to be essential. However, this is a major operation, physically and emotionally, will bring on instant menopause of course, and is still not guaranteed to end pain, if the endometriosis has spread outside the pelvis. You should weigh up the consequences very carefully before opting for such a radical step and certainly should try everything else first.

The usual advice to women these days after removal of the uterus and ovaries is to take hormone replacement therapy (HRT), an oestrogen and progestogen formulation designed to prevent the dramatic drop in oestrogen that increases the risk of osteoporosis. However, HRT should not be given immediately after surgery to women with endometriosis as the oestrogen component is likely to keep any remaining endometriosis in other parts of the body still active. Experts advise waiting six to nine months before starting HRT, by which time the residual endometriosis should have shrunk away.

• Complementary therapies •

Many women who suffer from endometriosis have tried alternative remedies such as homoeopathy, herbalism and naturopathy and found they have helped. Some also swear by vitamin and mineral supplements. These can be taken alongside conventional treatment and may even help reduce some of the side-effects of strong hormone treatments. Most often vouched for are vitamin B_6 (which may reduce depression and irritability), selenium ACE (which may reduce pain and improve the immune system), evening primrose oil (to reduce pain) and dolomite (a compound of calcium and magnesium) to help reduce period cramping. Taking zinc can help to increase fertility, where zinc deficiency is a problem.

It's not a good idea to end up taking too much of anything, which may do more harm than good and will certainly be expensive. The Endometriosis Society can give good advice if you want to try these methods.

• Fibroids •

Fibroids are benign, solid tumours which can grow outside or inside the uterus and are sometimes referred to by doctors as myomas or leiomyomas. They may affect between a fifth and a quarter of all women by the age of 40. Black women are particularly susceptible to developing them, especially before they have had children.

Fibroids are not necessarily anything to be bothered about. Sometimes they are tiny, the size of a pea, and unless they cause any symptoms can safely be left in place; but sometimes they keep on growing and reach the size of an orange or become even larger. They can then get in the way of other organs (see page 247).

Fibroids tend to increase in size more quickly if you are pregnant or if you are taking an oestrogen-containing pill, such as the combined contraceptive pill or hormone replacement therapy (HRT). They also tend to shrink away after the menopause if women are not taking HRT, so there clearly appears to be a connection with oestrogen levels.

Fibroids that grow on the outside of the wall of the uterus are known as subserous fibroids and those growing inside are known as intramural fibroids. Some protrude from the lining of the uterus into the uterus (submucous fibroids) or hang from the uterus by stems (pedunculated fibroids).

• Symptoms •

Small individual fibroids don't usually produce any symptoms at all, which is why so many of us have them without even knowing it. Large fibroids or a collection of a lot of little ones most commonly make periods much heavier; it is usually the subserous and intramural type which have this effect. Sometimes increased blood loss can be so heavy and so prolonged that there is a high risk of anaemia developing. This is most likely the case with intramural fibroids. However, the abnormal bleeding which fibroids cause only occurs at the time of menstruation. If you know you have a fibroid and experience bleeding at any other time in the cycle, do not attribute this to the fibroid: seek investigation.

Another common symptom is increased pain during periods, perhaps caused by a fibroid-induced increase in the production of prostaglandin, the hormone responsible for causing cramps during periods and contractions during labour. Stronger abdominal pain is more likely caused by a fibroid growing so large that its blood supply can no longer meet its needs. The fibroid then withers and severe pain is experienced. A pedunculated fibroid twisting on its stem can also cause pain.

Other symptoms may be caused by the pressure of large fibroids on other organs. The most common are backache, swollen abdomen, heaviness in the abdomen, discomfort during sex, painful urination and constipation. These are unpleasant symptoms but not dangerous. Of serious concern, however, is a fibroid that starts to obstruct the flow of urine because it is pressing on the urethra, the tube that takes urine from the kidney to the bladder. If the fibroid is not treated, kidney damage may develop.

• Consequences •

Although fibroids don't necessarily affect fertility, sometimes subserous or submucous ones can obstruct the entry to the fallopian tubes, preventing eggs getting inside and travelling to the uterus. Some experts believe that even very small fibroids inside the uterus may interrupt blood flow to the endometrium, preventing it from thickening properly and becoming able to support a fertilised egg.

When pregnancy does occur, the presence of a large subserous fibroid may occasionally increase risk of miscarriage but most cause no problem at all. A very large fibroid that swells the uterus during pregnancy may sometimes trick it prematurely into labour.

In very rare cases a fibroid may become a malignant very fast-growing tumour of the smooth muscle in the uterus, known as a leiomyoma. It grows so fast that the uterus seems to swell up incredibly quickly. You should see your doctor at once in the unlikely event this should happen. A hysterectomy is the usual treatment.

• Diagnosis •

Fibroids that are not tiny can be felt by a doctor during routine pelvic examinations. They can also be detected on smear tests. You should have another check six months later, if you have no symptoms, but only if they start causing a problem or have grown considerably do any further steps need to be taken.

If fibroids are suspected from symptoms, their position and size can be clarified by an ultrasound test. If your symptoms are abnormal bleeding and nothing else especially indicates a fibroid, you are likely to be referred for a hysteroscopy (see page 219) or, failing that and less desirably, for dilatation and curettage (D&C, see page 219).

Even tiny fibroids can be seen during hysteroscopy and can be treated this way too whereas a D&C may miss small fibroids and thus not put an end to heavy bleeding.

• Treatment •

The least drastic surgical solution is a myomectomy, removal of the fibroids without removal of the uterus. The more drastic is hysterectomy.

Myomectomy is definitely favourite for women who still want to have children, although there is no guarantee that fibroids won't re-grow afterwards (at least 10 per cent do so).

Myomectomy has traditionally been a major operation, however, requiring a large abdominal incision and with a higher complication rate than hysterectomy. The main problems are heavy scarring and the formation of adhesions (see page 238) which in themselves may adversely affect fertility or increase the risk of miscarriage. Also, traditional myomectomy may weaken the uterine wall, with the effect that a Caesarean may be necessary at childbirth if a woman does become pregnant. Scarring and adhesions can cause backache and pain during sex.

Fortunately, the advent of telescopic surgery has removed a lot of these problems. Fibroids inside the uterus can be removed via the hysteroscope (page 219) and fibroids outside the uterus can be removed via the laparoscope (page 218). These methods may be suitable when fibroids are not too large and are even becoming more of an option for some larger fibroids because of drug treatments which can help shrink them first.

For a few months prior to surgery, you are given a drug called Goserelin which suppresses the menstrual cycle and starves the fibroid of oestrogen. This helps it to shrink and makes it easier to remove (but isn't a treatment in itself as the fibroid will grow again after you stop taking the drug, which cannot safely be taken for more than six months).

At surgery a hysteroscope is positioned via the vagina or a laparoscope is inserted through the abdomen. The surgeon can view the pelvis by one of these means while using tiny cutting instruments or a laser (inserted via tiny incisions in the abdomen) to remove the fibroids. The scarring is much reduced, you can go home a day later, resume normal life within a week or ten days and your chances of future pregnancy are much increased. This sort of surgery is becoming much more widely available for gynaecological conditions as more doctors learn the techniques.

A new option which requires no surgery at all is the progestogen-releasing IUD which both works as a contraceptive for a five year period and appears to shrink intramural fibroids. Over this period of time, the fibroid may disappear altogether and perhaps may not grow again. It may therefore be of great interest to many women not yet ready to start a family and reluctant to risk needing repeat surgery.

Some doctors may recommend hysterectomy if your family is complete, arguing that the problem is then dealt with once and for all. But hysterectomy brings with it all the problems of premature menopause and certainly should not be undertaken without careful consideration and preferably a second opinion. Bear in mind, if you are nearing the menopause and do not urgently need treatment, that fibroids should then shrink naturally. If the fibroids are enormous or there are other complications, hysterectomy may be the only viable option.

• Benign ovarian cysts •

It is quite common for a benign cyst to develop on the ovary, usually when a follicle has started developing at the beginning of the menstrual cycle, grows large but neither ruptures and releases an egg nor disintegrates. Most cysts fill with fluid; others become solid.

Many cysts cause no trouble at all and often just disappear of their own accord within a couple of menstrual cycles. Others grow and grow and can become a problem. They may twist and cut off the blood supply to the ovary. They can burst, emptying their contents into surrounding tissue which may then become inflamed. Peritonitis, inflammation of the lining of the abdominal cavity, is a particularly severe consequence, causing extreme abdominal pain and shock. A very small percentage of ovarian cysts may become malignant.

• Symptoms •

You can often have a cyst without knowing it. Your doctor may discover it during a routine pelvic examination and it will probably be worth waiting a couple of months to see if it disappears by itself. If a cyst does give you symptoms, however, these may be pain during sex, pain or discomfort in the abdomen, a swollen abdomen and disturbed menstrual cycle.

• Diagnosis and treatment •

A cyst can be confirmed by ultrasound scan. Gynaecologists are likely to want to remove what they find because of the problems they may cause.

A little cyst can be removed by the telescopic surgical technique, laparoscopy (see page 218). However, this is only done if the cyst is definitely benign because it is quite easy to burst a cyst during laparoscopy and then the contents, if malignant, will spread. Larger cysts or questionable cysts must be removed by laparotomy, in which access to the pelvis is gained via an incision made across the abdomen and the surgeon has more room to work. Tissue is taken for analysis to find whether the cyst is malignant or not.

• Polycystic ovarian syndrome (PCO) •

This is an enigmatic syndrome in which one or both ovaries are covered with multiple small cysts. Textbook symptoms of PCO include an irregular menstrual cycle or loss of periods altogether with consequent loss of fertility, hirsutism and obesity. (Hirsutism means excessive hairiness in areas usually relatively free of hair in females, such as the upper lip, tip of the nose, chin, cheeks, ear lobes, upper pubic triangle, chest, abdomen and thighs.)

However, polycystic ovaries have very commonly been found in women with hardly any or none of these symptoms. Less than half of women diagnosed with PCO are obese. And nine out of ten women with only slightly excess hair have been found to have polycystic ovaries. One study completely upset old thinking a few years ago when it was found that as many as a quarter of healthy women with no menstrual disturbances at all had polycystic ovaries. Ultrasound screening now reveals that at least one in five women has them.

It has now been suggested that polycystic ovaries may in fact be a variation of a normal state, as so many women have them. (However, the position may be complicated by a relatively recent finding that one in three women found to have polycystic ovaries has a sub-clinical eating disorder – a tendency to try to over-control their eating and to have periodic binges, but not to the extent of having full-blown anorexia or bulimia.)

• Causes •

PCO is thought to be caused by an imbalance in the levels of the hormones LH and FSH, produced by the pituitary to stimulate the ovaries. There is more LH and less FSH produced than in a normal menstrual cycle. The increased LH leads to a higher than average secretion from the ovaries of androgens (male sex hormones which all women produce a little of) while reduced FSH fails to trigger the normal steady increase of oestrogen. (Oestrogen levels appear to be raised early on in the cycle but are derived from the conversion of the male sex hormones and do not increase in amount.) No ovulation occurs and no period follows. The excess facial and body hair which may accompany PCO is caused by the excess circulating male hormones.

• Diagnosis and treatment •

The syndrome can be diagnosed by ultrasound or by testing for a raised LH:FSH ratio and raised testosterone levels. LH continues to be produced in excess and the syndrome is self-perpetuating unless treatment is given.

For women with hirsutism, the usual treatment is with the anti-androgen, cyproterone acetate, combined with an oestrogen to ensure regular menstrual bleeding. The contraceptive pill Dianette has this formulation and may be prescribed for women with severe hirsutism and acne. Anti-androgens are not usually given without an oestrogen as, should a pregnancy occur, a male foetus would develop with feminine characteristics. Treatment needs to continue for at least six months to a year because hair follicles are influenced by hormone levels in tissue rather than in blood and these do not drop so quickly.

Taking the combined contraceptive pill can sometimes be sufficient to suppress androgen secretion that is stimulated by LH levels. However some progestogens are themselves androgenic and need to be avoided. The progestogen desogestrel is not androgenic and is for this reason usually recommended for hirsutism, although it may not be specially effective.

If these methods fail to control the hirsutism, nasal sprays of GNRH analogues, which suppress the activity of the ovaries altogether, may be tried.

These cannot be used for longer than six months because they reduce bone density, increasing the risk of osteoporosis.

About 20 per cent of non-ovulating women with PCO who are over-weight have been found to be secreting insulin in too high amounts. This can affect the ovary, making periods irregular. (Interestingly, three out of four women with bulimia have been found, at ultrasound, to have polycystic ovaries. They too have high insulin levels, which rise to bring down blood sugar when carbohydrate is eaten but are left with nothing to act on if the carbohydrate is then vomited up.) High insulin also affects blood fats, reducing those that are protective against heart disease.

The best way to reduce the effects of insulin on the ovary is to lose weight and to exercise. One study has shown that women with polycystic ovaries who lose weight also start to lose excess hair but it may be a year before this effect is seen, for the reasons described above.

Women with PCO who want to become pregnant can very often be helped by drugs which either reduce prolactin levels if they are raised, stimulate ovulation or adjust the LH:FSH ratio. Another possible option is for a wedge to be cut out of the ovaries, which very often helps the ovaries to start ovulating normally .

• Polyps •

These are little overgrowths of tissue or glands on stalks that protrude from the uterus (endometrial polyps) or, less commonly, the cervix. Cervical polyps are like little thin tubes, red at the end where the skin covering may have been rubbed off. The main symptom in either case is bleeding, usually intermittent and often after sex with a cervical polyp, and after a period or mid-cycle with endometrial polyps. Commonly, however, there may be no symptoms at all. A cervical polyp may be discovered during a routine pelvic examination.

Treatment may not be necessary for small cervical polyps that don't cause any bother. If symptoms develop or if they start to increase in size they can easily be removed under local anaesthetic. The polyp is twisted off by its stem and a heated instrument applied to the base to seal it.

An endometrial polyp can be diagnosed by hysteroscope (see page 219). Removal can also be carried out via hysteroscopy. If this method is not available, a D&C can be carried out (see page 219).

Very rarely are polyps malignant, but as they may mimic a cancer or produce the same symptoms (abnormal bleeding) it is usual to take a tissue sample to check.

• Pelvic relaxation •

Pelvic relaxation or prolapse is the term used when the muscles of the pelvic floor become weakened and cannot hold the pelvic organs in place any more, with the result that one or more of these organs fall forward out of position.

The uterus is most often the organ to prolapse and this is known as a uterine prolapse or, colloquially, as a dropped womb. The uterus drops into the vagina and, when the prolapse is severe, may fall as far as the entrance to the vagina, with the cervix protruding. If the prolapse is extremely severe, almost the whole of the vagina may be turned outward. This sensitive, exposed tissue will then often ulcerate.

When the lower front wall of the vagina has become slack, the urethra bulges into it and the condition is known as a urethrocele. When the upper wall of the vagina is slack, the bladder bulges into it and this is known as a cystocele. Often the bladder and urethra prolapse together. If the rectal wall has been affected, the rectum may bulge into the vagina, a condition known as a rectocele. If the vagina's top half prolapses, doubling over and with loops of bowel involved, this is known as an enterocele.

• Symptoms •

You may feel a lot of backache or general discomfort in the abdomen and lower back. There will probably be a heaviness or dragging down sensation in the pelvic area which you are particularly aware of after exertion, standing a long time, coughing or straining to pass a motion.

Sex is likely to be uncomfortable or painful if the uterus has prolapsed. Sensation is affected when the vagina has stretched and, if you use the diaphragm as your form of contraceptive, you may suddenly find it will not stay in place any more.

The pressure of the prolapsed organ or organs may cause a leak of urine when you cough, laugh a lot or do any exercise. This is known as stress incontinence and does not happen at any other time. (Urine that dribbles constantly or any other urinary symptom has a different cause.) However, sometimes a prolapse has the opposite effect and it becomes more difficult to pass urine.

Needing to urinate more often indicates a prolapsed urethra and experiencing pain or a burning sensation during urination may point to a prolapsed bladder. When the rectum is severely prolapsed, straining to pass a motion puts considerable pressure on the vaginal wall which can be exquisitely uncomfortable.

Mild prolapses of any of these organs are quite common, however, particularly after the menopause, and may give rise to no symptoms at all.

• Causes •

Pregnancy and labour are the main causes of pelvic relaxation and prolapse, although the condition may in rare cases be congenital.

During pregnancy, hormones are produced to make the ligaments more stretchy (to ease labour when childbirth occurs) but this also has the effect of increasing risk of injury. The abdominal muscles are stretched during pregnancy and during labour all of the pelvic floor muscles are stretched, often with some accompanying injury to the nerves that supply the pelvic floor and the urethra.

It used to be believed that making a cut in the perineum (an episiotomy) during labour helped prevent tearing and subsequent pelvic relaxation and prolapse but there has never been any evidence to support this.

Straining to pass bowel motions puts more pressure on the relaxed pelvic floor and can add to any muscle and nerve injury, as can chronic coughing. Being overweight makes pressure on the pelvic floor worse.

After the menopause, hormonal changes affect muscle. All muscles start to lose strength as we age, particularly if not exercised.

• Prevention •

Fortunately muscle stretched in pregnancy and during childbirth can recover its shape and tone naturally, if exercised properly. Pelvic-floor exercises are essential for strengthening the pelvic floor before labour, helping it recover its strength after childbirth and keeping it in good functioning order thereafter. Physiotherapists who specialise in working with pregnant women and new mothers recommend at least 50 pelvic-floor exercises every day for life after childbirth.

These shouldn't be performed all in one go, as this would be too tiring and by the end you wouldn't be exerting much muscle power at all. Preferably to do them in blocks of five throughout the day whenever you think of them. It often helps to associate them with routine aspects of the day, such as cleaning your teeth, combing your hair, standing at a bus-stop, and to regularly perform them then.

Alas, most of us probably don't do any such thing and forget about pelvic floor muscles for ages at a time, if we do them at all. Not doing them is not an instant recipe for a prolapse, if your muscles are in relatively good shape. But doing them as often as you can remember certainly increases your chances of keeping them strong and effective.

• Pelvic floor exercises •

1 To establish which muscles you need to be exercising, try stopping your flow of urine once started. The muscles you use are the pelvic floor muscles. If you can stop the flow fully and instantly, you are in great shape. If not, you can quickly increase your abilities in this direction with some daily exercise and, even if your muscles are very weak, may expect to see some definite improvement within three months.

2 You may find it easiest to start with if you lie on your back to do these exercises, with your knees bent and your feet flat on the floor. As you get more practised, you can do them in any position.

3 Concentrate your mind on the opening to your vagina and pull up on the muscles, as if you are pulling something up into the vagina. You will probably find yourself tightening your buttocks as well but make sure you are also tightening the muscles around the front.

4 Hold the muscles for a slow count of five, then relax them gently.

5 Test your progress by inserting two fingers into the vagina and squeezing your pelvic floor muscles. You should be able to feel a tightening around your fingers. If you have a male sex partner, squeeze his penis with your pelvic floor muscles during sex and ask him to let you know if he feels it happening.

• Self-help for prolapse •

1 Start pelvic floor exercises (see above) immediately you notice a problem, if you haven't been doing them before. If the prolapse is mild, strengthening your pelvic floor may help enormously and prevent you from needing any other treatment.
2 Minimise discomfort by wearing a supportive girdle and avoiding standing for prolonged periods or over-exerting yourself.
3 Coughing a lot will add to strain and to stress incontinence. If your cough is a chronic smoker's cough, try to give up smoking.
4 If you are overweight, make a dedicated effort to lose some.
5 Wear panty liners or thicker pads, according to the degree of your stress incontinence. But avoid wearing these all the time, however, as constant friction between the pad and the vulva as well as the increased heat and moisture may lead to vaginal itch and discharge.
6 Eat plenty of high-fibre foods so that you can pass bowel motions without strain.

• Treatments •

If your main symptom is stress incontinence, be wary of operations to correct prolapses of the uterus or vagina, as these are not primarily intended to improve this condition and may in some instances make it worse.

If you are in considerable discomfort with a prolapse, the least drastic option is to have a ring pessary inserted. This is a small plastic ring which fits around the cervix and helps support the uterus. It needs to fit really properly to be of any use. Its main drawbacks are friction, resultant irritation and increased risk of infections. For this reason it can't be worn for very long at a time and it must be removed and cleansed frequently. It should also be reviewed and changed every four months.

A surgical repair may be possible, the nature of which will depend upon the type of the prolapse. For example, redundant vaginal tissue may be cut away, affected ligaments may be shortened and the uterus may be lifted and reattached. A repair, which is carried out through the vagina may be able to help a fallen bladder and rectum too.

Most drastic and least desirable is hysterectomy. Some doctors may suggest this rather quickly as a solution whereas in fact it is often not necessary and should only ever be carried out in the most severe of cases.

31

HYSTERECTOMY

HYSTERECTOMY is the removal of the uterus, with or without other of the reproductive organs. More than 65,000 hysterectomies are performed in England and Wales every year.

• Why is the operation done? •

Hysterectomy is carried out for a number of reasons, not always good ones. There are several potentially life-threatening conditions which hysterectomy is usually considered essential treatment for. These include:

- Invasive cancers of the reproductive organs.
- Severe, uncontrollable bleeding.
- Severe, uncontrollable pelvic infection.
- Very severe prolapse of the uterus.
- Conditions of the uterus affecting the bladder or intestines, to the extent that they threaten life.

Hysterectomy is often carried out in conditions which are not life-threatening but which severely affect quality of life. These include:

- Severe endometriosis.
- Large fibroids which are causing symptoms.
- Prolapse.
- Some precancerous conditions.
- Severe adhesions (where scar tissue makes pelvic organs stick together, causing pain).

• Are there alternatives? •

Yes. In many cases where hysterectomy is not life-threatening, there are other treatments or less drastic forms of surgery which ought to be tried first. (See the entries for the relevant gynaecological condition.) If your doctor does not suggest any, ask why. Some gynaecologists don't believe the uterus is worth having after childbearing years, or they believe that taking it out, and perhaps other pelvic organs with it, brings the benefit of preventing the development of cancer in these organs.

However, the undesirable consequences of losing the uterus and other pelvic organs may make the benefits of protection against comparatively rare cancers seem less attractive to the woman concerned. On the other hand, there may be very good reasons why alternatives are not suitable for your particular condition or for you in particular.

You need to be very clear that you understand why the operation is being suggested for you and to think what it means for you personally. Many women would take the risk of an alternative not working rather than go for a hysterectomy straight away, while others are made so miserable by their symptoms that they don't want to mess about with treatments that may not work for them and which may mean prolonging their agony and putting them through additional surgery or treatment.

If the reason you are advised to have a hysterectomy doesn't seem reasonable to you, don't be afraid to seek or ask for a second opinion.

• Types of hysterectomy •

There are a number of different operations which may be referred to by surgeons as a hysterectomy, even though most involve removing more than the womb. Most of them have rather daunting names, so you need to be clear about what each entails.

Sub-total or partial hysterectomy Removal of the body of the womb, leaving the cervix in place. This operation is not very common now, because the cervix is viewed as a potential site for cancer and the thinking is that it might as well be removed at the same time. However, the surgeon doesn't have to cut into and then stitch the vagina, and it is quicker to recover from. Also, many women find the cervix plays a part in their sexual arousal .

If you are advised to have a hysterectomy but do not want to lose your cervix, ask for it to be left in place. Unless a surgeon has very good reasons for wanting the cervix removed, your views should be respected. Regular cervical smears are recommended whether or not you keep your cervix after hysterectomy.

Total hysterectomy Removal of the uterus and cervix. The most common form of hysterectomy performed in this country and normally performed to treat large fibroids, prolapse or heavy menstrual bleeding.

Total hysterectomy with unilateral/bilateral salpingo-oophorectomy This is removal of the uterus, cervix, fallopian tubes and one or both ovaries. This operation is sometimes also referred to as pelvic clearance and is more usually done when a woman is past the menopause, or when the ovaries or fallopian tubes are affected by the condition for which the hysterectomy is being carried out: for example some cancers, very large fibroids, extensive endometriosis or pelvic inflammatory infection.

Radical or Wertheim's hysterectomy Removal of the uterus, cervix, fallopian tubes, ovaries and the top of the vagina as well as some lymph glands in the pelvis. It may be performed for cervical or endometrial cancer, according to its stage. This operation is also called pelvic clearance.

• The importance of ovaries •

If you do not have to lose your ovaries but a surgeon suggests removing them anyway, you need to think carefully about the pros and cons, as you perceive them.

Once you have your ovaries removed, you have entered the menopause, whatever your age. You will no longer have periods and you may experience the type of symptoms often associated with the menopause, such as hot flushes and vaginal dryness. Most importantly, your oestrogen levels will fall and your risk of osteoporosis and heart disease will increase. You can, of course, be prescribed hormone replacement therapy to make up for the oestrogen deficit, as long as there are no reasons why this would be unsuitable in your case.

If your ovaries are removed, there will be no risk of ovarian cancer or the development of benign but bothersome ovarian cysts and you will cease to suffer premenstrual symptoms, if previously you had them.

If you retain your ovaries, you should carry on ovulating and, as the female hormones oestrogen and progesterone carry on being produced, you will continue to suffer any premenstrual symptoms suffered previously. It will, of course, also still be possible for you to develop ovarian cancer or ovarian cysts.

Even if you do keep your ovaries, however, there is some evidence that they start to fail earlier after hysterectomy and sometimes symptoms of the menopause may begin to be experienced within two years of the uterus being removed.

The decision whether to keep your ovaries or have them removed may be a difficult one to make but you need to make very sure that you are involved in that decision. There have been cases where woman have gone into hospital for hysterectomies only to come round from the anaesthetic to find their ovaries gone too, and not necessarily for what they themselves considered compelling reasons. If you do not want your ovaries removed, write in large letters on your consent form something like 'I do not want my ovaries removed unless it is a matter of life and death'. Preferably, establish before the operation any conditions in which removal of the ovaries might be found to be wise, so that you can agree that your surgeon proceeds accordingly.

• Methods of hysterectomy •

There are three main methods by which hysterectomy can be performed.

Abdominal hysterectomy   This is the traditional method (and anything other than a sub-total or total hysterectomy has to be performed this way). An incision is made across the bikini line or, sometimes, vertically from the navel to just above the pubic bone. It takes longer to recover from a vertical cut. Whichever way, the scar is long and, it is to be hoped, thin.

Vaginal hysterectomy This method brings the benefit of an invisible scar, as the incision is made in the vagina and the uterus removed this way. There is little post-operative discomfort, a hospital stay of only a few days and full recovery occurs within days instead of weeks. However, it is more difficult to perform; not all gynaecologists do it; and it is not suitable for all types of hysterectomy. One disadvantage is that the vagina may be slightly shortened as a result.

Laparoscopically-assisted vaginal hysterectomy This relatively new procedure enables a vaginal hysterectomy to be performed for conditions which would normally have had to be treated by abdominal hysterectomy. A laparoscope (see page 218) is inserted into the abdomen below the navel. Using this to see the pelvis, the surgeon can then use tiny cutting instruments, introduced into the pelvis through three tiny cuts around the bikini line, to remove the uterus. Even hysterectomies to treat early cancers of the uterus, ovaries and endometrium can sometimes be carried out this way. Recovery time is equivalent to that for vaginal hysterectomy and scarring only marginally more.

However, although interest in laparoscopically-assisted surgery is growing, this method will not necessarily be widely available yet.

• Recovery •

After abdominal hysterectomy you are likely to be in hospital up to a week, but for only a couple of days after the other methods. Initially you will probably be given an intravenous drip and maybe a catheter for passing urine. You will be encouraged to get up and about after a day or two to get your circulation back to normal and reduce the risk of thrombosis (blood clots). Make sure you are given adequate pain relief. You will have some light vaginal bleeding or discharge for a few days. Your bowels will probably take a day or two to start functioning again.

After an abdominal hysterectomy, you will need to try to take things more easy than usual for several weeks, avoiding over-activity and heavy lifting. Call in all favours from friends and family beforehand (or set yourself up for a few!) so that help is organised for your return from hospital and some time afterwards. You can start to resume most normal activities – but gently – after about a month and should be back to normal after six or seven weeks, although expect to feel far more tired than usual. Doctors usually advise avoiding sex for six to eight weeks, until healing is complete.

If you have had your ovaries removed, you need to consider hormone replacement therapy (see page 446).

• Cervical smears •

You should continue to have cervical smears even if your cervix has been removed because precancers can develop in the vaginal skin in the area where the cervix used to be (the vaginal vault) or in the vagina itself. If your hysterectomy was for reasons other than a precancer or cancer, you should have a smear once every three years. If you did have a cancer or precancer you will probably be advised to have an annual smear.

• Feelings •

Many women are surprised to find they feel depressed or sad after hysterectomy, even if they thought they were prepared for it. Try to allow yourself any feelings you may have about losing the ability to reproduce or losing the organs associated with reproduction and therefore femininity. Although you will be just as much a woman as before, having and coping with such feelings, if they exist for you, is important for coming to terms with them.

There will be particular emotional pain, of course, if hysterectomy has put paid to your chances of ever having a family, should you have wanted one. You may find it helpful to contact a support group (see page 492).

You are likely to feel more positive about the operation (and recover from it more quickly both physically and psychologically) if you were fully involved in the decision to have it and felt it would be right for you. For very many women who have been plagued by painful or disabling symptoms for years, losing their uterus is experienced as a liberation and, far from feeling prematurely 'old' or de-sexed, they feel full of energy and and youthful zest again.

• Sex •

Sex may or may not be different afterwards. If symptoms have made sex a painful activity reluctantly engaged in, hysterectomy is likely to improve matters no end. However, there could be a reduction in desire and in ability to be aroused if you have had your ovaries removed (and are not on hormone replacement therapy). See Vaginal Dryness (page 260) for ways to improve vaginal lubrication. You may also experience some discomfort if your vagina has been made a little shorter as a result of vaginal hysterectomy. Scar tissue from either method may sometimes cause pain.

Some women may find it less easy to reach orgasm or to achieve the same depth of orgasm as before if their cervix has been removed. However, it may just be a while before full sensation is recovered in the pelvic region and sex is as good as before.

32

VAGINAL DRYNESS AND IRRITATIONS

VAGINAL dryness occurs when there is not enough moisture in the vagina to keep it comfortably lubricated. It is estimated to affect 5,000,000 women at any one time, 3,000,000 of them after the menopause and 1,000,000 after hysterectomy. The effect is not only discomfort and soreness during sex but also chafing, soreness and/or itching when walking or when wearing jeans or other clothing that is tight around the crotch and causes friction. Using a tampon during a period may be painful too. Vaginal dryness can develop for a number of reasons, the most common of which is lack of oestrogen and the medical term for which is atrophic vaginitis.

• The role of oestrogen •

Oestrogen, one of the female sex hormones produced by the ovaries, has an important part to play in keeping the vagina moist and healthy. Just before and at the beginning of a period oestrogen levels are at their lowest. Some women may notice that it is uncomfortable to insert a tampon at this time.

As the monthly cycle continues, oestrogen is produced in greater amounts which triggers the glands of the cervix to produce a watery mucus. At the time of ovulation vaginal mucus can be plentiful enough to seem like a vaginal discharge. The mucus thickens in the second half of the menstrual cycle when progesterone is dominant but oestrogen is still produced until a few days before a period. The vagina itself also secretes a mucus that is dictated by the balance of oestrogen and progesterone.

The moisture produced as a result of the presence of oestrogen is slightly acidic, creating conditions least conducive to harmful micro-organisms which can cause infection. So women whose vaginas are dry tend to be more prone to attacks of thrush and other vaginal infections.

• What causes insufficient oestrogen? •

There are a number of possible causes for lack of oestrogen.

The menopause By far the most common cause is the menopause, when ovaries stop producing oestrogen or produce very little. It is estimated that one in three women past the menopause experiences some degree of vaginal dryness. However, degrees of vaginal dryness may first be experienced some years before the menopause is complete. This is a transitional period known as the perimenopause, in which the oestrogen production is slowing down.

Premature menopause   This is caused when a pre-menopausal woman has a hysterectomy. If the ovaries are removed along with the uterus, the menopause occurs at once. However, even when only the uterus is removed the ovaries commonly tend to start failing within a few years and a premature menopause is still likely to occur.

Cancer treatments   Radiation or chemotherapy treatments used to treat cancer may lead to insufficiency of oestrogen if the treatment adversely affects the ovaries.

Stress and fatigue   Stress can actually affect the balance of a woman's hormones and prevent sufficient oestrogen production from being triggered. In these cases ovulation will not occur either. Also, both stress and fatigue can reduce levels of circulating oestrogen as well as the blood flow to the vagina that is necessary for the production of the natural secretions.

Drastic weight loss and over-exercise   Excessive weight loss and too much exercise interfere with oestrogen production and usually also lead to loss of periods. You do not have to be emaciated for loss of periods to occur, just a little too far below your natural body weight.

The pill   Versions of the contraceptive pill that are low in oestrogen may cause dryness because they suppress the production of natural oestrogen but replace it only with lesser amounts.

Childbirth   Oestrogen levels are well below their norm for about two months after giving birth and so are very likely to have an effect on vaginal secretions. Nearly half of women experience vaginal dryness after childbirth but may not realise the cause and assume that they are dry because they are too tired or too sore after stitches for sex.

Breast feeding   The low-oestrogen effect lasts longer in women who breast feed after childbirth.

• Other causes •

Lack of oestrogen is not the whole story. Other causes include:

Lack of desire   When a woman is sexually aroused, the lubrication of the vagina increases considerably and very quickly. If there is insufficient lubrication, and the cause is not inadequate oestrogen production, the likelihood is that you are not sexually aroused. This could be because a partner has proceeded to penetrative sex without adequate time for foreplay – a problem that may be resolved once diplomatically discussed – or it may be connected with your own attitude towards sex or your partner.

Women who are uncomfortable about sex, have had bad or painful past experiences or are nervous or embarrassed may not be able to achieve arousal very easily. Not feeling happy with the partner you are with can have the same effect. Perhaps the relationship is not good or perhaps there is some unresolved or unexpressed bad feeling about something a partner has or has not done (probably nothing to do with sex itself). Sometimes, women who feel guilty about having an affair may unconsciously express this through lack of lubrication.

Vaginal dryness caused by psychological or emotional difficulties cannot be resolved without the difficulty being dealt with or at least acknowledged first. In some cases, an open discussion with your partner may sufficiently clear the air and open the way to change; in others, sexual or marital counselling may be most helpful.

Drugs Taking antibiotics can kill off benign bacteria called lactobacilli which live in the vagina and which help to create the healthy, slightly acid nature of vaginal moisture. Antihistamines, found in hay-fever remedies, may also cause vaginal dryness and so may some other drugs, so, if you are taking anything on a regular basis and are suspicious, check with your doctor.

Chemical irritants Inappropriate use of antiseptics around the delicate skin of the vagina, chemicals in perfumed bath oils, bubble baths, soaps, the detergent underwear is washed in and even certain spermicides used with the condom may irritate the vagina, causing vaginitis.

Vaginal infections Some vaginal infections, such as thrush, can cause vaginal dryness despite the fact that there may be a lot of discharge caused by the infection. The discharge is actually an irritant that may make the skin around or in the vagina painfully dry and sore.

• Treatments •

If the cause is one which can be remedied, for example by getting an infection treated, changing to a contraceptive pill with a dosage more suitable for you or by facing psychological difficulties, obviously this should be your first way of solving the problem.

For vaginal dryness that is due to a temporary lack of oestrogen, perhaps occurring before a period or during a time of stress, a vaginal lubricant will probably be helpful. However, using something not specifically designed as a vaginal lubricant, such as a baby lotion or other kind of gel, is not a very good idea as it may contain chemicals which irritate the vagina, compounding rather than curing the problem and, if oil-based, may damage the rubber of condoms or diaphragms.

It is safer and more effective to buy one of the vaginal lubricants available over the counter in pharmacies. Take advice from your pharmacist about any new ones for which particular benefits are claimed. The most familiar name to most of us is probably KY Jelly. Another option is Senselle, more like a liquid and similar in consistency to natural secretions.

Replens is a gel which, as it name suggests, replenishes moisture, and it also maintains a natural level of protective vaginal acidity. It has to be inserted into the vagina two or three times a week for it to be effective and it is not cheap, so may be more attractive when oestrogen deficiency is long-term). Your doctor can also prescribe a topical oestrogen cream or pessaries if this is deemed appropriate.

If oestrogen deficiency is chronic, oestrogen creams or pessaries may still help but will not deal with the increased risk of osteoporosis which occurs when oestrogen levels are very low. Prior to the menopause, oestrogen-replacement therapy is an option. This is similar to hormone-replacement therapy and must be prescribed by your doctor. Hormone-replacement therapy is usually a good solution for women who have passed the menopause unless there are factors which make this unacceptable.

A recent addition to treatments is the oestrogen-delivering vaginal ring, brand name Estring (available on prescription), which is inserted into the upper third of the vagina and worn continuously for three months. In trials it caused significant beneficial changes in vaginal skin and acidity after 12 weeks of use.

Women who have had endometrial or breast cancer, which are oestrogen-sensitive, should not have oestrogen replacement or hormone replacement therapy. The over-the-counter remedy Replens (see above) can be very helpful, however, as it creates a layer of lasting moisture in the vagina if used regularly enough and combats all the symptoms of vaginal dryness.

• Pruritis vulvae (itchy vulva) •

This is a general term used for itchiness around the genitals. The itch may be caused by skin diseases (see Vulvodynia, page 264), threadworm or whipworm which primarily make the anus itchy but can affect the vulva as well.

When the vulva is dark red and swollen as well as itchy, this may be a sign of diabetes.

Dryness after the menopause, sensitivity to chemicals and vaginal and sexually transmitted infections can cause itching (see Vaginitis, below).

Vulval itchiness can sometimes be a manifestation of anxiety, sexual frustration or unhappiness in a sexual relationship.

It is sometimes the only symptom of the very rare cancer of the vulva.

• Vaginitis, vulvitis •

This is inflammation of the vagina or vulva which may be accompanied by itching or stinging or abnormal discharge. It often occurs after the menopause, when skin in this area is more dry due to loss of oestrogen, and may be termed *pruritis vulvae* (see above). However, a number of vaginal or sexually transmitted infections may be the cause (see page 357) or you could be sensitive to certain chemicals in talcs, bath oils, soaps, etc.

Another possible cause is a forgotten tampon or diaphragm which, once removed, resolves the problem. If, however, a bacterial infection has had a chance to take hold while the object was still inside, treatment with antibiotics may be needed.

• Vulvodynia •

A medical term which may be used to describe irritation and burning sensations in the vulval area. A genito-urinary clinic is the best place to go for diagnosis. The skin conditions psoriasis and eczema can be a cause and, once diagnosed, can be treated.

Also, two auto-immune conditions which affect the skin – *lichen planus* and *lichen sclerosis* – may be responsible. *Lichen planus* mainly causes burning pain and rawness in the vulval area and inside the vagina as well as an itchy rash. Spots may be violet initially but fade to brown. *Lichen sclerosis* mainly causes itch but some rawness and pain as well. Both usually respond to steroid cream.

As there is a very slight chance that lichen in the genital area can develop into a skin cancer (the slow-growing sort that starts as an ulcer or small growth, not melanoma), doctors recommend annual checks after treatment.

33

URINARY-TRACT INFECTIONS

WOMEN are particularly prone to urinary-tract infections because the opening to the urethra is so close to the openings to the vagina and anus. (The most common infection is cystitis: see page 266.) Harmful micro-organisms – or organisms which may be harmful when out of their natural habitat – may easily be wafted or even assisted from the vaginal and anal passages into the urethra (during sex or masturbation, for example, or by wiping from back to front after going to the toilet). Another reason that urinary infection occurs relatively commonly in women is the shortness of the urethral passage to the bladder – only about 4cm (1½in) – leaving the bladder rather easy prey for ascending infections.

The most common cause of urinary-tract infection is *Escherichia coli* (most usually described as *E coli*), a bacterium which normally lives in the lower intestines and causes no problem there.

Other bacteria that live in the lower intestines may also be implicated, and sexually transmitted organisms, such as trichomoniasis and chlamydia, can cause infection in the urethra and bladder as well as the vagina. This is quite likely to happen if symptoms of a vaginal infection include a copious vaginal discharge or if, in the case of the usually symptom-less chlamydia, there is simultaneous infection with another vaginal disorder that does cause a lot of discharge.

These examples apart, drinking plenty of water to make sure of a healthy regular flow of urine is usually sufficient to keep the bladder healthy. Pregnant women are particularly susceptible to urinary-tract infections, however, because pressure from the expanding uterus against the bladder prevents the bladder from emptying completely, leaving any bacteria in urine more chance to grow.

Another risky time is post-menopause, when the drop in oestrogen and reduced acidity of the vagina also gives bacterial infection more chance to take hold. Also, damage to the urethra from birth or any surgery involving catheterisation may increase your risk of getting one.

Sometimes a prolapse of the urethra or the bladder, where these organs fall forward out of their normal position because of weakness in the pelvic muscles, may precipitate infection.

The most serious possible complication of a urinary-tract infection is pyelonephritis, a serious infection of the kidney which may occur when infection has been undiagnosed or uncontrolled. The symptoms of acute pyelonephritis are high fever, lower back pain, pain in the groin and often the abdomen, shaking, nausea and vomiting. The pain tends to be constant rather than intermittent, is worse when you move and is focused in one place. Urgent treatment with antibiotics is required.

Sometimes chronic pyelonephritis can occur when urinary-tract infections are inadequately treated, keep recurring and are inadequately treated again. Although this is pretty uncommon nowadays, the end result can be kidney failure.

• Cystitis •

Cystitis is the most common urinary-tract infection suffered by women, with probably four out of five suffering at some time in their lives.

• Symptoms •

There is an increased urge to urinate at very frequent intervals and a burning pain when you do. Quite commonly there is blood in the urine. Sometimes the urge to urinate is uncontrollable; often the urge is still experienced strongly even when there is nothing left in the bladder.

Because of the burning pain usually felt when acidic urine comes into contact with the bruised skin around the opening to the urethra, cystitis may sometimes be mistaken for genital herpes. (Conversely, cystitis may sometimes be diagnosed when the real cause is genital herpes.) However cystitis is not a sexually transmitted disease.

• Causes •

The three main causes of cystitis are infection, bruising or an allergic reaction to certain chemicals.

E coli Infection is most commonly caused by bacteria called *Escherichia coli*, which live happily in the colon but cause cystitis when they transfer to the urethra and bladder. This may occur during sex, during a bad attack of diarrhoea or from the ill-advised practice of wiping from back to front after using the toilet. Also, some women's urinary tracts are unfortunately just more receptive than others to *E coli*.

Sexually transmitted diseases If you catch a sexually transmitted infection such as trichomoniasis, gonorrhoea or chlamydia, the culprit micro-organism can also easily be transferred to the urethra to cause the additional problem of cystitis.

Friction and bruising Friction and bruising are important causes of cystitis. Sex can set off cystitis, particularly if you haven't had it before or for some time or if you are dry. However, cystitis is by no means uncommon in women who have sex a lot, often because of the above reasons or because of having sex at times when your bladder may be full enough not to cause discomfort but to be more susceptible to bruising during sex. (Having sex with full bowels may lead to the same effect.)

Another possible cause of friction and bruising around the urethral opening is the wearing of very close-fitting jeans. Leggings are comfortable and don't feel tight but, as with tights, block air circulation to the vaginal and urethral area and help create a moist, warm atmosphere conducive to bacterial growth.

Diaphragm   If you use a diaphragm as your contraceptive method and are prone to cystitis, ensure that the fit of the diaphragm is not too tight, otherwise it will press on the bladder and, as the diaphragm must be left in place for some hours after sex, you will have several hours when full release of urine from the bladder is blocked. Also, diaphragm users are more at risk of infection from *E coli*.

Not passing urine   Not passing urine often enough gives infections such as *E coli* a greater chance to take hold, whereas in normal circumstances they might be flushed out in a good flow of urine. Reasons for holding on to urine, intentionally or otherwise, include the tight fitting diaphragm mentioned above, pregnancy (when the growing foetus presses against the bladder and prevents it from emptying completely), a prolapse of the bladder into the vagina, not drinking enough fluids and being too busy to go often enough.

Allergy to chemicals   Allergic reactions to chemicals in, for example, some spermicidal contraceptive foams and creams, perfumed soaps and bath oils, coloured dyes in underwear and harsh washing detergents, may precipitate cystitis in many women.

Childhood kidney infections   A history of childhood kidney infections will leave you more susceptible to cystitis as an adult.

Menopause   After the menopause all women are more vulnerable to infection with it, as hormone changes mean the vagina is less acidic and less able to protect against infections.

• Diagnosis and treatment •

If you have more than just an isolated attack of cystitis which resolves itself, it is important to get a diagnosis. This means providing a urine specimen. You may be asked to provide an early morning specimen because, with the lack of urine passed at night, there are likely to be plenty of bacteria getting well settled in. However, some doctors prefer urine from later in the day, as this is more representative of how much the bacteria are really the problem.

It is important to try to eliminate any contamination from the skin around the urethral, vaginal and anal openings where other bacteria may be lurking. Use an antiseptic wipe or a clean swab of gauze wetted with clean water to wipe around the openings. Use a different wipe for each. Then aim for a mid-stream sample of urine, which means not collecting the first flow that emerges and letting that wash away any remaining organisms that may have escaped your swipe.

Start collecting from halfway through in a clean container that has not contained anything medicinal or chemical before. Your sample will then be tested for presence of infection and cultures will be grown to identify the culprit bacteria.

Usually a course of antibiotics is sufficient to cure cystitis, as long as you take the full course as directed. Exactly which antibiotic is prescribed depends upon the cause of your cystitis. Sometimes, however, cystitis is persistent and then further investigations are necessary for a cause. These may include:

- Intravenous pyelogram (IVP) in which a safe dye that shows up on X-ray is injected into a vein.
- Cystoscopy, in which an instrument like a telescope is inserted, under anaesthetic, through the urethra to view the bladder;
- Cystogram, in which dye is inserted into the bladder until it is completely full and X-ray records what happens when the bladder empties. For example, an obstruction may show up or urine may flow back up to the kidneys instead of down and out, indicating a faulty valve where the urine-collecting tube meets the kidney. Treatment may involve surgery: for example, to repair a prolapse.

• Prevention •

Fortunately, there is quite a lot women can do to help prevent cystitis from recurring.

1 Always wipe from front to back after urinating or opening your bowels and wash your hands afterwards.

2 Drink at least eight glasses of water a day to keep your system flushed through. If cystitis is a particular problem for you, drink considerably more.

3 Urinate when you feel the need to. Don't put it off or hold on to it any longer than you can help.

4 Pass urine before and no more than 15 minutes after having sex, and also wash. Encourage your partner to wash his penis before sex. This will all help keep any potentially problematic bacteria away.

5 Never have sex when dry. Use a vaginal lubricant. You may find the rear entry position or prolonged use of it is not good for you because it puts pressure on the urethra and may cause bruising.

6 Avoid tight-fitting clothes or a tight-fitting diaphragm, if you use one. Wear cotton underwear, to help air circulate and make the groin less attractive to bacteria.

7 You may find it is better not to use tampons during a period, as these can also press on the urethra. Whether you use tampons or pads, change them at least every four to six hours so that bacteria do not collect there, where it is moist and warm.

8 Avoid all potentially irritating chemicals, whether in soaps, bath preparations, detergents, coloured dyes in underwear, or spermicides. Some women say they react even to the coloured dye in toilet paper.

9 Be aware that coffee, tea, alcohol, citrus-fruit drinks, cola drinks and spicy foods can irritate the urethra for many women. Equally, some other food or drink may quite possibly be a problem for you, as the effects on individuals vary. Make sure, however, that you have a good balanced diet and that you eat regularly, to make sure your immune system has as much ammunition as you can possibly give it to keep you healthy.

10 Many women have found that vitamin-C supplements help, but do not exceed 500mg of vitamin C a day because this may increase urinary-tract problems; 1000mg of vitamin C changes a low-dose combined contraceptive pill into a high-dose one, with all the accompanying risks of thrombosis, etc: see page 402.)

11 You could try making urine more alkaline at night-time by taking 5ml (1 tsp) bicarbonate of soda mixed in water in the evening.

12 Herbal remedies may help. One recommendation is yarrow infusion, to be drunk warm three times a day. Make it by pouring a cup of boiling water on to 5ml (1 tsp) of dried yarrow and leave it to infuse for 15 minutes before drinking.

13 Make a point of drinking cranberry juice every day. It has long been folk wisdom that this helps prevent cystitis, but its effectiveness has also been backed up by research findings.

14 If you suffer from cystitis quite a lot, read *Understanding Cystitis: a Complete Self-help Guide* by Angela Kilmartin, the undisputed expert on the subject and one-time serious sufferer (see Further Reading).

• Handling a cystitis attack •

This is Angela Kilmartin's recommended method for aborting an attack of cystitis in three hours.

1 As soon as you feel an attack coming on, drink a pint of water to help dilute the acidity of your urine and make it less painful to pass it. Take two pain killers if you need them.

2 Mix 5ml (1 tsp) bicarbonate of soda in a quarter of a glassful of diluted orange squash (never concentrated juice) and drink it. Bicarbonate of soda is alkaline. Do this once an hour in the next three hours, but not more often.

3 Have a cup of strong black coffee each hour. Because it will irritate the bladder (not desirable when you don't have an attack) it will act as a diuretic, speeding up your need to pass urine and helping flush out the problem bacteria.

4 Swab round your urethra with cotton wool moistened in clean water every time you urinate.

5 Throughout the three hours drink half a pint of liquid such as weak tea or diluted fruit squash every 20 minutes.

6 Lie down with two hot water bottles, one behind your back and one wrapped in a towel between your legs so that it soothes the urethra.

Another option to try instead is to buy from the pharmacy a cystitis treatment specially designed to have a similar effect to the above. One such is
Cymalon, sachets of granules which should be taken in a drink every eight
hours for 48 hours. The granules make the urine less acid and also act as a
diuretic.

• When to seek help •

Whichever remedy you try, if your urine is cloudy or contains blood after
the course is over, or if you have fever, pain in the back and abdomen and
feel nauseous or vomit, call your doctor.

Fever can signify a serious kidney infection, pyelonephritis, most often
caused when infection has failed to be diagnosed or be fully controlled. It
requires urgent treatment with antibiotics as otherwise it can cause permanent
kidney damage.

CERVICAL CONDITIONS

NON-CANCEROUS conditions that can affect the cervix are described in this section. For information about cancers affecting the reproductive organs, please see the next chapter, page 272.

• Cervical erosion •
(cervical eversion)

This is a condition in which the lining of the cervix swells and can be seen on the outside of the cervix. The word erosion gives the impression that some of the cervical cells have eroded away, whereas in fact they are perfectly normal, just turned outward. For this reason eversion (turned outward) is now becoming the preferred term.

Some women are born with a cervical eversion and it is a common development during pregnancy or if taking oral contraceptives.

Myth has it that cervical eversion may cause backache, deep pain during sex, pelvic pain generally and even cystitis. There is no evidence for any of this and none of these symptoms has been found more often in women with cervical eversion than in women with a normal cervix.

Because the cervical tissue is naturally mucus-producing, you may notice more of a vaginal discharge but this should not be of an irritating kind. You may also notice a little blood in discharge after sex because of friction against the delicate tissue. However, you don't need to do anything about cervical eversion, although you do need to be certain that increased discharge is not due to a vaginal or sexually transmitted infection, or that there is not some other reason for the bleeding.

• Cervicitis •

This is an inflammation of the cervix usually caused by vaginal or sexually transmitted infections (see pages 357) but sometimes of no known cause.

Usual symptoms are increased vaginal discharge and maybe pelvic pain, backache, pain during sex and increased need to urinate. If there is an infection, treatment will cure the condition. If there is no obvious cause but a lot of abnormal inflamed tissue, doctors may recommend its removal by laser therapy, cryosurgery (a freezing technique) or cauterisation (a technique using extreme heat).

If you do not have an infection and your symptoms are not thought worrying and do not trouble you too much, you may wish to try some self-help measures before thinking about other treatments. Vitamin E oil, applied directly to the cervix, may help healing.

CANCERS OF THE REPRODUCTIVE SYSTEM

THE SYMPTOMS, risk factors and conventional treatments for the various cancers that can develop in the pelvic organs are described in this section. For information about alternative approaches to cancer treatment and organisations to contact for more advice, please see the general section on cancer, page 453.

• Cervical cancer •

Cervical cancer is the seventh most common cancer in women, affecting over 4500 women each year in the UK. Around 1500 to 1600 women die of it each year. However, cervical cancer is one of the few cancers which can be diagnosed and treated at a precancerous stage. Nearly all the women who die from cervical cancer have never had a smear test, the screening method most commonly used to detect it. As the percentage of women aged between 20 and 65 who have smear tests rises, so the number of deaths is falling: by 15 per cent in the last decade.

Cervical cancer affects mainly older women. While there was a large increase in the number of women under 35 diagnosed with a particularly fast-growing form of the disease between 1960 and 1980, numbers have stabilised and cancers in this age group make up only 15 per cent of all cases.

• Who is most at risk? •

There are a number of risk factors for cervical cancer. Women who have sex at an early age, when the cervix is not yet mature, are at higher risk. Starting from 21 and working backwards, risk increases the earlier a young woman has sex.

Women who have genital warts (human papilloma virus or HPV) are at increased risk, although it is unlikely that having genital warts is sufficient to cause the disease. There are four kinds of genital warts, known as HPV: labelled 6, 11, 16 and 18. Both 6 and 11 appear to be lower risk and 16 and 18 high risk. Genital warts are sexually transmitted (see page 371). The genital herpes virus was also once thought to increase risk, but it now seems that this virus is much less implicated, if at all, than the wart virus.

Smoking is an important risk factor because it lowers special immune cells in the cervix, making it more vulnerable to attack by the genital wart virus. The more a woman smokes, the more damage is done.

Women with low blood levels of folic acid may also be at increased risk, especially if they have other risk factors. American research found that women are at five times the normal risk if they have low folic-acid levels and genital warts, at twice the risk if they smoke, and at three times the risk if they are on the contraceptive pill. However, these particular figures are contentious, especially as the pill's connection with cervical cancer is hotly debated but thought to be minimal.

• Prevention •

1 Have a regular smear test (see next page). Women between the ages of 20 and 64 who have ever been sexually active should attend a GP surgery or family planning clinic for a smear at least every five years, preferably every three. How often you receive a smear will probably depend upon practice in your GP surgery.

   You should be invited by letter to attend for your smear but if the system breaks down and the requisite number of years has passed until your next is due, phone the surgery yourself to make an appointment. Keep up smears even if you are no longer sexually active because this cancer can very often take ten years or more to grow. Also smears can pick up certain cancers which are not associated with sexual activity, such as adenocarcinomas of the cervical canal; relatively rare but more commonly found in women over 60. If you have or had genital warts, an annual smear is recommended.

2 If you have casual relationships, even just occasionally, use a condom to protect yourself against genital warts.

3 Use a barrier form of contraception even if you are in a monogamous relationship; if your partner is not monogamous; or you suspect he might not be.

4 Try to give up smoking if necessary. Cut down if you can't because risk increases according to how many cigarettes you smoke a day.

5 Make sure your diet contains plenty of fruits and vegetables, particularly of orange, yellow and green colours. These contain beta carotene, which is thought to be protective. So too is vitamin C, found richly in citrus fruits, and vitamin E. Green leafy vegetables are also a good source of folic acid, as are nuts, pulses, yeast extract and wheatgerm.

• Having a smear test •

A smear may be carried out by your GP or by a nurse, if she has been trained to do it. You will be asked to remove your underclothes and lie on your back on a day bed with your knees bent and apart. To see into the vagina, the doctor or nurse must insert an instrument called a speculum which gently pushes the walls of the vagina apart (see page 217). Next, a wooden or plastic spatula or a special brush is passed through the speculum and wiped across the cervix to scrape off a few cells. You may feel this a little, but it is just like a little nip.

It is very important that cells are collected from the right place in the cervix, otherwise the smear will be useless and you will have to attend for another one.

It helps, therefore, if you relax as much as possible, to make the task easier. Once the cells are collected, the speculum is withdrawn and the smear is over. It all takes a matter of minutes. The sample of cells is sent away for examination in a laboratory under a microscope and you should be told – or enquire – when you are likely to get the results. Even if you are told that you will be notified, if more time elapses than you were led to expect, ring the surgery yourself to check whether results are in yet. Don't assume that if you hear nothing, all is well. Probably, all is indeed well but you cannot take the risk of it not being well and your not being informed because of an administrative error.

It is possible that you might receive a letter asking you to attend for a repeat smear. This is not necessarily because anything is wrong but because the smear taken was inadequate in some way and could not be read.

• Are smear tests really any use? •

Every so often the newspapers are full of scandals surrounding smears. A doctor or nurse has been found to be using the wrong technique or taking cells from the wrong place; administrative error means that a whole county of women has to be recalled for repeat smears; laboratory cutbacks mean too few staff are struggling to read too many smears, leading to increased human error, etc.

The smear test is far from perfect and better techniques are being devised (see below) but at present it is the screening method in most common use and it does mostly work. Statistics show that women who have never had a smear are most likely to develop cervical cancer. Regular tests are likely to show up precancerous changes at a time when they can be treated easily and be completely cured. Government figures released in 1994 showed that eight out of ten women between the ages of 20 and 64 had had at least one smear taken, and that the death rate from cervical cancer is dropping (from 2000 a year a few years ago to just over 1500.)

• New advances to detect cervical cancer •

Other, perhaps better, methods being developed for detecting cervical cancer cells include the Polarprobe, a pen-sized probe developed in Australia which can identify malignant and pre-malignant cells, and can be carried out instead of a smear by a GP. Once inserted into the vagina, the probe beams out light and an electrical charge at the cervix. It takes a minute to scan the whole cervix and results are instant. No cells need to be collected and no laboratory is involved. The inventors say the technology could even be incorporated into a computer chip for the GP to wear on a finger, eliminating the need even for a speculum. The probe is currently on trial in the UK.

Also under investigation is a staining technique which, with the aid of a computer, should mean easier detection of malignant and pre-malignant cells in samples collected via smears. This would cut down on laboratory error but obviously a smear would still be necessary.

A technique which caused some excitement a few years ago is called cervicography, a method of photographing the cervix. However, it has a high false-positive rate and has to be backed up by a smear, so is unlikely ever to be widely used.

• Results of your smear test •

Smear test results are usually described as positive or negative. A negative result means that nothing unusual was found and your cervix is normal. A positive result means that there is some change in the appearance of the cervical cells. This could be extremely minor through to major. Most abnormalities are minor.

If the abnormality is extremely minor, it will usually be termed 'borderline' or 'inflammatory'. In these cases, the cervical changes are very often caused by some vaginal infection present, such as thrush, bacterial vaginosis or trichomoniasis. If the organism can be identified just from the smear, the laboratory will identify it and you will be offered treatment by your GP. If it cannot be identified, you would be wise to attend a genito-urinary clinic for a check so that the infection can be correctly diagnosed. Any cell changes revert to normal after treatment.

Inflammation may be interpreted as a negative smear by some doctors and you may not be told about the inflammatory bit; but you need to know, so that you can get checked for infection or just keep an eye on things. Sometimes a laboratory may describe changes as inflammatory or borderline when another laboratory would have termed them CIN 1 (see below). It is wise, therefore, even if told your result is negative, to ask whether any inflammation was present.

If the cervical cells have undergone precancerous changes, this is known as cervical intra-epithelial neoplasia or CIN. There are three grades of CIN: CIN 1 being mild changes, CIN 2 moderate and CIN 3 severe, although all are precancerous. Instead of CIN, some doctors may use the terms mild dyskaryosis, moderate dyskaryosis and severe dyskaryosis.

• What happens next? •

There are over 300,000 abnormal smears reported each year in the UK. This is where there is some controversy. At present, if your result is borderline or CIN 1, normal practice is to invite you to attend for a repeat smear in six months' time and at six-monthly intervals for a while, if the result stays the same. No further investigations are usually arranged at this stage because some research has shown that half of all mildly abnormal smears revert to normal by themselves within two years and therefore enormous numbers of women would be subjected to the trauma of further investigation and perhaps even treatment for nothing.

However, more recent research studies carried out in London and Aberdeen have found that mildly abnormal smears are not likely to revert to normal in the majority of cases at all and that eventually, most women with this result will eventually need to be investigated and treated. There may, of course, be more research reported in due course which reverses this finding again but there is, in some experts' minds, a definite case for reviewing current procedure and, should resources allow, referring women for investigation after just one abnormal smear.

If the result is CIN 2, some doctors will refer you immediately for further investigation and others will carry on with the six-monthly smear monitoring, to see what happens. If the result is CIN 3, you will be referred immediately for further investigation.

• Further investigation •

If investigation is thought necessary, the next step is usually colposcopy which is carried out by a gynaecologist at an out-patient clinic (see page 220). You lie on your back on the colposcopy couch with your underclothes removed and your knees bent and apart. A speculum is inserted to hold the vagina walls apart and the cervix is wiped with a piece of cotton wool soaked in an acid solution that has the effect of staining the abnormal areas of the cervix and making them show up well as they are viewed via the colposcope.

If any abnormality is seen, a tiny piece of tissue is taken to be sent for examination in the laboratory. This is called a biopsy. You may feel a sudden brief pain, or nothing at all, as the tissue is taken. The whole process takes no more than 15 minutes but it may be a week or so before the results of the biopsy are ready.

Colposcopy is a very effective means of examination and usually the doctor will have an idea of the treatment you are likely to need, even before the biopsy results are back.

Many women find the idea of colposcopy alarming and therefore may find it hard to relax, particularly as they are going to be anxious about the outcome. You may like to bring a friend with you to the appointment, so that you have someone to be with afterwards. You may feel a little sore and you are likely to bleed a little.

• Cone biopsy •

Occasionally, if the abnormal area extends further into the cervical canal than the doctor can see, colposcopy is not sufficient and a cone biopsy has to be carried out in order to be sure of where the abnormality ends. This is a hospital in-patient procedure, carried out under general anaesthetic. As the name implies, a cone of tissue is taken from the cervix for examination. Before colposcopy became widely available, it was the routine means of investigating abnormal cells.

After a cone biopsy you will probably feel period-like cramps for a day and experience some bleeding for a few days afterwards. Usually, however, the operation is sufficient to cure any problem that is found and no further treatment is needed. One drawback, however, is that sometimes the outside opening to the cervix may become rather tight after this operation, causing periods to be painful.

• Treatment of precancerous cells •

If you are found to have precancerous cells in the cervix, you are likely to be treated however mild the cell changes are, although some gynaecologists may suggest a wait-and-see policy.

The treatments most often used to treat pre-cancer are:

- Laser (which destroys cells).
- Large-loop diathermy (burns away cells).
- Cryosurgery (freezing the cells).

Two other treatments based on burning may sometimes be used, but less commonly: hot wire or electrodiathermy and cold coagulation (not cold at all but less hot).

Laser treatment This is carried out under local anaesthetic by a laser attached to a colposcope and takes about five minutes. The laser destroys the abnormal cells. You may feel a mild cramping period sort of pain.

Large-loop diathermy A high-frequency electric current is passed through a large loop which is used to shave off the abnormal cells. The procedure takes a couples of minutes under local anaesthetic and is often carried out at the same time as colposcopy, originally as a further form of investigation, but now commonly as a treatment in mild cases because it is so cheap. You may have a period-type pain and some bleeding afterwards.

Cryosurgery A long instrument called a cryoprobe is inserted into the vagina so that the tip is on the cervix. Attached to the cryoprobe is a pressurised supply of carbon dioxide or nitrous oxide which becomes extremely cold when released on to the cervix. The affected area of the cervix is frozen in this way for a few minutes and then, after thawing out, the process is repeated for another few minutes. No anaesthetic is required because the freezing is anaesthetic enough, but you might feel a mild period type of pain. Two separate treatments may sometimes be necessary.

Hot wire and electrodiathermy Very very high temperatures are used to burn the abnormal cells away with wires or electrodes and so this procedure has to be carried out under general anaesthetic. There is no pain, of course, but you may feel after effects from the anaesthetic, although a very mild short-acting one is used. Afterwards, you may have a bloody discharge for up to four weeks.

Cold coagulation Similar to hot wire or electrodiathermy but with only a fraction of the heat. It takes a few minutes only and no anaesthetic is needed, although you may experience period-type pain. Afterwards you are likely to have a bloody discharge for up to four weeks. This method is more often used to treat CIN 1 and CIN 2, rather than CIN 3.

Whichever treatment is used, you will be advised to avoid using a tampon or having sex for some weeks, until the cervix has completely healed. For some precancers, cone biopsy, carried out for investigation purposes, may also be the treatment.

Sometimes a hysterectomy is recommended for precancer if a woman has other problems such as large fibroids or painful periods and has had or does not want a family.

• Feelings after treatment •

If you have one of the quick out-patient treatments, you may feel that you should be able to get up, go away and carry on as normal. But you will almost certainly feel quite shaky and should have someone with you to accompany you home. Many women also find having the treatment quite emotionally draining. There may be a range of reactions, such as feeling angry, invaded or embarrassed or even ashamed and guilty (perhaps over having had an affair or many sexual partners in the past).

Whatever treatment is given, some women have difficulty at first adjusting to what may seem a sexual assault or they may feel they are somehow changed sexually or as a woman. Depression is not uncommon for a while and desire for sex may be decreased for some months in such circumstances. Relationships may suffer in some cases.

It helps to acknowledge these feelings if you have them and to talk about them to someone you trust or to a professional counsellor at one of the cancer charities.

• Spread of cervical cancer •

Abnormal cells, if not detected by a smear, can start to spread beyond the cervix and this is when the actual term of cervical cancer starts to be used. Caught at an early stage they may only have spread into the uterus (stage 1). By stage 2, there is a spread slightly beyond the uterus. At stage 3 the spread is further into the pelvis and at stage 4 other organs in the body are affected. Some cancers spread more quickly than others. They also tend to spread more quickly in younger rather than older women.

• Symptoms •

Very commonly, with early cervical cancer, there are no symptoms at all. At a more advanced stage there is likely to be bleeding after sex or between periods and a vaginal discharge, but these may more commonly be symptoms of other far less serious disorders. Always, however, check out any abnormal bleeding or discharge.

• Treatment •

This will vary according to where the cancer is and how far it has spread and to find this out tests, such as X-rays of various organs, may have to be performed. If spread is minimal a cone biopsy may be sufficient treatment in some cases (see page 276) but more usually a hysterectomy will be advised, unless a woman still wants to have children. When a hysterectomy is carried out the pelvic lymph nodes are usually removed too but ovaries are left in place, if a woman has not yet reached the menopause.

Radiotherapy, given externally or internally, may be prescribed in more advanced cases or for more elderly women. For external radiotherapy, a woman attends the radiotherapy department as an out-patient and receives a calculated dose of radiation delivered daily by machine (except at weekends) for a few weeks. For internal radiotherapy, a radioactive rod is inserted into the vagina and the uterus and left in place for a few days. During this time the patient must be cared for in a separate room and visitors cannot stay long, for their own protection. Pregnant women and children may not visit at all. After the rods are removed, all radioactivity is gone and there is no risk to anyone.

Unfortunately radiotherapy is not without side-effects, as other organs such as the bladder and bowel may be slightly damaged, however well shielded during the treatment. After effects may be pain on urinating and a tendency towards diarrhoea or constipation, but these are usually temporary. The vagina can be adversely affected by the radiation too, shrinking and becoming less elastic.

The success of treatments for cervical cancer varies considerably, according to the extent of the cancer.

• Ovarian cancer •

Ovarian cancer is the fifth most common cancer in women, with more women diagnosed as suffering it each year than are diagnosed with cervical cancer. It also kills more women than all other gynaecological cancers combined. Tragically, because it is a mainly silent disease it is diagnosed late when treatment successes are fewer. Of 5000 new cases diagnosed each year in the UK, over 4000 women die. However, real advances are now being made in screening for early disease.

• Who is most at risk? •

Ovarian cancer mainly affects women over the age of 40, with 90 per cent occurring after the age of 45 and most usually after the menopause. Women in Northern Europe, Western Europe and North America are more likely to suffer it than Indian, Japanese and Chinese women, suggesting that environment and/or diet may play some part.

Although most women who develop ovarian cancer are well past their menopause, there is a different type which can affect women at any age and is most common (although altogether extremely rare) in young women aged 15 to 19. This kind of cancer arises in germ cells, any embryonic cells that have the potential to develop into eggs, and is known as a germ-cell tumour (GCT). Happily, it has a very high cure rate. GCT accounts for just 1 to 2 per cent of ovarian cancers.

In general, women who have most periods are at greatest risk of ovarian cancer. There are higher rates among women who have never been pregnant, whether through infertility or choice, whereas the more pregnancies a woman has the more protected she appears to be from this particular cancer. Also, those women who use the contraceptive pill for some appreciable period, who start menstruating late and reach menopause earlier or are sterilised appear to be less likely to suffer it.

Factors which have been associated with ovarian cancer but for which there is no conclusive evidence include obesity and using talcum powder in the genital region.

There is a small hereditary factor, with 5 to 10 per cent of women with ovarian cancer having a family member with it. You are at three times the usual risk if you have a mother, sister or daughter (known as first degree relatives) who developed ovarian cancer before the menopause. Anyone who has two first-degree relatives who developed the disease before menopause is estimated to have a one in three chance of developing it herself. This is the highest risk group, accounting for about 1 per cent of all ovarian cancers (about 50 each year). Fortunately, screening is now available for highest-risk women.

Women who have had breast cancer are at double the normal risk of developing ovarian cancer, while women with ovarian cancer are at three to four times the risk of developing breast cancer. Also, women with blood group A may be at higher risk: they have featured more often than average among ovarian cancer sufferers.

• Causes •

There is no certainty about causes of ovarian cancer but the menstrual cycle would appear to be implicated, as women whose monthly cycle is suppressed (such as during pregnancies or by the contraceptive pill) have lower rates of this cancer. Women who are infertile or who have a late menopause are exposed to many more monthly cycles and this may be one factor which increases susceptibility.

As women from different parts of the world have differing rates of ovarian cancer, with Western women most commonly affected, environmental factors may play a part. So too may the Western diet. Although no specific foods have been linked with ovarian cancer, there is a connection between ovarian and breast cancer, and high intake of animal fats is thought to be a possible risk factor for breast cancer.

• Symptoms •

Unfortunately, it is very unusual for a woman to have symptoms in the early stages. Most early cases are diagnosed in routine examinations or because of investigations for vague symptoms such as pelvic pain or swelling in the abdomen that are more often associated with other gynaecological conditions. The most common symptom is abdominal swelling. Other symptoms which may occur later include weight loss, nausea, change in bowel and urination habits, sometimes shortness of breath caused by fluid in the lungs and, rarely, abnormal vaginal bleeding. However, often there is no pain or discomfort at all until late stages.

• Diagnosis •

A suspected ovarian tumour will probably be confirmed by ultrasound scan, chest X-ray and blood tests plus an analysis of any lung or abdominal fluid that accumulates. Surgery is then necessary to establish the nature of the tumour and its spread.

• Treatment •

If the growth of the tumour is limited to one or both ovaries (stage 1), or has spread from the ovaries but is still inside the pelvis (stage 2), surgery alone can be an effective treatment, with up to 70 per cent of women surviving at least five years. However, the cancer is found at these stages in only 10 to 15 per cent of women with ovarian cancer.

If the cancer has spread to the abdomen (but not the liver) it is referred to as a stage 3 cancer. Stage 4 is when it has spread to the liver and other organs. For these late-stage cancers, chemotherapy is the mainstay of treatment after extensive surgery has removed as much of the cancer as possible. Radiotherapy is not commonly used because of the need, in this type of cancer, to irradiate the whole of the abdominal area.

First-line chemotherapy is a drug containing platinum, such as cisplatin, with or without other cancer-killing drugs. At least 70 per cent of women treated with it improve initially and 20 per cent may survive ten years or more. But the tumour does tend to recur. In this event a second course of platinum is given, which reduces the tumour size in over half of women whose disease has recurred more than two years after first treatment and in a quarter whose recurrence was within a year.

Women whose disease advances within six months of platinum therapy are not usually helped by a second course of it. However a new drug may help in these and other advanced cases which are resistant to conventional treatment. The drug, paclitaxel (Taxol), is derived from bark extracts of the Pacific yew tree and is the first in a new class of anti-tumour agents called taxanes. Although it has the same effect as other types of cancer drugs, stopping the cancer cells dividing and growing, it has a different mode of action. It encourages the stabilisation and proliferation of 'microtubules' within cancer cells, and by preventing their breakdown, causes the cancer cell to die. However, some studies have shown treatment with paclitaxel keeps the cancer at bay only for about six months and helps only about a fifth of women treated; but in a few cases there has been no sign left of disease after the treatment.

Another approach that is looking hopeful is treatment using monoclonal antibodies (antibodies which a high-tech method enables to be reliably reproduced in large numbers) in addition to surgery and chemotherapy. Radioactive molecules can be attached to these antibodies and directed at the cancer cells wherever they have spread. When they arrive they deliver the required radiotherapy dose. In one small trial at Hammersmith Hospital in London, 80 per cent of women treated by this means were alive after two years whereas previously only 10 per cent would have been expected to survive. Further trials are in progress.

Monoclonal antibodies with radioactive markers can also be used to show whether and where the cancer has spread and to help a surgeon ensure that all cancer deposits are removed during surgery.

• Screening for ovarian cancer •

Ovarian abnormalities can be detected by conventional abdominal ultrasound but the disadvantage of this type of screening is that surgery then has to be performed to check whether a growth is cancerous or not. If this kind of screening was routine, numerous women would undergo unnecessary surgery.

More sophisticated approaches are being developed which are making it possible to identify malignancy without investigative surgery but these are still at the experimental stage (although available in some hospitals to women at highest risk) and still need refining.

One of the most successful methods so far is combined transvaginal ultrasound screening and colour blood-flow imaging. A probe is placed in the vagina and allows a clearer view of any growth in the ovaries than conventional abdominal ultrasound. The probe can also detect changes in the blood supply to structures within the ovary, indicating which tumours are more likely to develop and spread. This research is being carried out at King's College Hospital in London.

Another line of research is the identification of protein markers produced by ovarian tumours and development of a simple blood test to test for raised levels. One blood test for a marker known as CA 125 has been tested on over 20,000 women and has led to diagnosis of a number of cases of ovarian cancer before the women had any symptoms. However, it also failed to signal a problem in some women who developed the cancer within 12 months of taking the test.

Other protein markers are looking more hopeful. The most recently discovered marker is OVX1 which, together with CA 125 and ultrasound, is undergoing a nationwide trial involving 120,000 women. Pilot studies have shown that testing women for both OVX1 and CA 125 and screening them with ultrasound is more than 90 per cent sensitive. Marker tests combined with transvaginal ultrasound and colour blood-flow imaging may be an even more promising screening approach.

Some leading researchers engaged in the search for reliable and cost-effective screening believe ovarian screening could eventually become routine in the older age groups. Others remain sceptical about its value and claim that there is no conclusive evidence as yet that screening will improve survival rates.

• Endometrial cancer •

This cancer is also known as cancer of the uterus or uterine cancer. It starts from a growth in the lining of the uterus, the endometrium, that has become malignant (a precancerous growth may be present for some years previously), invades the wall of the uterus and may spread to other pelvic organs and beyond if not caught in time.

There are fewer than 4000 new cases of this type of cancer each year in the UK and the survival rate is higher than with any other of the gynaecological malignancies.

• Who is most at risk? •

Endometrial cancer mainly affects women who are past the menopause and three-quarters of sufferers are over 50. Women who are heavily overweight are at extra risk as are those who suffer from diabetes, high blood pressure or fibroids, or who have not had children.

If a woman has been exposed to high oestrogen levels not balanced by progesterone, she is at greater risk: sometimes the case, for example, if her menstrual history is one of long gaps between periods, or failure to ovulate, or if she has been given oestrogen therapy for menopausal symptoms without a progestogen component.

• Symptoms •

The main symptom is bleeding. Women who are still having periods may have heavier periods or spotting between periods. Women who are past the menopause will notice slight bleeding. There may also be cramping pains like period pains, increased need to urinate if the tumour is pressing on the bladder and possibly a vaginal discharge, which might range from watery and pinkish to thick, brown and unpleasant-smelling.

• Treatment •

Growths in the endometrium can be detected by ultrasound. A D&C or hysteroscopy may be performed (see pages 218 and 219), during which the growth may be removed and checked for malignancy. If cancer is present, treatment may include surgery, radiotherapy or chemotherapy and some cancers may respond to hormone treatment.

Usually the uterus, fallopian tubes and ovaries are all removed (total hysterectomy) and four to six weeks of radiotherapy are given but if cancer has spread further, surgery may have to be more radical. Radiotherapy may sometimes be given as a radium implant, before or after the operation (see more about radiotherapy under cervical cancer, page 279, and breast cancer, page 322).

When this cancer is caught before it has spread beyond the endometrium, the cure rate is up to 90 per cent. It is less than 50 per cent after it has spread beyond the uterus, however.

• Cancer of the vulva •

This is a very rare cancer, hardly ever found in women under 60. Its causes are not known but if the vulva has been irritated over a long period by too harsh chemicals or infections that have not been properly treated or keep recurring, it may be more susceptible to disease.

The first sign is a small, hard lump which grows very slowly and usually itches. Eventually it becomes an ulcer, with raised edges and red and sore in the centre. It is either painful or itchy. A tissue sample will reveal whether the lump is cancerous and if so, simple removal of the growth and some of the surrounding skin should be sufficient to effect a cure in the early stages.

In more advanced cases, the tumour may have spread to the vagina, urethra and anus or, more seriously still, to the lymph nodes in the groin from where there may be further spread. Treatment is usually surgery or chemotherapy followed by radiation.

• Vaginal cancer •

This previously extremely rare cancer has become slightly more common because of a link between its development and the taking of DES (diethylstilboestrol), a synthetic oestrogen once sometimes prescribed to pregnant women to prevent miscarriage. Although the drug didn't even work, it continued to be prescribed by some doctors till 1970, most commonly in America. Women who took the drug are themselves at higher risk of vaginal cancer and so too are their daughters, who may develop it even prior to adolescence. The main symptom is a vaginal discharge that looks like mucus.

If you took DES yourself or your mother did, see your doctor to arrange for regular checks. The cancer can be detected on smears but may also be missed on them. Colposcopy (see page 220), is the most reliable form of diagnosis.

Surgery and radiation have been used with some success in treatment (the vagina may be able to be reconstructed after removal of the cancerous part). Also, researchers are investigating whether progesterone suppositories may halt the disease or even be capable of returning the vaginal cells to normal. All further exposure to synthetic oestrogens should be avoided after treatment.

· ALL ABOUT ·
BREASTS

36

BREAST DEVELOPMENT

UNDERSTANDING something of the structure and development of the normal breast and the great variety in normal breast appearance can help us worry less about things that aren't a problem but be more aware when something really is amiss.

· Development up to adulthood ·

When a male or female foetus is about six weeks old, nipples develop along two lines or ridges that run from either side of the groin up the front of the body, over what will become the breasts and into the armpits. By three weeks later, all of these nipples have usually disappeared except two where you would expect to find them on the chest.

Occasionally, not all of these primitive nipples disappear, and then women, or more commonly men, may be left with one or more extra nipples along these lines. Very occasionally the nipples in the breast area disappear along with the rest, leading to complete absence of breasts for which there is no treatment except, for appearance only, cosmetic surgery.

When the foetus is three months old, milk ducts begin to form and open on to the nipple via reservoirs called sinuses. Nothing much more happens until puberty when the surge of female hormones produced by the ovary, oestrogen and progesterone, causes the breasts to grow.

Oestrogen, which is present first, makes the milk ducts elongate and increase in number by branching out. Fatty and connective tissue also form. As more milk glands form, the areola, the wrinkled skin around the nipple, starts to develop and become pigmented.

When progesterone comes in, it stimulates the milk-producing glands at the ends of the ducts to grow. No milk is produced, however, until a woman is pregnant or breast feeding. Puberty occurs, on average, at the age of 12½, although it is not abnormal for it to occur as early as nine or as late as 18. The breast carries on developing milk lobules, areas which contain milk-producing cells, until about the age of 25.

• Structure of the adult breast •

Women's breasts lie partly on the ribs and partly on the chest wall over the pectoral muscles, which move the arms. There is a little tail of breast tissue, under the skin, that extends into the armpits. Each breast has a large number of milk-producing glands. There are about a dozen milk ducts which open on to the nipple and at the other end of each is a lobe containing numerous lobules which in turn contain large numbers of milk-producing cells.

Around these milk glands is fatty tissue and also fibrous bands or ligaments which separate the milk glands off from each other and also support the weight of the breasts. In between are blood vessels, nerves and lymphatic channels (see below), but no muscles except for the minuscule ones in the nipple to make it erect.

The milk-producing cells surrounded by fat often feel lumpy when you feel with your fingers but this is perfectly normal. The fibrous ligaments stretch as they age. When there is a malignancy in the breast, they often pull inward, giving the characteristic dimpling to the skin that is one of the signs to be aware of when examining the breast.

The lymphatic channels carry a fluid called lymph which collects any unwanted material or germs which are then filtered out by lymph nodes in the armpit (axilla). If infection is present, these lymph nodes may become inflamed while the filtering process is occurring. If the foreign body is a cell from a cancerous lump, the lymph nodes may be able to destroy it. If not, the nodes may enlarge.

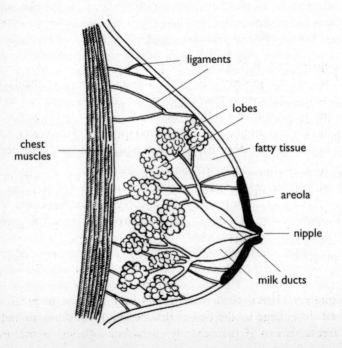

ligaments

lobes

chest muscles

fatty tissue

areola

nipple

milk ducts

• Shape and appearance •

Breasts can be a variety of shapes and look different even from each other. Some are very large; usually the plumper a woman is, the larger her breasts. Some are naturally very small. Some appear to be set high on the chest, others low. Even the position of the nipple may vary, either sitting on the edge of the widest part of the breast or else just below this, which may give the appearance of a sagging breast when the breast isn't sagging at all. Gaining a lot of weight and then losing it may leave the breasts sagging, as the fibrous tissue will have stretched. Sometimes the areola appears to increase in size with weight gain too but this goes back to normal when the weight is lost.

The size of the breast is not much affected by exercise. Exercise may cause the muscle underlying the breast to enlarge, pushing the breasts forward a bit. If you tend to exert the arm on one side much more than the other – for example by constantly washing windows, scrubbing pans, etc – the muscle on that side of the chest may develop more than the other, creating the appearance of a slightly larger breast on that side.

• Changes of the breast •

Monthly changes Breasts are influenced by the hormones produced by the ovaries. It is very common to feel more sensitivity or tenderness in the breast at ovulation, midway through the menstrual cycle. Towards the end of the cycle, before a period, fluid collects in breast tissue and they may feel swollen and painful, sometimes so much that treatment is necessary for the intense discomfort. For more mild discomfort, sleeping in a properly supportive bra for a few nights before a period may be helpful.

The contraceptive pill When taking the pill, your own hormones are suppressed and your cycle is governed by artificial ones in the pill. Usually, taking the pill lessens any previous breast discomfort you may have had. If not, ask to try a different brand or a different type. When taking the pill, if you are fair-skinned you may notice that your nipples darken. This is a common side-effect and mimics what often happens to the nipples during pregnancy.

During sex When a woman is sexually aroused, the tiny muscles in the nipples contract and the nipples become erect, but not necessarily simultaneously. Smaller nipples appear to increase in size more than larger ones but this is only because the effect is more noticeable. The breasts swell and may be covered with a flush.

Some women are very sensitive to stimulation of their nipples, others less so or hardly at all.

During pregnancy Breast tenderness occurs very early on in pregnancy. The breasts start to enlarge by the end of the second or third month and the nipple and areola darken – permanently. Sebaceous glands in the areola develop, giving the appearance of raised nodules. A clear discharge may emerge from the nipples during pregnancy.

After breast feeding The hormone oxytocin produced by the pituitary gland stimulates the ducts to squeeze out milk. Breasts enlarge considerably at first but then reduce a little again, even though milk is still being produced. At first, breasts may feel sore and a bit lumpy until feeding settles down. When a woman stops breast feeding, sometimes the breasts become engorged which is very painful. Stimulating the breasts so that the milk can be expressed helps. Sometimes giving the baby one last unexpected breast feed after an interval of a few days can help the breasts empty naturally without them producing more.

After stopping breast feeding, breast size will inevitably reduce. Some women find their breasts shrink to a size smaller than that pre-pregnancy, others that they return to their normal size. If fibrous ligaments have been stretched a lot by the increase in fatty tissue or milk during pregnancy and breast feeding, the breasts may appear to sag somewhat after stopping.

At the menopause The ovarian hormones oestrogen and progesterone stop production at the menopause, with the result that any monthly breast swelling, tenderness or pain ceases too. However, without these hormones, some women find that their breasts shrink in size, although in very many women breast size stays exactly the same as before. But breasts may tend to drop, because the fibrous ligaments are less elastic. In the decade before the menopause and carrying on till after it, fatty tissue in the breast is increasingly replaced by connective fibrous tissue.

• Common cosmetic concerns •

Women often worry that their breasts, or some aspect of them, are abnormal. However, as mentioned earlier, there is great variety to the normal. When abnormalities do occur, most of these can be altered.

• Small breasts •

Some women have breasts which stay as just small discs of tissue behind the nipple and areola rather than developing into normal rounded breasts. During pregnancy, however, breasts like these may develop dramatically and function normally.

As mentioned, exercises cannot significantly alter the size of breasts. Any change is very minor, caused by development of the muscle underneath the breast. Good posture can help in the same limited way. The only option for any woman truly concerned and upset about having small breasts is to have breast enlargement, a cosmetic surgery procedure often called breast augmentation (see page 295). It needs very careful consideration because there are as many problems as there appear to be benefits.

• Large breasts •

Very large breasts, which hang below the waist, can be a source of great embarrassment and physical discomfort. They may be very tender and the skin between them may chafe easily or itch because sweat collects there and causes a rash. The skin should be kept scrupulously dry and powdered to prevent such problems.

It is helpful to pad bra straps at the shoulder so that the weight of very large breasts does not make them bite into the skin. Women embarrassed by very large breasts very often round their shoulders to try to conceal them, but this just adds the problem of poor posture and resultant muscle tension. If breasts are excessively large, breast feeding is usually not possible.

Cosmetic surgery to reduce breasts is an option some women choose (see page 302). It is technically possible to breast feed afterwards, if the surgeon does not cut through the main milk ducts or remove too much of other tissue important for milk production. However, it is probably simpler to breast feed first and then have a reduction, unless breast feeding is impossible anyway because of size.

• Breasts of unequal size •

This is very common, as few women have breasts exactly the same size, but some women have one normal sized breast and one abnormally small. The small breast will develop normally during a pregnancy. However, for cosmetic reasons, women may choose to have their breasts evened up by surgery. This usually means an enlargement of the smaller breast and sometimes a reduction in size of the larger breast.

• Inverted nipples •

These are nipples that lie flat on the breasts, sometimes with the appearance of a fold, instead of protruding from them. They are quite common, occur when the milk ducts are too short and are no cause for concern if they have been this way since puberty. However, if a nipple which normally stands out appears to flatten and retract this should be investigated promptly as it may be a sign of breast disease.

There is no need to do anything about inverted nipples unless you want to breast feed. However some women do not like their appearance and it is often possible, with commitment, to encourage naturally inverted nipples to turn outward. The manipulation method involves placing a finger on either side of each areola and stretching the nipple. Then change the position of your fingers so that one is above the nipple and one below and then stretch again. You need to do this repeatedly, two or three times every day, until you see some change.

If this doesn't work, you could try with breast shields, one way that you can often make breast feeding possible with inverted nipples. Breast shields are plastic or rubber discs which you wear under your bra. The nipple is gradually pulled by suction through the hole in the middle of them. You need to wear breast shields first for an hour or so at a time, to get used to them, and then for increasingly longer periods. If you are pregnant and hoping to breast feed, the earlier you start this the better, so that you can manage quite long periods towards the end of the pregnancy. If the method fails, however, breast feeding may not be possible. A newer option is a device called Naturally Niplette by Avent. It is easy to use, and wearing it painlessly lengthens the ducts. It is available from pharmacies in packs of one or two.

There is also a surgical operation to change inverted nipples but unfortunately many women are still unable to breast feed after having it. The operation is a minor one, carried out under local anaesthetic, and involving a tiny incision either side of the nipple.

• Hair around the nipples •

Hair around the nipples is perfectly normal. If you have quite a lot of hair on your body, you are likely to have some hair around your nipples too. It may be more noticeable if you are dark-complexioned. Hair around the nipples appears to bother many women, in the same way that hair under the arms or on the legs may bother them. In this case, it is perfectly safe to remove the hair by any of the usual hair-removal means. Some say that plucking stimulates more growth. Certainly, care needs to be taken, as the skin around the nipples is very sensitive.

• Taking care of breasts •

Choose a bra that fits properly A bra that fits poorly is a very common cause of breast pain and discomfort. One survey by a woman's magazine

_____ MEASURING BRA SIZE _____

To measure your bra size as accurately as possible, put a tape measure around your body just under your breasts. Then add 4 to an even number and 5 to an odd number. The result is your bra size in inches. For example, 28 plus 4 equals 32in; 31 plus 5 equals 36in.

To determine your cup size, measure over the fullest part of your breasts, then subtract the bra size you have just worked out from the full breast measurement. Then use that figure to calculate your cup size from the following:

−1 = AA cup	3–3.5 = D cup	
0 = A cup	4–4.5 = DD cup	
1–1.5 = B cup	5 = E cup	
2–2.5 = C cup		

For example, if your bra size is 34 and your full breast measurement is 35, the difference is 1 and you probably need a B cup.

found that 58 per cent of women measured were found not to be wearing the right bra. A bra that cuts into your back or wraps tightly is too small. A bra that rides up or is loose is too large.

When you put your bra on, always slip the straps over your shoulders first, hold the bra from both sides at the bottom and then lean forward to let the breasts fall into the cups. Make sure the bra is centred properly when you straighten up. And once you have got a bra that fits well and is comfortable, make sure the clothes you wear on top are comfortable too: for example, not so tight that your breasts get uncomfortable again.

Walk tall   The more you keep your shoulders up and your upper body stretched, the more room you have to breathe and your breasts to fall comfortably.

Avoid fluid retention   A number of things contribute to fluid retention, which bloats the breasts before a period. Stress increases it, so build relaxation into your daily lifestyle. (Stress and tension also exacerbate breast tenderness.) Overweight increases it, so watch your diet. Also, be aware of what you eat, as certain foods and drinks, such as animal fats, salt, tea and coffee, increase fluid retention and others, such as fruits and vegetables – particularly grapefruit, apples, cucumbers and potatoes – help reduce it.

Stimulate your nipples   Stimulation of the nipples is a good thing, (according to Australian professor Tim Murrell of the University of Adelaide) because it appears to help protect against breast cancer. He suggests that partners do it or women do it themselves using fingers or a rough flannel, for two or three minutes twice a week. His theory is based on the fact that the hormone oxytocin, which is produced during breast feeding, is also produced when the nipple is stimulated and at orgasm, causing breast cells to contract and expel any milk or other breast fluid. Women who have breast fed are known to be at lower risk of breast cancer.

Of the 5000 women who enrolled in Professor Murrell's nipple stimulation programme at his university clinic, none had developed breast cancer after three years whereas statistically two or three cases of cancer would have been expected.

• Breast self-examination •

Breast self-examination remains controversial in that one study follows another with conflicting conclusions, finding first that self-examination doesn't lead to earlier detection of cancers or doesn't increase survival from breast cancer, and then that it does. However, experts involved in breast screening and cancer care do advise self-examination. The current favoured term is breast awareness, but it all comes down to the same thing: women need to keep an eye on their breasts, know what their breasts look and feel like when healthy and be able to spot any deviations from the norm which may warrant investigation.

The problem is that the idea of breast examination scares many women. They would rather not look than risk finding a lump. Or they don't like the thought of examining their breasts and then feel guilty for not doing it. But it also isn't the answer to become obsessive about it and check for nooks and nodules every day. You only need to check your breasts once a month and, if making a performance of it puts you off, try having a relaxed look while in the bath or shower. If breast self-examination particularly bothers you, you could ask to have your breasts checked periodically by your doctor or at a well-woman's clinic.

• How to examine your breasts •

1 Check your breasts once a month, preferably just after a period as at this time of the month breasts are least naturally lumpy and least tender. If you do your check at the same time each month, you will know what to expect, whereas if you do it at different times during the menstrual cycle, you will feel more or less lumpiness at different times and not have any norm to gauge changes by. If you don't have periods, choose any convenient time for your checks that you are most likely to remember, such as the beginning or end of every month.

2 Face the mirror, undressed to the waist, with your arms swinging comfortably by your sides, and study your breasts. Establish what is their normal appearance: is there a difference in size, are the nipples at slightly different heights, etc? Each month take the same stance and look at both breasts for any unusual differences in size or in nipple height.

3 Look at each breast individually to see if there is any
   • dimpling in the skin
   • unusual irregularity in shape
   • drawing in or uncustomary retraction of the nipple
   • changes in skin texture
   • changes in skin colour
   • veins standing out more than usual.
   Do this first with your arms by your sides. Then repeat with your hands on your waist, then with your arms raised straight up above your head and finally with your hands clasped behind your head.

4 Squeeze each nipple gently to check for any unusual discharge or any bleeding.

5 Lie down comfortably or do the next bit in the bath. You are going to feel your breasts carefully for any unusual lumps. Lie on your back and put the arm on the side that you are examining behind your head. Use your right hand to examine your left breast and vice versa. Do one breast at a time.

6 Use the flat of your middle three fingers to work around each breast, moving your fingers in small circles and feeling what is underneath them. You may like to divide each breast mentally into quarters and work around each in turn or prefer to move your fingers in small circles all around the

Step 2

Step 4

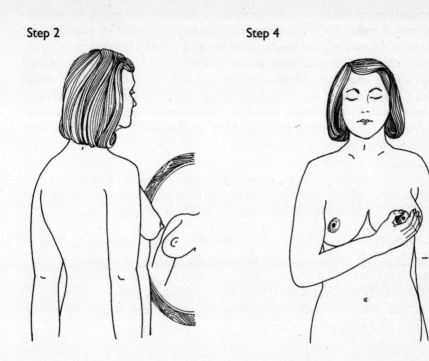

Steps 5 and 6

Step 7

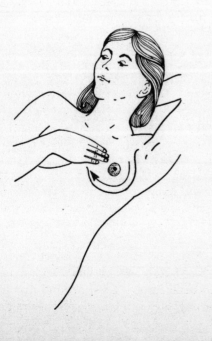

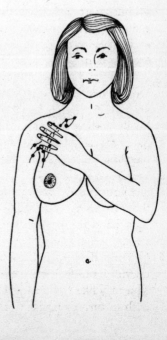

outside of each breast and then move inward until you reach the nipple. You are looking for any lump at least the size of a pea that you can feel with the flat part of your fingers (false lumps are easily felt with the finger-tips), that moves up and down and from side to side with your fingers and that is fairly clearly a separate entity, as opposed to a lumpy bit of normal breast tissue. Cancerous lumps are usually firm, irregularly shaped and clearly defined. If you think you have found something suspicious, feel in the same position on the other breast. If you can feel the same there, it is more likely to be part of normal tissue.

7 Finally, feel your armpit for any lymph nodes. Put your left arm down by your side and slide your right hand into the armpit as high as you can reach, then bring it down over the ribs. Repeat on the other side. Any lump which might warrant investigation will be larger than a pea.

If you do find a worrying lump, don't panic but arrange to see your doctor within a few days. Nine out of ten breast lumps are not cancerous. There are numerous benign breast conditions (see page 305) which cause lumps and which can easily be dealt with. There are many which cause tenderness and pain as well, both of which are far more commonly associated with benign conditions than with breast cancer.

37

COSMETIC BREAST SURGERY

BREASTS tend to generate strong feelings in women. They are an integral part of a woman's sexual and biological identity, whether she is comfortable with them or embarrassed to have them. They are always on display, even if covered with clothing. And they may seem to others to make a statement about their owner, even if it is not one she herself is trying to express.

Most women are willing to accept their breasts, whether they come up to their own idea of perfection or not, although probably few are completely happy with their size, shape or other aspects of their appearance. But some women have their lives adversely affected by their feelings about their breasts: they may be unwilling to participate in any activity that might require them to show their breasts, such as trying on clothes in communal changing rooms, getting undressed to go swimming or even having sex – at least certainly not with the light on. Some women, for these reasons, may consider surgery to enlarge or reduce their breasts.

Women who are comfortable with their breasts may experience a severe and deep blow to their sense of body image if they have to lose a breast through breast cancer. Many will choose to come to terms with not having a breast. But breast reconstruction is a realistic option for others. (See page 336.)

Whatever the reason for choosing cosmetic breast surgery, a woman who is seeking it is emotionally vulnerable. It is important to be clear about the pros and cons of each type of cosmetic operation and to find a person you trust who is competent, experienced and qualified to carry it out (see Cosmetic Surgery, page 128).

• Breast enlargement •

Breast enlargement (or breast augmentation) is the insertion of a silicone implant behind breast tissue to give the appearance of fuller breasts and also to lift them a little. Very many women seek this operation every year because they are embarrassed by what they consider to be too small and unsexy breasts. Or their main concern may be to look more attractive. It is important to be really sure that your expectations are realistic if you seek this procedure, as it is not one of cosmetic surgery's greatest success stories in terms of technical outcome. For example, having larger breasts doesn't mean instant sexiness, as that comes from the person you are, not the way you look.

Yet it has to be acknowledged that many women do feel more sexy after breast enlargement because, for the first time, they feel attractive (however attractive they might always have seemed to others) and are confident about themselves. It is not the breasts that make them sexy but their own feelings about having them. Having larger breasts does not, however, help mend ailing marriages or bring back wandering partners.

• Be realistic •

If you are definitely set on seeking breast enlargement, it is important to be realistic about what can be done. The size of breast you end up with has to be related to the size of breast you have started out with, as skin will only stretch so far and the smaller your breasts, the less skin there is to go around your new ones. If your breasts are different sizes, an implant can help to even them up. But implants can only alter size, never shape.

• When to do it •

You need to think carefully about the timing of a breast enlargement. No reputable surgeon would consider doing one for a girl still in her teens, as the breasts have not yet stopped growing. Also, it is only after adolescence that we start to come to terms with our adult appearances and a breast size which may have seemed an unconquerable catastrophe then might not even be a source of embarrassment by our early twenties.

Another consideration is whether you want to breast feed children. It is perfectly possible to breast feed with implants but any breast infection caught while breast feeding – certainly not an uncommon occurrence – might cause problems to the implants and damage them. So if you haven't yet had children or think you might want more and definitely want to breast feed, it is probably worth waiting until you consider your family complete before paying a considerable amount of money for breast enlargement. In fact, quite a common reason for seeking breast enlargement is the shrinkage in breast size that often occurs after childbirth.

• Decisions to make with your surgeon •

You should discuss with your surgeon at the outset the enlarged size of breast that is realistic and suitable for you. If you have an implant that is too big, the breasts will be pushed forward making your own skin stretch too much. The pressure this creates will cause some of the fatty tissue in the breast to be reabsorbed, leaving even less natural breast tissue than when you started out. This might not appear to be a big problem once you have breast implants but it could become one if something goes wrong and the implants have to be removed.

You will probably find it easiest to get an idea of the implant that will suit you if you look at before and after pictures of others, which your surgeon should be able to show you. It won't help to say that you want a 36C or a 38B: implants are not bras and don't come in bra-cup sizes. Ask also for a photograph to be taken of your own breast before the operation, if the surgeon doesn't suggest it. It is easier then to assess your satisfaction with the outcome of the procedure. For example, many breasts are not exactly level but it is easy to forget this and think the implants are uneven afterwards, if you have nothing to look back to.

• Implants •

The materials used for implants are very realistic sphere-shaped silicone bags filled either with silicone gel or sterile saline. They feel rather like plastic bags filled with water and when you lie down, they flatten and spread, just as normal breast tissue does. Silicone gel feels more natural, however, whereas saline can feel rather cold and heavy.

A silicone implant with an outer covering made of polyurethane foam, to avoid some of the problems associated with silicone coverings described below, was introduced in around 1980. But the manufacturers have voluntarily withdrawn these because of scares over links with liver cancer in mice, even though there has never been any proof of this effect in humans. However, as thousands of woman do have the polyurethane covered implants, their benefits and problems are still included here. Silicone implants are now made with either a smooth or textured surface; the latter with the aim of gaining some of the benefits of the polyurethane-covered version, without the risks.

• The procedure •

The operation to insert implants is usually carried out under general anaesthetic, although a local can sometimes be used. It lasts about one hour. (Polyurethane ones take half an hour longer.)

Discuss with your surgeon beforehand where he or she plans to make the incision. It can be made under the breast crease, the easiest place for the surgeon because bleeding can more easily be controlled there, but the scarring will be more noticeable than if the incision is made either under the armpit or through the nipple. If the incision is made through the nipple, the cut should be continued behind the breast tissue, not across it. A cut which goes across is quicker for the surgeon but means that the breast tissue there is unnecessarily separated from its milk ducts.

If the incision is made under the breast, you will have a scar either just on or just under the breast and it will be about 5cm (2in) long and visible. Scars in the armpit and around the nipple will be the same size but less visible; around the nipple least so.

The implant is always placed behind the breast tissue, either between the breast and the chest muscle that lies beneath it or under the chest muscle, so that it lies between the muscle and the ribs. Discuss which your surgeon thinks is best for you. Appearance is often better when breasts are very small if the implant is placed under the muscle, but there may also be the disadvantage that this can push the breasts up too high and make them move up and down in a rather unnatural manner whenever the muscle is being used (when riding a bike, for example). Saline implants may be more comfortable when placed under the muscle.

• Afterwards •

After surgery, you will probably feel very bruised and your nipples may feel as if they are burning. It is usually more painful if the implant has been placed between the muscle and the ribs. Only a day's stay in hospital afterwards is usually necessary but you have to keep bandages around the breasts for at least five days after the operation, and then wear a good supporting bra for at least three weeks, day and night.

Don't judge the outcome of the operation by the size of your breasts at this stage. They will still be swollen and this won't all disappear for at least six weeks. Your breasts will be extremely tender for three weeks but after four weeks, you should be able to go back to your daily routine.

• Possible complications •

Occasionally one implant is placed higher than the other, because it is difficult always to be absolutely accurate when positioning implants in someone who is lying down. However, as mentioned above, it may not be the implants which aren't level but the natural position of your breasts. Refer back to your 'before' picture to check. If the implants are indeed at different heights, the operation will need to be repeated to set them right.

The operation will also have to be repeated if blood collects around the implant and makes the breast swell up like a balloon. Normally, excess blood is drained away through drainage tubes inserted during the operation and removed a day later. However, if blood collects, the implant has to be removed, the bleeding controlled and then the implant reinserted, but this isn't a common event.

USING FAT INSTEAD OF AN IMPLANT

Another technique which has been used, but uncommonly in this country, is the injection of fat taken from the buttocks or thighs instead of an implant. However, fat very often degrades when moved to another part of the body without its natural blood supply, and the fat cells may die (fat necrosis). Critics say the fat will then calcify and inflammatory effects may make it difficult for a breast cancer to be spotted. As well, the calcified fat may be mistaken for a cancer during mammography. Nuclear magnetic resonance or biopsy are likely to be necessary to distinguish a cancer from calcified fat. But the fat necrosis will still have to be surgically removed.

Also uncommon, occurring in about one in every 100 women undergoing the procedure, is an infection developing after surgery. The implant once again must be removed and may only be replaced about three months later, when the infection has had a chance to be cleared properly with antibiotics and doctors are confident it will not recur

The most common complication, and very common it is too, is a hardening around the implant which fixes it in position like a cricket ball. This occurs when a fibrous capsule of scar tissue forms around the implant as the area is healing. The capsule of scar tissue may be so hard and tight that doing any physical activity or even just lying down is unpleasantly or excruciatingly painful. About half of all women fitted with the older silicone implant are likely to experience this unfortunate occurrence. If caught early a very hard squeeze can be sufficient to crack the capsule but this hurts quite a lot. It is also quite alarming to experience because of the fear that the implant will break, although in fact it is only the capsule which cracks. More usually, however, the cracking will have to be done under general anaesthetic.

Alas, once cured, the problem is extremely likely to recur and many women find themselves having to have their capsule cracked under general anaesthetic every two or three months. It is, of course, not desirable to have so many general anaesthetics because of the risks, however slight, to say nothing of the nuisance of it all. Quite a number of women give up and choose to live with implants that sit like cricket balls in their chests.

This disastrous scenario is less likely to occur if the implant is placed under the muscle, but this choice has to be balanced against the possible piston effects mentioned earlier.

Only about 5 per cent of women fitted with polyurethane-covered implants suffer capsule formation, probably because the breast tissue is irritated by the polyurethane and reacts with inflammation which then causes the scar tissue to be irregular rather than smooth. Irregular tissue is less likely to contract and form a capsule. The disadvantage of this is that an on-going inflammatory reaction behind the breast is quite probably not such a good thing and we don't yet know the effects of it because the polyurethane-covered implants are so much newer than the silicone ones.

A second disadvantage is that these implants are more difficult to remove in the event of an infection. The newer rough-textured silicone implant has been found to cause hardening in about 10 per cent of cases. It is probably best if a textured implant is used when the implant is placed directly under breast tissue. If placed under the muscle, however, textured implants are less desirable because they cling to the adjacent tissue and can't move (for example, fall naturally when lying down).

Implants filled with saline solution have been known to burst suddenly, with the obvious embarrassing consequences. (It is important when having a breast X-ray to mention if you have saline filled implants as the pressure of this procedure can provoke a rupture.) And all types of implant can leak. Particles of silicone have occasionally been found in the breast tissue or lymph nodes of women fitted with implants, and even further afield in the body, but it isn't known whether this could cause problems later. Even if there is no real cause for concern, there may be alarms because stray bits of silicone are likely to be walled off by the body's defence system and these could then look similar at screening to a breast lump.

This list of possible problems seems pretty daunting and certainly needs careful consideration before going ahead with breast enlargement. On the other hand, most women who have it done genuinely seem happy with the outcome if nothing goes wrong, and only six in every 100 women who have the implants are dissatisfied enough to have them removed.

• Is silicone safe? •

There have been a number of scares as to whether silicone implants may increase the risk of breast cancer, slow down its detection or be linked with a higher incidence of auto-immune disease. Unfortunately, much of the evidence is conflicting.

Concern about the safety of implants was fuelled a few years ago when breast implants were reclassified by the Food and Drug Administration in America so that they would, for the first time, be regulated in the same way as new drugs, thus requiring all manufacturers to provide proof that their implants were safe. Until the issue was decided, manufacturers were also asked to stop shipping implants and doctors were asked to stop implanting them. However, this ban was lifted in early 1992 when no evidence could be found to support it.

The main concern was over the polyurethane-coated implants. When an implant is inserted, the body treats it as a foreign substance and attacks it. In this case it could have the effect of making the polyurethane break down chemically to release tiny amounts of a substance called TDA which can cause liver cancer in animals.

Those experts who believe these implants safe claim that the particular type of tumour caused is peculiar to rodents and never found in humans. They cite two studies that suggest implants may protect breast-cancer-prone mice from malignancy. Even the FDA says that, should there be in humans a polyurethane breakdown rate similar to that in laboratory rats, the added cancer risk would be very small: less than one in a million for a woman who has had two implants for a period of 35 years. In the unlikely event of the polyurethane breaking down all at once, the risk would be about one in 12,000.

Results of one major Canadian study, the largest ever conducted, reported in 1992, found that women with implants in general did not have any increased breast cancer risk, and in fact had fewer cancers than would have been expected in a group of over 11,000 women. This finding was similar to that of an earlier American study. However, the researchers were keen to point out that they could find no reason why having implants would reduce cancer risk and certainly didn't recommend them as a protective. Critics claim that it may just take more years before increased cancers show themselves.

Certainly it is not seen as a very good idea to rush off and remove polyurethane implants which are already in place, because there is a relatively high risk of infection and disfigurement. However, many thousands of American women and over one thousand in the UK have indeed had their implants if not altogether removed at least replaced with the less contentious saline versions.

• Impeding screening •

On the issue of implants impeding breast screening, there are some areas of agreement and some of disagreement. The conventional thinking has always been that mammography and self-examination should not be affected by the presence of implants which are always placed under breast tissue. When implants are placed under the muscle, 96 per cent of the breast can be seen in a mammography compared with 80 to 85 per cent when the implant is over the muscle, according to one piece of American research.

Another study found that women who had had implants tended to have more advanced breast disease by the time they were diagnosed, although the cause is unknown and may not be related to the implant at all. Yet other studies have shown stage of detection of cancer in women with breast implants to be almost the same as that in other women.

Both silicone gel and saline-filled implants might make the detection of early breast cancer a bit more difficult because they can distort the appearance of the breast and because calcium deposits which form around the implants may make the interpretation of a mammogram harder. It is important to tell staff at a breast screening unit if you have an implant, so that they know to take account of them.

• Risks of silicone leakage •

Silicone and polyurethane have both been used in surgery other than breast enlargement for very many years without appearing to cause problems. However, recent laboratory tests have revealed that silicone is not an inert substance and can irritate the immune system in animals. Also, tests of 100 Californian women with implants found that 35 were making antibodies against their own collagen (connective tissue).

There is therefore a worry that leakages of silicone, in tiny amounts or because of implant rupture, could increase risk of auto-immune diseases such as rheumatoid arthritis, lupus and scleroderma. However, another and larger study, at the Mayo Clinic in New York, has found no evidence of an increased risk of auto-immune diseases. In an unrelated study of almost 100 women in which nearly a quarter experienced a rupture of their implant, the silicone remained within the capsule made by the implant and didn't spread anywhere beyond.

Leakages from saline-filled implants are less likely even to be thought to be a problem (and the saline type is more prone to rupture) because salt is not a foreign substance to the body. However even saline-filled implants are covered with silicone, so if there is indeed any problem there might still be a minor risk with saline.

As yet the relevance of the presence of antibodies to the development of disease is not known and there is nothing to prove that women with implants who developed auto-immune diseases would not have developed them anyway. The Department of Health, having reviewed the evidence, decided it was inconclusive.

One rather alarming development since, however, is the discovery of abnormalities in the oesophagus in six out of eight children, aged from 18 months to 13 years, who were referred to specialists for abdominal pain and who had been breast-fed by women with implants. None of the other children referred for the abdominal pain had similar abnormalities nor did three bottle-fed children of women with implants. However, the affected children were not found to have any abnormal antibodies.

Because of all the uncertainty and anxiety about silicone implants, the names of all women who have breast implants inserted now have to be placed on a national register so that they can be contacted easily should there ever be a need. Doctors have also been asked to supply names of women who have already had implants: over 100,000 in all.

• Breast reduction •

Breast reduction leaves a lot of unsightly scarring but for the most part this is all too willingly borne by women whose breasts are so large that they cause them real physical discomfort. Very large breasts may reach as far as the pubic area and be a severe source of embarrassment. Smaller but still large breasts can cause enormous strain on the neck and back and a lot of chafing and skin rashes where breasts meet each other or fold over other skin. While many women are happy and proud to have large breasts, others dislike the comments they may attract and the assumptions some men may make about their owner's sexual inclinations.

• Issues for consideration •

By removing breast tissue, an operation for breast reduction can result in smaller breasts similar to their previous shape. However, long breasts cannot be made full if they were not full before. The considerations regarding timing of such an operation are similar to those in breast enlargement. For example, it is thought best to wait until your family is complete if you want to breast feed as it is not usually possible after this operation – but sometimes it is impossible to breast feed anyway if the breasts are too large.

Whereas implants would not be given to a teenage girl, breast reduction might well be done at this age if breast size is an enormous cause of embarrassment and if she is willing to accept that a repeat operation will possibly be necessary when her breasts have finished growing. So, if the money is available, an operation is indeed not to be dismissed out of hand. Also, breast reductions in severe cases may be available on the NHS but the waiting lists could be offputting.

You can have as much breast tissue removed as you like in breast reduction. However, a good surgeon is likely to try to persuade women out of anything drastic, although many are so disenchanted with their chests that they may say they want as little breast tissue left as possible. Be guided by your surgeon as to how much tissue removal will leave the best shape.

• Breast-reduction procedure •

The operation takes about three hours. As well as removing the excess breast tissue, the surgeon must reposition the nipple and the areola. If the breasts are not too large, these can both be moved up to a new central breast position while still attached to living breast tissue. But if breasts are very large or the blood supply to the nipple isn't good, the nipple and areola have to be removed and then sewn back on again as a skin graft.

Noticeable scars are unavoidable, one circling the areola and then coming down to the bottom of each breast, and another crossing under the breasts (and maybe hidden in the breast skin fold). The appearance of scars varies from person to person and according to where they are on the body. These scars could be narrow or wide, flat or thick, and in colour they could range from white through to pink or brown.

Naturally, you will have some pain initially and will need to wear bandages around the breasts, followed by a firm supporting bra, day and night, over a period of some weeks. For about six weeks, there will be swelling, so don't imagine that virtually nothing has changed. Lifting, stretching and doing anything that jiggles the breasts will be out of the question for a while but after about three weeks your life should be back to normal.

• Possible complications •

There are not anywhere near as many problems with this procedure as with enlargement, although it is a far more major operation. Sometimes heavy bleeding during surgery will cause clots, which must be removed at once, as well as swelling.

Sometimes skin will slough off around the nipple if the blood supply to the nipple and areola in their new position isn't strong, and the new skin beneath may be lighter. The nipples themselves may lose some or all sensation, occasionally permanently and more commonly just for a few months. If this happens, it is important not to get burnt, if sunbathing topless.

One woman in ten may develop little lumps of fat which harden because of poor blood supply to the area. They are harmless and usually disappear after a while but may cause a scare if felt and presumed to be a malignant breast lump.

One in ten may suffer the formation of a painful ulcer at the point where the vertical scar down the breast and the horizontal one under it meet. With careful dressing it usually heals within a couple of months.

A very unpleasant but fortunately extremely rare complication can occur when there is a complete failure of blood supply to a nipple that was moved while still attached to breast tissue. The nipple dies and a large hole is left in the breast which has to be dealt with by skin grafts from elsewhere on the body.

• Breast lift •

This procedure is often considered if breasts appear to droop, which may happen when there has been a significant increase in breast size followed by significant decrease but with the breast skin less elastic than before and less able to spring back into position. This often occurs after breast feeding or after general weight increase and then weight loss.

• Issues for consideration •

The breast lift is a procedure that changes the shape of breasts by removing the stretched and excess skin, as well as any stretch marks on the section of skin that is removed but none that are on the skin that is left behind. The size of your breasts stays the same as previously. It is pointless to have this operation if you are still open to the idea of having more children. It is also a very temporary solution at the best of times, so it probably isn't worth having if you have a very minor droop, especially as the scarring will be out of all proportion to the benefit. The older you are the more quickly the droop will return, too.

• Breast-lift procedure •

The operation, under a general anaesthetic, takes about two hours. Excess breast tissue is removed and the nipple is repositioned. Unlike in breast reduction, the nipple is always kept alive in this procedure because no breast tissue is removed. However, the scars are similar in appearance, running around each nipple and down to the bottom of each breast where they will cross another scar that runs around underneath the breasts. Though the same in position, these scars are less obvious than those from breast reduction and may fade more.

You don't have much pain after this operation. You will still need breast bandages and then a support bra to wear day and night for a few weeks but you will be back to normal within a month, if you have not overdone it in the intervening time.

• Possible problems •

The only really likely problem is one that afflicts one in every ten women having a breast lift: skin separating at the point where the scars cross and an ulcer forming. It usually gets better within a couple of months, during which time you have to wear dressings inside your bra.

38

BENIGN BREAST DISORDERS

EXPERTS now tend to view most benign breast disorders (that is, non-cancerous ones) as conditions which arise as a result of the normal processes that occur in the breast from puberty through to the menopause: first, breast development, then cyclical changes associated with the menstrual cycle and then shrinkage of breast tissue (involution) that occurs towards the menopause. These phases in fact overlap: development takes place on average between the ages of 15 and 25; cyclical changes between 15 and 50; and involution from 35 to 50.

Because so many benign disorders are clearly understandable in terms of these three stages, some experts prefer the term ANDI (aberration of normal development and involution) which recognises them as a consequence of the normal, rather than as abnormalities. Not all breast disorders fit these categories of course, but apparently most do.

• Breast lumps •

The following disorders have lumps as a main or major symptom but there may also be other important symptoms too.

• Fibroadenoma •

This is a benign breast lump which develops from a single lobule (there are numerous lobules in each breast which each contain milk-producing cells) and is made up of fibrous and glandular tissue. There may well be more than one of them, in either or both breasts. About one in five women with the condition has more than one lump in both breasts. Where one breast only is affected, it is more usually the left. In the West, the average is two to four lumps in one or both breasts, whereas black and oriental women often have a lot more. There is a hereditary element to the likelihood of having them.

Fibroadenomas tend to occur most often in the 15 to 25 age group, when technically the breast tissue is still developing. But they may not be diagnosed until much later, for example when changes in the breast after pregnancy or the menopause make the lumps more easy to feel. Some experts suggest that fibroadenomas could probably be found in all breasts if one looked hard enough, and they are certainly so common that they could well be regarded as normal. They respond to changes in the breast in the same way as normal lobules, growing during pregnancy, producing milk if a woman is breast feeding and shrinking at menopause. Very, very rarely does a cancer develop in a fibroadenoma, and even then it is the type that stays put and doesn't ever spread.

Growth up to a size of 5cm (2in) is considered within the normal range for a fibroadenoma although most usually they don't extend beyond a diameter of 2 to 3cm (¾ to 1¼in), staying the same size from then on. During the growth period, the lump doubles in size in six to 12 months. One that develops beyond 5cm (2in) is called a giant fibroadenoma and is considered abnormal. Giant fibroadenomas, while rare, are most often seen in adolescence, but sometimes also develop towards the menopause.

There is uncertainty about the role of the contraceptive pill in fibroadenoma. There is no evidence that use of the pill has increased incidence in general and some studies have suggested that long-term pill users are less than half as likely to get them. However there is also a suggestion that an increased incidence of multiple fibroadenoma now being seen could be linked with pill use.

Fibroadenomas feel rubbery and firm, very mobile and smooth, with well defined edges. They are often called by the rather unpleasant name of 'breast mice' because of their tendency to slip away from the fingers when grasped at. The exception are ones that lie behind the nipple, where surrounding ducts restrict their movement.

Although the fibroadenoma may not be discovered until later in a woman's life, it cannot at that stage be confidently predicted to be a fibroadenoma because breast changes have made the lump less well defined and mobile by this time. A biopsy (removal of a small piece of living tissue) can be carried out simply by inserting a needle into the lump and drawing some fluid into a syringe so that cells can be examined under a microscope (cytology).

Before the age of 25, a fibroadenoma can easily be diagnosed clinically and, in fact, because of the nature of the breast at this age, cytology can even be misleading.

• Treatment •

It is usually recommended that fibroadenomas are removed, although some authorities now suggest keeping an eye on one in a woman under 25 and only removing it after six months if it has grown and she wishes it removed. After 25, no one would recommend leaving it and, indeed, most women prefer removal because a fibroadenoma of 3cm (1¼in) can produce a lump that is quite marked when looking at the breast. The operation is a simple one and may even be carried out under local anaesthetic if the lump is close to the surface of the breast. Ability to breast feed is not affected.

Giant fibroadenomas are usually deeper in the breast and may have taken over a vast amount of breast tissue, so surgery under local anaesthetic is not

BREAST-CANCER LUMP

This is obviously not a benign lump but is included here as a comparison. A lump that is cancerous is usually hard and painless and is felt most often in the upper, outer area of the breast, although it could be located anywhere. It is likely to be irregular, firm, be clearly distinguishable from other breast tissue and move quite easily underneath your fingers. It may be close to the surface of the skin or feel as though it is deep down.

As well, there may be nipple discharge, a pulling inward of the nipple; and dimpling of the skin as the tumour pulls on the fibrous tissue of the breast, which can happen even when the lump is still relatively small. Sometimes the skin of the breast may get puffy or thicken. Although pain is rare, it does occasionally occur with a cancerous lump.

Of course, these symptoms also occur with other conditions that are not cancerous, so, while they need investigation, they are not in themselves instant cause for fear. Conversely, even a lump that doesn't fit with the above description could still be a breast cancer, as symptoms can vary or be uncommon. It is therefore important, for both safety and for peace of mind, to see a doctor as soon as possible if you find any kind of breast lump at all.

---

appropriate. Breast tissue usually grows back to normal once the giant fibroadenoma has been taken out.

In some European countries, hormonal treatments such as danazol, tamoxifen and progestogen are often used to shrink them but this isn't recommended here, especially because of side-effects of these treatments, both known and – in the case of tamoxifen – not fully known. The lumps may recur after surgery or may grow again somewhere else, necessitating more surgery, but if a lot keep appearing, repeated surgery is obviously not a good idea and management will be on an individual basis.

• Phyllodes tumour •

This is a rare disorder, variously known also as *Phyllodes sarcoma* and *Cystosarcoma phyllodes*, although these terms are very often not strictly correct. The term 'sarcoma' (a cancer of the connective tissue) should only really be used in the occasional cases where the tumour is malignant. There aren't always cysts involved either.

The phyllodes tumour is usually benign and is related to the fibroadenoma, with women often having both, although it is not known whether the phyllodes tumour arises from the fibroadenoma or both occur simultaneously or separately. It is far less common, with about one being seen by doctors for every 40 fibroadenomas diagnosed. It is rare before the age of 20, when it is always benign, and is most likely to occur, if it occurs at all, between the ages of 35 and 55. It hardly ever appears in both breasts.

Phyllodes tumours are softer than fibroadenomas and can grow quite large, sometimes taking up most of the breast. Large dilated veins show on the area of breast skin that covers them.

• Treatment •

The tumour can be excised but usually needs a good margin taken around it, as otherwise it is quite likely to recur. In a small tumour (less than 4cm or 1½in), 1cm (⅜in) of normal breast tissue is likely to be enough. However, with very large or recurring phyllodes tumours, taking a wide margin may mean virtual mastectomy. Simple mastectomy and immediate breast reconstruction, if wanted, is usually recommended in such circumstances, so that it does not recur and because recurring tumours have slightly more of a possibility of becoming malignant.

• Fibrocystic disease •

This is a not too helpful term which some doctors use to describe any benign growth in ducts and lobules of the breast. It could therefore cover fibroadenomas, cysts, fibroadenosis and many other conditions described here. It may also be used to describe small clusters of cysts surrounded by fibrous tissue which make the breasts feel lumpy and painful particularly just before a period, and which commonly affect women in the 35 to 50 age group. This condition is also often called adenosis, fibrosing adenosis, cystic mastitis, mastodynia and cyclical mastalgia, the last being the most accurate name and the one under which this condition is described in the section on breast pain. (See page 313.)

• Fibroadenosis •

Lumpiness that can develop in the breasts as a result of an increase in fibrous and glandular growth, making them painful and tender. Women in their forties and fifties are the most likely to have this.

• Fibrous disease •

As the breast ages, the lobules containing milk-producing cells are gradually replaced by fibrous tissue. Sometimes this occurs over-enthusiastically, creating a firm lump, not hard and without clear edges, usually in the upper, outer area of the breast. Fibrous disease occurs most often in women over 50 but can be seen in the younger breast, as involutionary changes (the shrinkage of tissue) may start as young as 35 and even earlier in unusual cases. It is not unknown for the condition to occur in the twenties. Excision is difficult and, unless desirable for a clinical reason, is usually avoided.

• Sclerosing adenosis •

This is an increased growth and hardening of glandular tissue which forms a lump: the name literally means excessive growth of and hardening of glands. This condition can occur from the mid-twenties until after the menopause, but most commonly affects women in their forties and fifties. There is a firm lump usually not bigger than 2cm (¾in), with poorly defined edges. Quite often, it causes pain which may be worse premenstrually or when pressure is applied. Sleeping may cause discomfort in such cases.

Sclerosing adenosis is rarely cancerous and the lump can simply be excised.

• Cysts •

Cysts are collections of fluid which form in a duct or lobule and are the most common breast disorder for which treatment is sought. Probably about 7 per cent of women develop a breast cyst at some time, most commonly after the age of 35 and before the age of 50. They are slightly more common in the left breast than in the right and tend to appear either in the upper outer or upper inner area of the breast. After the menopause they disappear quickly and it is thought that there is some hormonal cause for them, most probably an over-production of oestrogen, but this has never managed to be proven and hormonal treatments are not used for cysts, except maybe in recurrence (see below).

Cysts can be tiny, but they can also be quite large – 5cm (2in) in diameter – clearly affecting the shape of the breast. They often appear in a cluster over an area about 2.5cm (1in) wide and are dome shaped. Multiple cysts are more often found in larger breasts and single cysts in smaller ones.

The fluid can be yellow, green, grey, brown or almost black according to its contents, such as various hormones, proteins or lymph. Small cysts are usually impossible to feel because they are not hard, but just a very small increase in fluid volume can increase the pressure inside a cyst enormously and suddenly it can become extremely easy to feel and can be very hard indeed. They can be very painful: the pain usually arises from leakage of fluid from the cyst into surrounding tissue or the complete rupture of the contents into a duct. Occasionally there is a discharge from the nipples.

• Treatment •

Treatment is very simple. A needle attached to a syringe is inserted into the cyst and the contents aspirated. Once the contents used to be looked at under a microscope for any suspicious material but now this is not done unless there is any blood in the fluid, which might indicate a tumour although even a tumour in such instances is normally benign. If there is any evidence of blood (black fluid does not necessarily mean blood) only 1 to 2ml of the fluid is taken out, for examination. Otherwise all the fluid is taken, on average 5 to 10ml (about 1 to 2 tsp), and you see the lump disappear before your eyes as the fluid is drawn up into the syringe and the breast returns to its normal unbumpy shape. Often, however, the cyst doesn't disappear completely but reverts to its previous state, when it couldn't be felt in the breast and caused no bother.

• Recurrence •

Cysts can recur but it is not common. Probably no more than one in ten refill with fluid sufficiently to feel like a lump again. The cyst is simply aspirated once more, repeatedly if necessary. It is rare for one to fill more than two or three times. However, up to half of women who have one cyst aspirated develop another somewhere else in the breast or the other breast. A third are likely to have more than one develop elsewhere. Repeated aspiration may be a nuisance but there is nothing sinister about it; a breast X-ray, called a mammogram may be done to check for other problems. However many cysts need aspirating, the contents are only investigated further if there is blood present.

Some early studies have shown that a short course of the hormonal drug danazol markedly reduces recurrence of cysts and may perhaps be tried when recurrence is a significant problem. Beware any surgeons who suggest mastectomy for extensive breast cysts or recurrent ones, and seek a second opinion, because individual circumstances would need to be exceptional for such drastic measures to be justified.

• Galactocele •

This is not a very common type of cyst that is entirely filled with milk, is caused by a blocked duct and may occur in women who were breast feeding a few weeks or months previously. It is thought more common when breast feeding is stopped suddenly and the milk supply is dried up by artificial means. A galactocele isn't painful and feels like a smooth lump that moves with the fingers. It is usually near the areola and, in such cases, it may be possible to move it towards the nipple with the fingers where it may discharge itself. It may also possibly be found anywhere in the breast. It is easily aspirated and usually doesn't recur.

• Duct ectasia •

This is a benign condition sometimes known as duct ectasia/periductal mastitis complex. It is a dilation of ducts in the breasts, usually three or four of those closest to the nipple, which then fill with thick fluid, sometimes as thick as toothpaste, that is a mixture of cream, green and brown. Symptoms are odd-shaped lumps, pain or a burning and itching sensation and often nipple discharge: small amounts of fluid the same colour and consistency as described above, but sometimes containing blood. When the dilated ducts are around the nipples, they may feel like a tangle of worms. Horrible though the symptoms sound, they are probably very common in a milder form, with up to one in ten women having some dilated thickened breast ducts but never realising it.

The problem is thought to be caused when waste products become blocked in the ducts and the duct walls become inflamed, both by irritation from the waste chemicals and/or by infection caused by invading bacteria. (Or it may be that inflammation caused by bacteria sets the whole problem off.) It is the stagnant waste that makes the fluid so thick. Ulcers may sometimes form and the waste leaks into tissues around the ducts, causing massive inflammation inside the breast and maybe an abscess. When leakage into surrounding tissue occurs, the affected area of the breast is hot, swollen, red and extremely tender. Any blood in nipple discharge is thought to be caused by ulceration.

The inflammation around the ducts may cause scarring and as this scar tissue contracts and becomes hard, it draws the nipple inward, often leaving the surrounding skin dimpled and reddened. Nipple retraction happens in about a third of women with duct ectasia.

It seems that women with this condition have different symptoms at different stages. Women in their twenties and early thirties are most likely to suffer the inflammatory complications, with women born with inverted nipples the more frequent sufferers. But they do not usually experience nipple discharge which tends to occur at around 40 and is the age at which women usually experience pain, lumps and discharge. Once women are past the menopause, they may have nipple retraction but without ever having had any nipple discharge or inflammatory complications severe enough to have come to notice.

• Treatment •

In some cases, the condition may resolve itself and no treatment at all is necessary. If pain is not severe and the discharge is not too thick, antibiotic treatment with metronidazole and flucloxacillin may be tried. It is not effective when inflammation is greater and discharge is thick because the antibiotics then cannot reach the bacteria in the heavily blocked ducts. Fluid can be drained surgically but if there is heavy pus, repeated aspiration will not work and will only damage breast tissue, affecting the appearance of the breast after surgery. In the more severe cases, surgical removal of tissue containing the problem ducts is usually necessary. This is done under general anaesthetic and should leave a normal-looking breast and nipple. Surgery to correct a retracted nipple is also possible.

• Intraductal papilloma •

These are one or more little warty growths which may occur in one of the major ducts under the areola and nipple. They aren't very common and tend to appear, when they do, in a woman's forties. Some may be tiny and regress spontaneously; others may grow up to 5mm ($^2/_{10}$in) in diameter and feel like a pea. The main symptom is discharge from the nipple, which may clearly be blood or else a greenish fluid. Occasionally the pressure of the fluid build-up in the duct may cause tenderness. Pressing on the areola over the area of the papilloma often pushes the fluid out (and relieves the pain) and this is usually how a doctor will locate the papilloma.

• Treatment •

Intraductal papilloma can occasionally become malignant. Single ones are found almost always to be benign whereas two or three in a duct have more of an association with cancer. All papilloma are removed under general anaesthetic. An incision is made down the side of the nipple so that the surgeon can locate the duct with the papilloma and then that duct alone is removed. Both breast and nipple look normal afterwards. Regular check-ups should be advised as a woman who has had one duct papilloma is more likely to develop another.

• Fat necrosis •

This means death of fat cells, and may occur if a severe blow is experienced to the breast. The blow has to be severe enough to burst blood vessels in the breast, causing bruising, and also burst fat cells. In the elderly, the condition may arise when the hurt is less apparently severe because the older breast, with less fat and more fibrous tissue, is less able to absorb a blow without adverse effect.

When fat leaks out of the cells, the body attacks it and walls it off because, not used to its being there, the body thinks the fat is foreign matter. Scar tissue then forms, making a firm, irregularly shaped lump that can very easily be mistaken for cancer, especially as contraction of scar tissue then pulls on breast ligaments and dimples the skin.

In younger women, usually in their forties, fat necrosis is more likely to occur after an accident in which the breasts were quite badly hurt. At this age, the lump looks and feels more like a cyst and may be painful. A mammogram can easily confirm what it is and then it can be aspirated. An oily fluid will emerge. In the older woman, the fat necrosis appears as hard white tissue and must be cut out and examined, to ensure it is not cancer, as both look similar on a mammogram. Recovery is quick and painless.

Fat necrosis is rare. In fact breast cancer is far more common than fat necrosis, so it is unwise to dismiss a suspicious lump as the result of an injury experienced previously. Although it might be the harmless outcome of a blow, it equally might not be; especially if the lump was already there but was only felt when an injury necessitated examination or massage.

• Lipoma •

A lipoma is a lump made up of fat cells which can develop anywhere in the body, and sometimes in the breast. It is well defined, painless and harmless. However, it can mimic in appearance a certain type of cancerous tumour and so has to be carefully investigated to ensure that it is not cancerous. Usually a mammogram will show it up quite clearly as a see-through area with a clearly defined rim, which is the thickened capsule of tissue that surrounds it. A lipoma can quite safely be left untreated, the only concern being that if it grows more it may cause a noticeable change in breast shape. In this case, and in any cases of doubt, it will be removed.

• Breast pain •

More than half of women who are referred to breast clinics for help for a breast disorder come because they are in pain and probably between two-thirds and three-quarters of all women experience some degree of breast pain at some time. If it is pain that persists, it should never be ignored. Although pain is unusual as a main or accompanying symptom of breast cancer, it does happen sometimes, probably in 5 to 10 per cent of women.

Breast pain falls into two main categories. Pain that is linked with the menstrual cycle is called cyclical breast pain and the rest is called non-cyclical breast pain. About 15 per cent of women who suffer breast pain suffer so severely that they cannot sleep comfortably, nor can they cuddle their children or their partners without excruciating agony. As the pain may be easily diagnosed and respond to treatment, it is worth seeing your doctor rather than struggling on and putting up with severe discomfort.

• Premenstrual syndrome •

Breast tenderness is a common symptom of premenstrual syndrome, the group of physical and mental changes which may occur at or after ovulation and for varying lengths of time up until two or three days after the start of a period. It is estimated that close to half of all women of reproductive age suffer uncomfortable or painful premenstrual symptoms and half of these have significant breast discomfort for at least two and possibly as many as 14 days before a period. Women aged between 20 and 45 are the most frequent sufferers but it isn't unknown for symptoms to persist beyond the mid-forties.

The symptoms may be mild swelling and painfulness of the breasts or very severe swelling and exquisite pain, making it impossible to hold anyone or anything close to the body. It is thought that increased blood flow to the breasts is part of the cause of the swelling. Normal daily life obviously becomes badly disrupted in such cases and for many women marital problems develop as well.

When symptoms are mild, it may be enough to take a multivitamin and mineral supplement, containing 50mg vitamin B_6 (pyridoxine), magnesium and zinc. Cutting down on saturated fat intake may also help and very possibly cutting down on caffeine, although not much evidence supports this at all.

If your symptoms are severe, you should see your doctor who may prescribe gamolenic acid (the essential fatty acid found in evening primrose oil and some other substances) to take daily. If this helps, you should feel the difference in a few weeks but sometimes it takes as long as five cycles to have any real effect. Only in extremely severe cases would strong drugs such as bromocryptine or danazol be prescribed as they have unpleasant side-effects (see Cyclical Mastalgia, below).

Diuretics do not work at all, indicating that breast swelling is nothing to do with fluid retention. Some synthetic progestogens used in the oral contraceptive pill appear to increase breast discomfort. Norethisterone and dydrogesterone, for example, affect some women badly. You may feel better if you try a different brand.

• Cyclical mastalgia •

This is an extreme version of the normal lumpiness and mild swelling that is common before a period. Usually there is pain and lumpiness (nodularity) in both breasts and pain may even be experienced in the armpits and down the arms. One survey found that 69 per cent of well women over the age of 35 who were attending for breast screening reported cyclical mastalgia of a degree sufficient to cause discomfort or misery and interfere with their daily routine.

A questionnaire survey of 585 female Marks and Spencer employees in South Wales revealed that nearly half had experienced mild mastalgia and a fifth severe mastalgia, yet less than half in the severe group had ever sought medical help. It can affect women at any time in their reproductive years, although most commonly in the early to mid-thirties. It can come on out of the blue or, in some cases, after excision of a breast lump.

Two-thirds of cases of breast pain, not caused by disease which are referred to specialist clinics, can be accounted for by clinical mastalgia. In most cases, reassurance that the pain is not caused by anything sinister is sufficient and no treatment is required but, for 15 per cent, drug treatment is necessary to restore a decent quality of life.

Unfortunately, cyclical mastalgia is not taken very seriously by many doctors, the pain being viewed as just something to put up with or even all in the mind, as nothing is organically wrong. However, interest in the condition is gradually increasing, more is being written about it in medical journals and, at the time of writing, there are even specialist mastalgia clinics in London, Manchester, Nottingham, Edinburgh and Cardiff.

Normal procedure at a specialist clinic is first to establish for sure that the pain is caused by cyclical mastalgia (that is, related to the menstrual cycle) rather than non-cyclical mastalgia. This is simply done by asking you to keep a breast-pain diary for at least two menstrual cycles. (Mammography is not useful as a means of diagnosis.) Cyclical mastalgia has a regular pattern associated with the menstrual cycle and is usually at its most severe before a period. Obviously the experience of pain is subjective but if it causes loss of sleep and interferes with work life and sex, that is usually taken as severe enough to warrant trying treatment.

• Causes •

There have been many theories as to causes. The old beliefs that fluid retention was to blame or that women who suffered it were more neurotic have both firmly been laid to rest, although there may unfortunately still be doctors who don't know that. There is clearly a hormonal cause but quite what form this takes is still somewhat uncertain.

Early theories were that too much oestrogen or too little progesterone were being produced by the ovary, or that too much of a hormone called prolactin was being produced by the pituitary gland. Now, these theories have been proved wrong, as the levels of these are not apparently different in mastalgia sufferers from those in non-sufferers. However, it does seem that cyclical mastalgia sufferers are abnormally sensitive to levels of these hormones which all have an effect on breast tissue (see Breast Development, page 287). It is now thought that low levels of an essential polyunsaturated fatty acid, gamolenic acid (GLA), caused by low intake in the diet, may have an adverse effect on prolactin synthesis. (Or it may be that dietary levels are sufficient but the body cannot for some reason convert them for use efficiently.) Also, high levels of saturated fatty acids appear to increase the effects of hormones on the breast and make these effects last longer.

Severe mastalgia does not appear to be linked with use of the oral contraceptive pill and some studies have in fact found a beneficial effect. Sometimes, women experience mastalgia on starting a new brand but this usually settles down very quickly. If, however, severe mastalgia does develop for the first time when starting to use the pill, it is worth trying a lower dose (if there is one) or a different brand or, if the discomfort is severe enough, changing to a different type of contraception and seeing if there is any improvement.

Hormone replacement therapy is known to cause mastalgia which can usually be stopped by using a low dose combined preparation.

• Self-help •

Sometimes cyclical mastalgia can settle down on its own, so doctors are unlikely to recommend any heavy drug treatment unless you have been experiencing pain for at least six months. There are a number of drug treatments which can be useful but, unfortunately, the most effective often have severe side-effects. The first line of approach, therefore, is to alter your diet and, if necessary, to take gamolenic acid (GLA). Women may also benefit from changing their bra or having one properly fitted by a trained bra fitter.

Dietary approach This involves cutting down on saturated fats and, if over-weight, trying to lose some of the excess. One six-month study found that cutting down on total fat, but particularly saturated fat, and deriving more calories from carbohydrates instead did help to reduce breast tenderness.

Gamolenic acid This is now recommended as the first prescribed treatment to try for cyclical mastalgia, particularly in younger women wishing to become pregnant or whose symptoms keep recurring. It can be effective in mild to moderate cases. It is usually taken in the form of evening primrose oil and is available on prescription as Efamast. It can help up to 70 per cent of carefully selected women – that is, women whose symptoms are not too severe – although one study found it useful to only slightly less than half. The treatment unfortunately takes a while to reach maximum effect. In one trial, GLA taken at levels of 240–320mg per day slowly reduced breast pain, tenderness and lumpiness but maximum benefit only occurred after four months' treatment.

The good thing is that side-effects are minimal, mainly mild gastrointestinal symptoms if anything at all, and even when used for as long as a year nothing further untoward appears to occur. Fish oil is also a good source of essential fatty acids and early trials indicate it may be as effective or even more effective than evening primrose oil, again with minimal side-effects. For severe pain, however, these measures will not be enough.

Danazol Most effective is danazol, a powerful drug which acts on hormones produced by the pituitary and the ovaries. It helps at least 70 per cent of women with very severe pain. The usual dose is 100-200mg twice daily but, while the higher dose works more quickly in relieving breast pain, tenderness and lumpiness in the breasts, it is accompanied by more severe side-effects in about a quarter of women.

These can include, most commonly, weight gain, irregular periods, headaches, nausea and vomiting. Less common but not altogether infrequent are rashes, acne, bloating of the abdomen, depression, hair loss, increased hair growth, depression, reduced breast size and a slight lowering of the voice. Voice pitch changes can be permanent if treatment isn't stopped or altered at once but are noticed by only a very small proportion of women to whom it happens and more usually are reversible on stopping the drug.

A side-effect which affects about a third of women is loss of periods altogether, and tests of progesterone levels in the second half of the cycle would suggest that ovulation is suppressed.

Normal practice is to try to keep dosage of this powerful drug down as low as therapeutically possible. Experts advise prescribing 200mg per day to begin with, starting on the second day of the menstrual cycle, switching to 100mg after two months if the effects are beneficial and then, after a further two months, using a maintenance dose of 100mg on alternate days or for just the one or two weeks before a period, if this is sufficient to keep symptoms in check and reduce unwanted side-effects. At these lower doses there is no effect on menstruation. Some doctors may prefer to start the other way around, beginning with 100mg a day, increasing to 200mg a day if there is no effect after one cycle and keeping to the higher level for a further two cycles before introducing a maintenance dose. Danazol at the higher doses would not normally be prescribed for longer than six months; at the lower maintenance doses, treatment can carry on longer.

Bromocriptine Another strong hormone-suppressing drug used for cyclical mastalgia, which acts on prolactin levels. Lowering prolactin levels has the effect of reducing prolactin-induced glandular activity in the breast. Six months of 2.5mg of bromocriptine twice per day has been found to improve breast pain and tenderness but side-effects are not inconsiderable. One study found that side-effects of nausea, headache, giddiness and constipation were experienced by a third of women, severely by 15 per cent. It has since been found that unwanted side-effects can be reduced if treatment is started at 1mg taken at night and then increased gradually.

With both danazol and bromocriptine, after six months of treatment about half of users need no further treatment at all and for most others, even if symptoms recur, they are milder and can be dealt with by simple analgesics.

Tamoxifen This is one of two other treatments that may be useful (see also goserelin below), but because they have significant unwanted side-effects and may not be better than existing treatments, are generally not prescribed for cyclical mastalgia. Tamoxifen is an anti-oestrogen, currently of use in the treatment of breast cancer, which is as effective as danazol in mastalgia. It has the side-effects of hot flushes and menstrual irregularity but of most concern are both possible association with increased incidence of other female cancers and also osteoporosis. Cyclical mastalgia is not covered by the product licence but tamoxifen can be prescribed by a GP on a named patient basis if thought appropriate when a person has severe symptoms that haven't responded to any other treatment.

Goserelin This is a drug which acts on the female reproductive hormones and creates menopausal side-effects. One UK trial has found it worked within a month. It may be useful for severe or recurrent symptoms that have not responded to any other treatment and its use will probably be restricted to this until clear comparisons with other existing treatments have been made.

• Inappropriate treatments •

Not useful in cyclical mastalgia are antibiotics, vitamin B_6 (pyridoxine), diuretics and synthetic progesterone (progestogens).

Antibiotics are often prescribed, wrongly, because cyclical mastalgia is often termed mastitis, which means inflammation of the breast. Biopsies (taking a tiny piece of tissue for examination) have clearly shown that there is no inflammation with cyclical pain, therefore treatment with antibiotics is always inappropriate.

Vitamin B_6 is often prescribed but although it may be of some benefit for premenstrual breast pain, it has not been shown to have any beneficial effects when the symptoms are more severe.

The pain and swelling in the breasts are not due to fluid retention: one study of total body-water measurements found absolutely no difference between women with cyclical mastalgia and women without. Therefore prescribing diuretics is pointless. And two controlled trials have found both progestogen cream and oral progestogen ineffective.

· Non-cyclical mastalgia ·

This is breast pain which is constant or intermittent but does not have any relationship to the menstrual cycle. It can occur pre- and post-menopause and the average age of onset is the early forties. The pain seems to be different from cyclical pain, occurring mainly in one breast and often specifically under the areola or on the inner area of the breast. Terms used to describe the pain might vary from burning and drawing to pricking or stabbing. The pain may last for minutes at a time or days. One study found patients rated the intensity of non-cyclical pain as less than that of cyclical pain, and usually lumpiness is less apparent and there may not be anything unusual to feel at the place where the pain is experienced.

Non-cyclical pain may be experienced with conditions such as breast cysts, duct ectasia, intraductal papilloma, a blow to the breast, sclerosing adenosis and fat necrosis. All of these conditions are described fully earlier: see Breast Lumps (page 305). A poor-fitting bra also can cause pain, particularly if it is too tight or has too much uplift. Having a bra fitted by a trained fitter might be helpful.

Non-cyclical breast pain for which there is no clear cause may sometimes respond to the same treatments used for cyclical pain: danazol, bromocriptine or evening primrose oil. These will, however, help less than half of women and it is mainly danazol which brings any benefit. Studies have indicated that in the main, bromocriptine and evening primrose oil are no more effective than placebos.

Sometimes breast pain may be the symptom of Tietze's Syndrome, a painful swelling of a rib where it joins the breast bone. It is felt in the breast because the breasts lie over the costal cartilages which connect the ribs to the breast bone and are the source of the pain. The pain is more intense when the affected cartilage is pressed. The cause isn't known and the condition usually sorts itself out, although sometimes local steroid injections are necessary.

Up to 13 per cent of women who seek specialist help for non-cyclical breast pain have not a breast problem but a musculo-skeletal problem of some kind which will usually respond to steroid injections. Sometimes the heart, lungs or gut may be the real source of the problem and sometimes shingles may first be felt as breast pain. When the shingle rash appears, however, it is easily diagnosed correctly.

Pain can occur with cancer, but it is uncommon that this is the only sign or symptom. However, no persistent pain should be ignored. When pain is caused by cancer, it is in one breast only (unless, presumably very rarely, there are lumps causing pain simultaneously in both breasts), is persistent and its position doesn't vary. One study has found that pain as the only symptom of cancer is mainly associated with smaller tumours.

• Nipple problems •

Nipples can be the source of a few problems too, and these, explained below, shouldn't be ignored.

• Nipple discharge •

This is not an uncommon occurrence and can have many manifestations and many causes, most of them benign.

First, of course, is milk. This is to be expected when you have given birth but might be a cause of alarm if you are not pregnant. Often, however, milk production can be stimulated by taking certain drugs, such as oral contraceptives, oestrogen, some tranquillisers, drugs for high blood pressure and tricyclic antidepressants. The discharge is clearly milky in appearance and will stop when the drug is stopped. A blood test to measure levels of prolactin, the hormone that stimulates milk production, can quickly confirm that the problem is galactorrhoea: milk secretion unrelated to breast feeding.

Sometimes milk production carries on a long time after stopping breast feeding, usually because of attempts to express remaining milk which then leads to more being produced. Leaving it alone will allow it to dry up. Sometimes a little milk is discharged at the menopause if the breasts are squeezed but this is no cause for alarm. If no drugs associated with increased prolactin are being taken and the other circumstances so far described do not apply, there is a slight chance of a pituitary tumour, so investigation is necessary.

A thick or thin discharge ranging in colour from white, cream or yellow to green, brown or even black is likely to be caused by duct ectasia (see page 310). This happens more often in later reproductive years. The lighter coloured discharges are likely to be the thick type, the dark ones more fluid. In fact, the discharge may be multicoloured, different types emerging from different ducts.

Bloody discharge can have various causes. It can happen in pregnancy, usually in the second or third trimester and can emerge from both nipples. It is merely something that may happen as breasts undergo development during pregnancy and sorts itself out, usually at the latest by two months after delivery. Friction between clothing and nipples when running can sometimes make nipples bleed (see Sore Nipples, page 320).

A cloudy discharge that is bloody or serous (discharge containing serum) can be yellow, pink, red or brownish and is usually caused by duct ectasia (page 310) or intraductal papilloma (page 311). If there is serum in the discharge, it is sticky. Sometimes either kind of discharge may indicate cancer or a pre-malignant condition. It is unusual for this to be found in women under 50 and very rare under 40. A biopsy is taken when a woman is over 40 but nothing may need to be done if a woman is younger and the discharge clears up on its own.

A watery discharge is unusual. When it occurs, the discharge is clear and there is a lot of it. It may be associated with multiple papillomas and be benign but it may also be associated with breast cancer.

A minor discharge can be left alone, once it has been correctly diagnosed. Usually mammography is advised if a woman with nipple discharge is over 30, particularly if the discharge is bloody, serous or watery. If there is infection, antibiotics will be necessary. If the discharge is profuse and extremely bothersome, excision of the affected duct(s) may be advised.

• Sore nipples •

Becoming more common is 'jogger's nipple', where friction between the nipple and clothing when a woman (or man) runs causes extreme soreness. Often the nipples will bleed. This unpleasant problem can be avoided by wearing a firmly supporting bra and putting tape over the nipples.

Eczema can occur on the nipples, in which case the nipples are red and sore along with other areas of the body. Moisturisers may help but sometimes steroid cream may be necessary. As with eczema elsewhere on the body, you need to be cautious about any perfumes, bath oils, bubble baths, etc, that may be causing or exacerbating the problem. Also, you might avoid washing in harsh detergent all bras or any swimsuits or tops that will be placed directly against the breasts.

One rare cause of sore nipple which mustn't be overlooked is Paget's disease of the nipple, which is caused by a cancer in a breast duct. If you have soreness of the nipple on just one breast and it doesn't clear up, it should be investigated to exclude the possibility of Paget's. This disease caught early can be successfully treated.

• Raynaud's •

This condition, which affects the extremities, most usually the hands and feet, can also affect the nipples, which show the characteristic Raynaud's colour change of white to blue to red, or at least two of these. Even when warmly dressed, the nipples may feel extremely cold to the touch. See page 481 for a full description of Raynaud's.

• Swellings and growths •

Polyps, little growths on stalks that look like skin tags often seen elsewhere on the body, can grow on the nipple. They may be up to 2cm (¾in) long. They are not sinister but they may feel uncomfortable rubbing inside a bra and can easily be removed under local anaesthetic. Cysts may develop on the nipple too and can be removed the same way.

Sometimes small circular swellings appear on the areola. These are sweat glands which may enlarge during pregnancy and are called Montgomery's tubercles. Sometimes a cyst forms inside them but there is usually no need for any treatment.

• Viruses •

Sometimes the herpes virus and genital wart virus can show up on the nipple. In addition, a sexually transmitted pox virus called *Molluscum contagiosum* produces a small lump on the nipple that may ulcerate.

• Nipple retraction •

This occurs when a tumour pulls the nipple inward, so should be investigated promptly. However, duct ectasia can also cause it, so the condition does not always signify cancer.

• Breast infections •

Breast infections are not common if you are not breast feeding. The bacteria which usually cause them, staphylococci, live harmlessly on the skin and only tend to get inside the breast if there is a crack in the nipple while breast feeding.

However, love bites to the breast and nipple are one of the other major causes of breast infection unconnected with breast feeding. Other bacteria can be the cause, commonly anaerobic bacteria (a type of bacteria that doesn't need oxygen). As well, infections are commonly to be found in duct ectasia and cysts may also become infected. An infected breast becomes inflamed. It looks red, it swells and it hurts. If it gets worse, an abscess filled with pus may form. Symptoms will then include throbbing and a high temperature.

• Treatment •

If an infection can be caught before an abscess develops, antibiotics should get rid of it; but once an abscess has formed, the pus will need to be drained. Sometimes it can be drawn out into a syringe with a wide needle. If not, surgical removal under general anaesthetic will be necessary. Usually the wound is left open to allow the abscess to drain fully and daily dressings are required for a while. Seeing the open wound isn't very nice and it may seem dauntingly big but it should heal without problem.

Sometimes the skin in the folds under the breast, or between them if breasts are heavy, may become red and sore, because of friction and sweatiness. This then encourages infection with bacteria or fungi that normally live harmlessly on the skin. The cure is simple: a better fitting and firm bra to keep the skin from rubbing. Also, an antiseptic skin cleanser can be helpful. Other odd infestations or infections may very occasionally occur on the breasts, but so rarely as to not be worth describing.

• Tuberculosis •

This is a condition which, although rare, does warrant mention because incidence of this disease is increasing in the UK and sometimes breast problems are the first symptom. It may show itself as an ulcer, a cold abscess (one with swelling but little pain) or as a contracted breast and, although drug therapy for tuberculosis will cure the illness, there is a risk that the breast may be left deformed or scarred.

39

BREAST CANCER

BREAST cancer is caused by abnormal cells developing in breast tissue, forming a lump or tumour. Why this should happen we don't really know but women whose mother or sister had the disease are at increased risk, especially if they had the disease before the age of 45 or in both breasts. Also with a higher than average risk of breast cancer, according to the statistics, are women who started periods late, reached the menopause late, had no children or had children late on, but most women fall somewhere between these categories and the actual overall increase in risk is slight. Eating a diet high in animal fats may also have a bearing on who develops breast cancer.

About 26,000, or one in 12 women, are diagnosed with the disease in the UK each year. It is the most common cancer in women and the single most common cause of death of women between the ages of 40 and 50 (accounting for one-fifth). However the rate of death from this cancer has been falling for the last 20 years in women under 50 and for 10 years in women under 60, with overall death rates down from the usually quoted 15,000 a year to just over 13,500. There is no sign of increased breast cancer rates in women who are now middle aged and who took the contraceptive pill when they were young. Taking the pill for several years from a young age can slightly increase the risk (rare) of developing breast cancer before the age of 36.

A breast-cancer tumour is able to spread from the site where it originally grew. Some cells may break off from the original tumour and travel via the lymph system or the blood to other parts of the body where they may form another tumour (known as a secondary or a metastasis).

• How do I know if I have it? •

Nine out of ten women first discover a lump somewhere in their breast, but although this is the most common symptom of breast cancer, nine out of ten breast lumps are actually benign. Other signs to be alert to are:

- a change in breast size or shape
- dimpling or thickening of the breast skin
- swelling in the armpit or upper arm
- a lump on the nipple
- the nipple turning inward.

Very occasionally a discharge from the nipple or a rash around the nipple can signify cancer. Usually however, these symptoms have other causes. Some women feel breast pain with breast cancer but the majority don't.

• Detecting breast cancer •

Suspicious breast lumps are usually first detected by women themselves. Also, GPs may find them during routine well-woman examinations or they may show up through mammography, (see below). Mammography is offered at three-yearly intervals in the UK to women aged 50 to 64 (for the reasons explained below).

• Self-examination •

In the UK, women are advised to be 'breast aware'. Most breast cancer experts recommend regular self-examination (see page 291) but, even if you don't like the idea of this or just keep forgetting to do it, it is a good idea to at least pay attention to your breasts when bathing, showering or dressing, so that you become familiar with how they feel at particular times of the month (sometimes they are lumpier than at other times) and what is normal for you. In this way, you may notice very quickly if there are any suspicious changes. If you do find a lump or notice any breast changes that bother you, see your GP.

• Mammography •

Women aged between 50 and 64 are routinely invited to have a mammogram – a special kind of X-ray in which the breasts are compressed between two plates so that a picture can be taken of them – every three years. There is some debate over whether women in their forties should be offered this form of breast screening. The strong belief in the UK has been that mammography for women under 50 could do more harm than good because younger breast tissue is more dense and cancers are therefore more difficult to detect accurately by this means, leading to a high false positive rate (a higher diagnosis of cancer when in fact there is none). Also, many cancers diagnosed by mammography at this stage are likely to be ductal carcinomas in situ, a kind of cancer which progresses to invasive cancer in less than half of all cases. Once discovered, however, they are likely to be treated because it isn't possible to know at that stage which ones could safely be left. The result, therefore, could be considerable unnecessary trauma and over-treatment.

Fortunately, the value of screening for women in their forties is now to be decided scientifically. In a study established by the UK Co-ordinating Committee for Cancer Research in 1995, 65,000 women aged 40 or 41 will be screened annually for seven years and 130,000 will act as controls (that is, not be screened). At the end of this large study it should be clear whether screening for women in their 40s is of any benefit.

Mammography for the over fifties is also not without some critics. Because the whole point of screening is to discover cancers at an earlier stage when treatment has a better chance of success, some cancers that are discovered (and treated), even in the over-fifties, may turn out to be of a type that have a low potential for malignancy. In other words, some women may go through the trauma of breast cancer treatment because of a lump so slow growing that it was actually unlikely to become dangerous to her in her natural lifetime. On the other hand, mammography definitely discovers many cancers at a stage when treatment can be given with the best chance of success.

What can be said with some certainty is that the compression of the breast that has to occur for mammography to be carried out does not make an inactive cancer (such as a ductal carcinoma in situ) active. Women do tend to find mammography uncomfortable, though. Fortunately, the procedure only takes a few moments.

• Familial breast cancer •

About 5 per cent of breast cancers are due to a gene or genes which can be inherited. There are already genetic tests available which can predict whether someone has inherited a gene that increases the likelihood of developing breast cancer but currently it is only available to women in families where there have been four or five cases of breast cancer, some of them occurring before the age of 50, because only in such cases can the gene be proved to be responsible for the clustering. However as research continues and gene testing becomes more specific, the test will become available to more women.

Having the test, however, and finding oneself with a 50:50 chance of developing breast cancer may be a very terrifying event. Many women may prefer not to know. Others may prefer either to know they have not inherited the gene and therefore need no longer worry about being at higher risk or to know where they stand and attend very regularly for screening. Preventive treatment with an anti-oestrogen (tamoxifen) may be recommended to reduce risk of development of breast cancer. Some women may opt for the drastic solution of a double mastectomy (removal of both breasts), preferring to be free of all fear.

In Britain, there is an increasing number of specialist cancer family-history clinics to which women can be referred by their GP if there is a strong history of certain cancers in the family, such as a mother or sister having breast cancer before the age of 40, or a mother or sister developing it before the age of 65 and another relative on the same side of the family developing breast, ovarian, endometrial or colorectal cancer before the age of 50. At the clinics, professionals are available to discuss individual risk, (which varies widely and particularly according to age), testing, annual screening and possibilities for prevention. They also offer emotional support, as well as carrying out valuable research.

• Prevention •

Breast feeding Young women who breast feed for at least three months have some protection against breast cancer, the amount increasing according to the length of time they breast feed.

Diet   There is some evidence that reducing the amount of animal fat consumed in the diet may help reduce risk of breast cancer. It also seems that eating broccoli, cabbage and brussels sprouts can help prevent breast cancer. These vegetables belong to the brassica genus, members of which contain a chemical by-product that can inhibit oestrogen. Oestrogen can encourage cancers to grow.

Nipple stimulation   Somewhat contentious, but interesting and certainly harmless, is the conviction of Professor Tim Murrell of the Department of Community Medicine at the University of Adelaide that stimulating the nipples for two or three minutes twice a week helps protect against breast cancer. (See page 291.)

Preventive drugs   Becoming much more of a reality is the possibility of giving 'safe' drugs to young women to prevent breast cancer ever developing. Tamoxifen, the anti-oestrogen used as a treatment for breast cancer for post-menopausal women and being tried as a preventive in younger women at increased risk of breast cancer, cannot be given on a more general basis because of a slightly increased risk of endometrial cancer. However, a drug similar to tamoxifen, that is not cancer-causing and would not be dangerous if taken when pregnant is under development.

So too is a new oral contraceptive which would suppress ovulation by blocking the action of the ovaries but would provide low-dose oestrogen to prevent oestrogen deficiency. Women using this contraceptive would also need a three-monthly injection of progestogen to induce menstruation, although the eventual aim is to combine the whole regimen into a single three-monthly injection.

• Diagnosis •

If you find a lump you should see your GP who will examine you and, unless there is no need for concern, should refer you for further investigations. Do not be fobbed off with reassurances from your GP that all is well if you are deeply concerned about the nature of a lump you have found. If nothing changes, wait only a little while before going back and asking again to be referred to a hospital for tests. Cancer experts now agree that women with breast cancer should be treated at specialist units. The Cancer Relief Macmillan Fund publishes a directory of specialist breast-cancer services which is sent to every GP in the country. So do ensure that your GP sends you to the most appropriate place.

At the hospital, you may be given a mammogram, a special X-ray of the breasts to confirm the suspicion of a cancerous lump. If you are under 35, however, breast tissue will be too dense to allow an accurate X-ray picture to be taken, in which case you are likely to be offered ultrasound. This doesn't hurt at all and the procedure will be familiar to any woman who has had a child, only in this case a gel is spread on the breasts, not the abdomen. An instrument which emits sound waves is passed over them and a picture of the inside of the breasts is created by computer from the way these sound waves bounce off the structures in the breasts.

If the content of the lump needs to be examined, this may be done in one of three ways, depending upon the nature of the lump. In most cases a fine needle and syringe can be used to draw up some cells from the lump for examination in the laboratory (needle aspiration). This can be done on an out-patient basis. Sometimes a small piece of tissue has to be taken from the lump. This is called a biopsy. It is usually done with a hollow needle under local anaesthetic but in some cases the whole lump may need to be removed for examination and this is done under general anaesthetic.

When tests show positive for breast cancer, other tests such as liver scans and bone scans may be necessary to try to ascertain whether the disease has spread to other parts of the body.

Results of the tests that are carried out will reveal not only whether a lump is cancerous but the stage of development of the cancer. This is important for doctors to know, as it will have a bearing on the treatment recommended.

Breast cancers are grouped as follows:

- Stage one: The tumour is small – less than 2cm (¾in) – and has not spread.
- Stage two: The tumour is between 2 and 5cm (¾ and 2in) but has not spread; the tumour is under 2cm (¾in) and hasn't spread but the lymph nodes in the armpit are affected; the tumour is between 2 and 5cm (¾ and 2in) and the lymph nodes in the armpit are affected but there is no spread.
- Stage three: the tumour is larger than 5cm (2in) and, usually, the lymph nodes in the armpit are affected but there is no spread.
- Stage four: the cancer has spread to another or other parts of the body. This is known as secondary breast cancer, regardless of the size of the tumour or whether the lymph nodes are affected.

• Feelings •

Most women are devastated to be told that they have breast cancer, even if they have suspected the truth. It is often very hard to take in more than those two words, although a doctor may then carry on to talk about treatment options and plans. A doctor may also be keen to get treatment started, leaving a woman little time to gather her thoughts and come to terms with what is happening to her.

After learning a diagnosis of breast cancer, there are a variety of emotions which you – and your partner – may experience. Besides shock and an inability to take in much of what anyone is saying, some women may feel panic and fear, some feel anger or resentment that this has happened to them, some feel guilt and shame, imagining that they themselves must be to blame. Or all these feelings may be experienced at different times.

Fortunately, there is increasing understanding from medical staff about the impact of a diagnosis of cancer. There are also increasing numbers of hospitals that employ specialist breast-care nurses who are there to support women through every stage of their breast cancer, right from diagnosis.

Also, it is now government policy to move towards the treatment of breast cancer in patient-centred specialist cancer units in district hospitals, linked to specialised cancer centres in larger general hospitals. This will gradually bring an end to the undesirable situation where a general surgeon more used to operating on varicose veins will occasionally operate on breast cancers but without necessarily being up to date with the most preferred treatments or how breast cancer sufferers feel. However, this network of services will take some years to build up and, even with better training in communication, there will always be professionals who are not easily able to handle others' strong emotions.

It may be best to take someone with you to the appointment at which you will be told the outcome of tests. Or find out beforehand whether the hospital has a breast-care nurse who will be present at the appointment. Do not let yourself be rushed into anything you don't want to do or don't understand. You may prefer to make another appointment to discuss treatment options and likely outcomes, and take a few days first to come to terms with the diagnosis of cancer, share thoughts and feelings with friends and family, and seek out information for yourself from support charities such as BACUP and CancerLink (see Useful Contacts).

You do not usually have to rush into starting treatment. A breast cancer will have been growing for some years before it is discovered. A few days or even weeks is unlikely to make a significant difference and it is far more important that you feel ready to cope with the treatment, physically and psychologically, before you embark upon it. When you see your doctor to discuss treatment, again it may be helpful to have someone you trust with you, so that there is less likelihood that what is said is forgotten and so that you feel supported. It is also a good idea to write down all the questions that have previously popped into your head to ask. It is all too easy otherwise to forget them on the day.

• Treatments •

Research is going on into breast cancer all the time and there are likely to be radical changes in treatment soon as medical science and technology become ever more sophisticated. However, current conventional treatments for breast cancer are still surgery, chemotherapy, radiotherapy and hormone therapy, singly or in combination.

There are many different types of breast cancer and the treatment that will be deemed most suitable for you may not be the same as the treatment other women you know or meet at the hospital have been offered for their breast cancer. If you are uncertain why certain treatment is recommended for you and not others, ask why. It may be to do with the type of tumour, its position in the breast, the severity of the disease, your age or your general state of health.

As well, we are all different, not only in the treatment we may need but in how we approach it. Some women want to trust that their doctor knows best. They do not want to have to make any choices for themselves about treatment options. Others want to play a very active role. If this is you, you may be happier if another specialist sees you and also gives an opinion on what treatment would be best for you. It is not at all uncommon for women to do this, so do not be embarrassed to tell the doctor who is looking after you that this is what you want to do. He or she may be happy to recommend someone or you may prefer to go to someone else whom you find yourself or through your GP.

All of the current orthodox treatments for breast cancer are aggressive and some women decide at this stage that they would rather explore gentler treatments for breast cancer, turning instead (or as well) to complementary therapies. Trained staff at BACUP and CancerLink can tell you where to go to find out more and, while they cannot advise you, can discuss with you the general benefits and disadvantages that are known.

• Surgery •

Surgery for breast cancer may take the form of:

- Lumpectomy: removal of the lump and a small amount of surrounding tissue, leaving a small scar and, sometimes, a small dip in the breast. Hospital stay is likely to be just a few days but usually radiotherapy is required afterwards.
- Segmentectomy: removal of the lump and rather more surrounding tissue, again with a hospital stay of just a few days and later radiotherapy.
- Simple mastectomy: removal of all of the breast tissue, leaving the chest flat on one side and with a long scar running either across the chest or diagonally down from the armpit. Hospital stay is likely to be a week to ten days.
- Modified radical mastectomy: removal of the breast tissue and lymph nodes and maybe also some muscle from the chest wall. Hospital stay is likely to be up to ten days.
- Radical mastectomy: sometimes known as Halstead mastectomy, after the surgeon who devised it, this is a drastic operation rarely done nowadays as other methods have a good or better outcome. It entails removal of all breast tissue and chest wall muscles and hospital stay is about ten days.

• Lymph node removal •

Whichever operation is carried out, it is likely that some lymph nodes will be removed from the armpit to check whether the cancer has spread to the lymphatic system. There is some controversy over how much is enough. Some surgeons believe that all the lymph nodes in the armpit must be removed for investigation (known as axillary clearance), as there is no such thing as a representative sample. Others think that taking a few is sufficient to give a reasonably accurate picture.

One possible benefit of removal of all lymph nodes is that this reduces need for radiotherapy and also reduces the likelihood of lymphoedema occurring (see page 340). This is something you may wish to discuss with your own surgeon.

• Timing of the operation •

Another area where there is still some controversy is over timing of the breast cancer operation. Researchers at Guy's Hospital in London have found that pre-menopausal women have improved chances of survival if surgery is carried out in the second half of their menstrual cycles: that is, at the time when oestrogen levels are opposed by progestogen levels instead of circulating on their own. But many other surgeons feel the evidence is not yet strong enough to warrant changing their normal practice.

• Which operation? •

Lumpectomy and segmentectomy are becoming increasingly common as the primary surgical treatments for breast cancer but mastectomies may still sometimes be necessary in specific instances, for example when the tumour is directly under the nipple and impossible to get at otherwise.

However, new advances bring changes all the time and it has now been found that large primary tumours, which might have needed mastectomy because of their size, can be shrunk sufficiently with pre-operative chemotherapy (cell killing drugs) to allow the breast to be saved and lumpectomy to be carried out instead. It even appears to lessen likelihood of spread. The role of pre-operative chemotherapy is now also being evaluated in less advanced tumours.

Not all women necessarily want lumpectomy rather than mastectomy, however. Usually women who feel happier about mastectomy want the reassurance that the cancer cannot come back in the affected breast. However, recurrence rates are no higher after lumpectomy, in the cases where lumpectomy is the recommended treatment.

Research over recent years has also shown that post-operative treatment of early cancers with hormonal drugs or chemotherapy significantly improves survival after surgery. There is also strong evidence that radiotherapy after surgery can improve length of survival because modern forms of the treatment do not cause damage to the heart with consequent increased risk of heart disease, a hazard of older versions.

• Radiotherapy •

This is usually a follow-up to surgery, carried out as a back-up after you have fully recovered from your breast operation, although for a few types of cancer it can be the sole form of treatment.

It is a means of destroying cancer cells by directing high energy rays at the areas in the breast and armpit where cancer cells may still be lurking. It can be given by a special machine that delivers gamma rays or X-rays on to the designated areas or it can be given internally, via radioactive wires which are implanted in the breast after the surgery is completed.

For the first method, you attend the hospital radiotherapy department as an outpatient for a course of usually daily treatment, except for weekends, for a number of weeks; the exact length of time will be decided according to your own breast-care needs.

The treatment has to be very carefully planned so that radiation is delivered exactly to the areas needed. You will be asked to lie under a machine called a simulator which takes X-rays but doesn't deliver radiation so that these exact areas can be planned out. Sometimes guiding marks may be made on your skin. You will be given advice about how to care for this area of skin during your treatment.

The treatment itself lasts only a few minutes per session and doesn't hurt, but you must lie very still while it is occurring. You will be on your own in the room, as those not receiving treatment mustn't be near it, but the radiographer (the person who operates the machine) will be close by.

If you have radiation as an implant, you have to stay in hospital for a few days. Because of the radioactivity while the wires are in place, you will be cared for in a room on your own, although you can have visitors for short periods of time but not pregnant women or children. Once the wires are removed, you pose no risk to anyone else.

• Side-effects •

There are some side-effects to radiotherapy, whichever form you may have. The skin in the irradiated area may become red and sore for a while and some women experience nausea. There is almost always tiredness and this may persist for quite a long time after treatment, which can be alarming if you don't realise why, and fear you are not recovering as you should be. Some women find the treated breast feels harder, becomes smaller or bigger than before or spidery red marks become apparent, due to tiny broken blood vessels (telangectesia).

Serious side-effects are now rare, due to advanced machinery, but occasionally however there are horror stories of machines set wrongly and giving too much radiation (or too little to do any good), with consequent suffering of symptoms such as pain across the shoulder and neck, swollen limbs and burns to the skin and lungs. There is a self-help group called RIPS (Radiotherapy Injured Patients Support) which supports women who have been hurt in this way.

• Adjuvant therapies •

These are therapies which are given in addition to surgery and radiation. They are hormone therapy, ovarian ablation (preventing the ovaries from working) and chemotherapy.

• Hormone therapy •

The female hormones, oestrogen and progesterone, act on all breast cells, including cancer cells. Oestrogen can encourage cancer cells to grow, so hormone therapy is directed towards suppressing its activity. Tamoxifen is a synthetic anti-oestrogen which is very commonly given to post-menopausal women after surgery or radiotherapy, but may also be given to younger women. It can help prevent recurrence and stop disease developing in the healthy breast. Because it has been so successful in adding healthy years on to life, it is now being tried as a preventive treatment for women at high risk of breast cancer. It does have side-effects, however, similar to those of the menopause – such as dry vagina, hot flushes, weight gain, growth of facial hair, lowering of voice pitch – and also menstrual irregularities in pre-menopausal women. It also slightly but significantly increases risk of endometrial cancer.

• Ovarian ablation •

This is the term used to mean stopping the ovaries from working, and it can be achieved by various methods. Least popular is surgery to remove the ovaries or irradiation of the ovaries, both of which have permanent effects and mean you cannot have any or more children. Also, losing the ovaries tends to bring on an early menopause, with its increased risks for osteoporosis and heart disease.

Drugs known as LHRH analogues have the same effect of knocking out the ovaries but their effects are reversible. They are usually only given for limited periods, however, as they also cause menopausal and also masculinising symptoms such as acne, weight gain and deepening of the voice.

• Chemotherapy •

This is the use of cancer cell-killing drugs (cytoxic drugs), very often used in addition to surgery or radiation, particularly as survival is shown to be increased when they (or hormone treatments) are given. They can also improve survival in older women when given as well as hormone treatment. Chemotherapy is a systemic treatment, meaning that it affects the whole body and may therefore kill cancer cells that have spread. But, by the same token, it also affects healthy cells in the body although these have more chance to recover.

The doctor in charge of your case will decide which combination of drugs is most suitable for you. They may be given orally or intravenously, by a drip. You may have treatment as an out-patient or, if you are receiving intravenous treatment which will probably last a few days at a time, you may require a short hospital stay. After the treatment a number of weeks will elapse before your next one, to allow your body to re-gather its strength. Courses of treatment may last from a few months to up to a year, according to the drugs used.

Reactions to chemotherapy   Chemotherapy has a very bad image, not surprisingly, as very powerful drugs are acting on all the cells in your body. But it is important to be aware that reactions vary, according to the nature of the drugs used and individual response, and some people do not find the experience even particularly unpleasant.

You may experience nausea and vomiting, although special drugs (anti-emetics) can be prescribed to prevent this. Some people have diarrhoea, some find their mouth is sore or ulcers develop in it. Hair loss or hair thinning may occur but not always, depending upon the drugs used. You will be very vulnerable to infection while having the treatment (because of a lowered cell count in your blood) and very tired. Afterwards, some people feel depressed for a while and there may be loss of interest in sex.

Do ask your doctor what kind of side-effects are likely with the particular drug combination prescribed for you. It may be a relief to know, for example, that in your case hair loss is unlikely. On the other hand, you can start to prepare yourself mentally if you know hair loss will occur. It does grow back after treatment is finished. Free wigs are available on the NHS should you need and want to take advantage of this, although many women prefer to wear scarves or dramatic hats.

Feelings   It doesn't really help to base your expectations on those of others who have been through chemotherapy because their experience may be very different from yours. Some women find they are so tired that they can hardly carry on functioning in between treatments; others find they can carry on their jobs and run their homes and families without problem. Some people find chemotherapy unremittingly awful, only starting to feel normal again just as the next lot of drugs is due. (Not surprisingly, many who experience this decide to stop treatment, preferring a better quality of life in the present than the possibility of a longer life ahead.) For others, there may be absolutely no side-effects at all.

SCALP COOLING

Keeping the scalp very cool during chemotherapy treatments can help to prevent hair loss. Some methods of achieving this can be rather unpleasant – such as wearing a freezing pudding basin over wetted hair – but there is also available a custom-made pre-cooled lightweight plastic cap, the Penguin Cold Cap system (manufactured by Medical Specialties of California: see Useful Contacts). It is filled with gel and fits comfortably over the head with a chin-strap, looking a bit like a bicycle helmet.

Cooling methods do not work for everyone but many women may feel they are well worth a try. Unfortunately, many hospitals do not even offer these methods or aren't receptive to their use, as they entail extra time and effort.

BACUP can provide more information about scalp cooling methods. See Useful Contacts.

If your own experience is not a good one, do tell your doctor and/or breast nurse, to see if anything can be done. Airing your feelings is important anyway as is the realisation that you are not alone or unusual in the way you feel, even if your neighbour sailed through similar treatment. As more drugs are developed and combined, there may be a greater chance of side-effects lessening in general.

Chemotherapy in the future In the future, for some slow-growing cancers and some advanced cancers, chemotherapy may be able to be given instead of surgery. Researchers at Nottingham City Hospital are working on a computer-assisted means of analysing the nature of individual tumour cells, enabling chemotherapy to be tailored to the individual.

• Complementary therapies •

Complementary care may include approaches such as taking vitamin and mineral supplements, massage, aromatherapy, acupuncture, homoeopathy, reflexology and healing; and psychological strategies such as counselling, visualisation techniques, deep relaxation and meditation. Many women choose to try one or more of these approaches in addition to conventional treatment in order to help boost their immune systems and to enable themselves to feel some positive control over their health and bodies again. Some choose not to have conventional treatment and to put their commitment and trust into complementary methods alone.

No one can decide for you which method, if any, would be best for you. You need to gather as much information as you can in order to assist your decision and to take into account practicalities such as the expense of certain complementary therapies, the practicalities of journeying to visit a therapist regularly, your commitment to the method etc.

The charity CancerLink publishes a booklet on complementary care and cancer which raises the issues you need to think about and helps you weigh up your choices.

The Bristol Cancer Help Centre, a pioneering centre for complementary approaches, strongly believes that, whatever treatment you opt to have for a cancer, a programme of vitamin and mineral supplementation can help cancer therapies to work and prolong survival. They believe the scientific evidence is now there, although conventional cancer specialists may remain sceptical. Contact them for details of their book *Cancer and Nutrition: the positive scientific evidence.*

• After treatment •

You will probably experience some pain after any kind of surgery and your arm may be stiff after mastectomy. Specific exercises for your arm should be recommended.

If you have had lymph nodes removed from under your arm or you have had radiotherapy, you are at higher risk of a condition called lymphoedema, which is the swelling of the arm or hand on the side on which you had breast cancer. Lymphoedema cannot be cured but it can be prevented or reduced and controlled which is why it is so important to take all the recommended precautions. See page 341 for details.

If you have had a mastectomy, you will be given a temporary prosthesis (artificial breast) made of very light foam which you can put inside your bra. When the chest area has recovered from the surgery, you will be able to be fitted for a permanent prosthesis if you want one. What you get on the NHS varies from hospital to hospital and may depend on who fits you: the appliance officer who deals with all kinds of prostheses or a breast-care nurse. If you do not receive sympathetic treatment from an appliance officer and do not feel happy with the type of prosthesis you are offered, you may prefer to buy one. The charity Breast Cancer Care can advise on choosing a prosthesis and where to get one and also sells both permanent and temporary prostheses, as well as bras, at a very reasonable price. They can also advise on swimwear and any other aspects of choosing clothes.

You may, however, prefer to think about reconstruction. This can be done at the time of the original breast surgery, although most surgeons aren't keen, or at a later date. See page 336 for details of techniques.

• Life after breast cancer •

Having treatment is not the end of breast cancer for most women. It is an enormously traumatic disease and a capricious one. For very many women it may never recur but for most there is always the nightmare that it will. And together with this fear for the future, there may be much difficulty emotionally in coping with day-to-day feelings.

Losing a breast or having surgery for breast cancer, even without losing a breast can deeply affect a woman's sense of her own sexuality, femininity and identity. There may be a deep sense of loss which it is best not to try to deny or ignore because emotional healing is so much quicker when pain is acknowledged and faced.

If you have had treatment which has affected your fertility, there may well be an additional strong sense of loss, even if you have had your family. You may feel such sadness is irrational if you have had children, but it is an emotional response and none the less valid for that.

There may be many conflicting emotions. Relief that the cancer is treated, anger, resentment, grief, anxiety and even shock, now that it is all over. Some women feel ashamed of their bodies and are reluctant to let their partners see them – or even to see them themselves. Others are lucky to have understanding and supportive partners who make it clear from the outset that their feelings remain unchanged. However, it may be impossible for some women even to trust reassurances like this if they themselves feel loathing for their changed body.

Some women may lose interest in sex because of their changed feelings about their bodies. This may make it harder for partners to be understanding because they still feel desire and are frustrated. There may be other physical changes to handle too, such as skin burns or hair loss, weight changes caused by different treatments and possibly a swollen arm. It is an awful lot to cope with. Sometimes it isn't easy to talk to a partner about feelings about such things because their way of coping may be to deny any problems and to believe that they are being helpful by acting as if you are exactly the same as you ever were. This might be a very loving response, but may not necessarily be the most helpful one for everyone.

Fortunately, there are many very helpful and sympathetic people around who can help on the coping side. There are charities (see Useful Contacts) to advise, support and just listen, and which can put women in touch with others who have been through breast cancer. If you are lucky enough to have a breast-care nurse at the hospital where you have been treated, she also will provide a listening ear for as long as you want it, for anything which may concern you.

As time goes on and confidence starts to return, a worry which may remain at the back of the mind, or even the front of it, is recurrence. It is not unusual to fear that any unexplained lump or bump anywhere or any sudden pain is a sign of cancer returning. The breast-care nurse or a counsellor on the end of the phone at one of the cancer charities may be able to advise when panic isn't necessary, and when a visit to your doctor would be a worthwhile precaution.

There is often a lot written about the link between how we react to events in our lives and the development of particular cancers. Although taking a positive attitude and doing everything we can to keep generally healthy certainly gives our immune systems the best chance, research shows that experiencing stressful life events does not make breast cancer more likely to occur nor more likely to come back.

Terrifying though it may be, the experience of breast cancer need not necessarily be all negative. For many women, breast cancer may have provided them with their first real opportunity to take stock of their lives, see what it really important and perhaps make some very positive changes. Some women learn to value themselves for the first time and make their own needs a priority as well as those of their family. It can be a time for learning a lot very quickly about inner resources, personal power and love, however much we would all rather learn this a different way.

40

BREAST RECONSTRUCTION

ALMOST all women who have had a breast partially or completely removed will be able to have breast reconstruction if they wish it. If you have had or will be having a mastectomy, breast reconstruction may be helpful for you if you are finding it difficult to accept the loss of a breast or to contemplate carrying on through life without one. You may find the idea of a prosthesis repugnant or not wish to be reminded every single day by its presence that you have had breast cancer.

• Issues for consideration •

Breast reconstruction, although it can never contrive a breast exactly equivalent to the one lost, may be a means of restoring lost confidence. You will look just as before when clothed and can certainly look good in a swimsuit or bikini. You have to be aware, however, that breast reconstruction cannot restore breast sensation. What you should have is a breast mound that feels like a natural breast and is a similar shape, size and colour to your other one, but it will not look like a natural breast.

You can have a breast reconstructed at the same time as having your operation for breast cancer but the wisdom of this needs careful discussion with your doctor. Many doctors prefer to wait for a year or more, so that they can be sure the cancer treatment has been successful or so that they have the option to prescribe radiotherapy or chemotherapy treatments as well, if necessary. Breast reconstruction cannot be carried out during these treatments as they adversely affect healing after the cosmetic surgery. You also may benefit from a waiting time, to see how you really do adapt to not having one breast. Some women find themselves far less concerned than they had imagined; others are as certain afterwards that they will not adjust to having only one breast.

Those who are in favour of breast reconstruction at the same time as breast cancer surgery, when appropriate, argue that the need for a second operation is averted and also the negative psychological effects of losing a breast may be minimised.

If further treatment for cancer is not needed, breast reconstruction can easily go ahead within six months of the breast surgery, if your doctor agrees.

You can also decide to have reconstruction years after breast surgery, if you so choose.

There are various approaches to breast reconstruction. The one that is chosen will mainly depend upon the kind of operation you have had.

• Silicone implants •

If you have had a simple mastectomy, you will probably have sufficient breast skin and muscle left to enable the surgeon to put a silicone implant in. For fuller details of this operation, see Breast Enlargement, page 295. Women who have had radiotherapy will not be able to have the option of an implant under the chest muscle.

• Tissue expansion •

This method takes longer than the ordinary insertion of a silicone implant, but tends to give a better cosmetic result. A silicone bag is inserted under the chest muscle, and once a week, under local anaesthetic, it is inflated with saline solution through a valve.

After about eight weeks of this, when the false breast is slightly larger than the real one, the valve is removed and then, after three months, the saline-filled bag is taken out and replaced with a permanent silicone implant. This method allows the false breast to develop a fall similar to that of the real breast. Sometimes this effect may be achieved by inserting a silicone implant from the start, in a deflated condition. The rest of the procedure is the same.

Many but not all women who have had radiotherapy may also have this procedure. But it may need to take longer with longer gaps between inflations, because the skin is not as elastic after radiotherapy and the final results are not as good as when women have not had radiotherapy.

• Muscle and skin flaps •

When a mastectomy is more extensive, underlying muscle as well as almost all the breast tissue is taken out, leaving too little skin over the area to enable anything to be inserted underneath. The solution is to take a strip of skin and muscle from another part of the body, usually the back, and move it so that it can be stretched across the chest, but while still connected to all its nerve and blood supply at the back of the armpit.

The implant is inserted under this skin and above the skin already stretched over the chest. Sometimes surgeons will take the skin and muscle from the abdomen, along with some fat from the abdomen and then use this fat instead of an implant. It is more problematic, however: about 45 per cent of women are recorded as experiencing complications with it, even when the operation was carried out by an experienced and skilled surgeon, but this is starting to change with increasing use of the method.

Although you might end up with a flatter stomach the method is probably out of the question altogether if you have ever had abdominal surgery. Either of these procedures can, as appropriate, be used for a woman who has had radiotherapy that prevents her from having any of the procedures described so far.

The operation will leave a scar across the breast that is not unlike the mastectomy scar (or one that runs right around the breast area, if more complicated surgery is required) and one on the upper back or across the bikini line.

Surgery that entails moving strips of skin and muscle from the back or abdomen is major surgery and will necessitate a stay in hospital of ten days to recover. You will probably have some pain for a week and will have to wear bandages across the chest and then a good supporting bra day and night for some weeks.

It is imperative not to do too much too quickly and to avoid lifting or even just moving the arms any more than you have to. You will, of course, feel sore in your back or abdomen, where skin and muscle have been taken, and you need to give these areas time to heal properly as well. It will be a good six weeks before life approaches being back to normal.

• Nipple reconstruction •

Nipple reconstruction, if desired, is usually carried out in a second operation at least three months after the first, to give the breast time to heal and settle into its natural position. Then the new nipple can more easily be positioned level with the one on the other breast.

The procedure involves making a new nipple from skin taken from the other nipple or from the earlobe. A new areola is usually made from skin from the inner thigh and is likely to end up lighter than the other areola because skin from skin grafts fades. The operation only takes an hour and for brave souls can even be done under a local anaesthetic.

However, you might feel you have had enough of surgery and, as the cosmetic results are far from perfect, that you would rather settle for ready-made or specially moulded stick-on nipples.

After nipple reconstruction, there will be a barely noticeable scar on the other nipple and a scar on the inner thigh.

Recovery after the operation for a replacement nipple is quite swift, although your nipple and thigh, where the skin has been taken from will, not unsurprisingly, feel tender for a little while. You must avoid anything rubbing the nipple that skin was taken from, as friction will adversely affect healing. Sex is best avoided for a few weeks because the skin of the inner thigh mustn't rub either if it is to heal well.

• Possible complications •

It is important to be aware that complications can occur, however infrequently, because some of them may make further surgery necessary at a time when you might feel very reluctant to have more surgery.

The complications of silicone implants are fully described under Breast Enlargement (see page 298). For the more major surgery, the biggest problem is when muscle is moved from the abdomen. In some cases, the blood supply to the muscle may be damaged and the strip fail to survive. Then a skin graft becomes necessary. (This only happens in 3 per cent of cases when muscle is moved from the back instead.) If muscle is moved from the abdomen, another possible complication is that the muscle that is left behind is weakened, causing a hernia. If fat is used to create the 'implant' a possible consequence is that fat may seep out of the breast – in the form of a yellowish oil. Gradually, if this happens, the 'breast' will start to disappear.

Whichever method is used, there is always a slight risk that the new breast will be set at a slightly different level from the other, appearing higher or lower. In this event, any adjustments are going to have to be made to the healthy breast, which could be a worrying prospect. So it is very very important to discuss in detail all possible procedures and outcomes for breast reconstruction and be sure that you are ready to go ahead. It is worth bearing in mind that very many women who have had breast reconstruction are very happy indeed that they did and have not been daunted by any associated problems. But the decision must be yours.

41

LYMPHOEDEMA

L YMPHOEDEMA is an unpleasant possible consequence of breast cancer; a severe swelling of the arm on the side of the affected breast. It is completely unexpected by most women and often not even mentioned as a possibility by their doctors. It is a tragedy that lymphoedema isn't routinely discussed along with protective measures, as much can be done to prevent its development or to minimise the misery if it does occur. Fortunately, the pioneering work of the British Lymphology Interest Group, made up of involved professionals, and the tireless efforts of the Lymphoedema Support Network, whose members are sufferers, are making the condition much better understood.

• What is lymphoedema? •

Lymphoedema is a swelling of tissues under the skin which occurs when lymph, a colourless fluid that forms in body tissues, fails to be drained away properly.

Lymph is a fluid formed in all of the body's tissues all the time. It contains water and proteins and is carried along lymph vessels which normally drain it back into the blood circulation. Dead cells, abnormal cells, bacteria and other such undesirable elements in the lymph are filtered out by the body's lymph nodes. The network of lymph vessels and lymph nodes – the lymphatic system – is an important part of the body's immune system. However, when the lymph vessels or nodes are damaged or blocked, the lymph cannot drain.

There are many reasons for damage or blockage but the main cause in Britain is surgery or radiotherapy to treat cancer, probably as a result of the formation of obstructive scar tissue. (Lymphoedema of the leg may occur after treatment for pelvic or bowel cancers and occasionally it can occur elsewhere, such as the chest or genitals.)

Until relatively recently it was thought that the fluid trapped under the skin in lymphoedema was high in proteins. However, research has now shown that protein levels in the blood are lower in women with lymphoedema than in non-sufferers, suggesting that the condition is caused by a disturbance in the way protein is dealt with in the circulation or tissues of the arm, along with restricted lymph drainage. This may eventually have an impact upon treatment possibilities.

Lymphoedema may not occur immediately after treatment. Sometimes even 20 or 30 years may pass before symptoms first occur in some people, although this is not usual. Common precipitating factors include insect bites or sudden exertion.

· Doctors' attitudes ·

Traditionally, doctors have not been very interested in lymphoedema because it was thought that little if anything could be done to solve it. Attempts to debulk the affected limb by conventional surgery (the swelling is not just made up of fluid but of solid material too) have not shown any lasting success. Drugs do not seem to help, nor do diuretics of course, as the swelling is not straightforward fluid. Patients are commonly told that they just have to live with it; sometimes even that lymphoedema is little to put up with, having had the cancer successfully treated.

However lymphoedema, untreated, is not little to put up with. The affected arm, in the case of breast cancer, can be enormously painful and lifting can be difficult. Sometimes the hand may even be affected. In extreme cases, the arm itself may become hard and distorted, with thick folds of loose, leathery skin. For many sufferers the painful swelling is a constant reminder of having had breast cancer, they have the misery of trying to disguise it with outsize loose clothing (all of which may sap confidence) and, importantly, they may easily suffer infections in the arm because of reduced immunity to infection caused by the blockage in the lymph system.

· Who suffers? ·

Some doctors may still believe that lymphoedema is relatively rare. In fact, it is horribly common. One of the earliest findings in this little-researched area revealed that 38 per cent of 200 breast-cancer patients at the Royal Marsden Hospital in London suffered lymphoedema after having both surgery and radiotherapy to the armpit. A quarter of those who had just one of the two treatments developed it.

A more recent survey of 1249 women in the Worthing area who had had a mastectomy generated a 90 per cent response rate, with 29 per cent of respondents having suffered lymphoedema after treatment, on average three years afterwards. Those who had had a radical mastectomy (see page 328) were more likely to develop it and to suffer more swelling than those who had a wide local excision. Radiotherapy treatment was found to double the risk but treatment of both breasts for breast cancer did not increase the incidence of lymphoedema.

· Protective self-help measures ·

There are a number of practical steps you can take to help prevent lymphoedema occurring or keep it minimal.

1 Don't let the skin on your arm get dry and cracked, when it will be more prone to infection. Moisturise it well. Always dry between your fingers thoroughly to prevent fungal infections such as athlete's foot which thrive in moist warm conditions.
2 Don't have very hot baths, as this can increase any swelling.

3 Keep clothing in the affected area comfortable, not tight, and avoid any jewellery, even a wedding ring or watch, on a swollen arm.

4 Always use an electric razor or creams to remove hair from the armpit on the side where you have had cancer treatment, never a razor blade. A tiny nick will provide entry for infection.

5 Protect yourself from cuts and scratches as much as possible. Wear gloves for gardening and washing up. Use nail clippers or a nail file on nails rather than a scissors.

6 Take great care not to let your arm burn in the sun.

7 If you do get any cuts, always clean the area thoroughly and apply an antiseptic. See your GP immediately if your arm becomes hot, red or sore, as this may be a sign of infection.

8 Don't have injections in the affected arm, blood samples taken from it or your blood pressure measured on it.

9 Always use insect-repellant if you are somewhere where you may be bitten. Mosquito bites are particularly a problem.

10 Don't avoid using your arm because normal exercise is an important part of helping lymph to drain normally. However, sudden intense exertion, such as heavy lifting or carrying heavy weights should be avoided.

11 Rest your arm whenever you are able to, keeping it slightly raised and supported.

12 Don't try to reduce your fluid intake. The swelling in lymphoedema is not related to how much you drink.

• Treatments •

However careful you are you can never completely avoid accidents or events which may trigger lymphoedema. Or it may just happen seemingly out of the blue. If swelling does occur, always check that lymphoedema is indeed the cause before embarking on any self-help measures. Swelling may, for instance, be due to an infection or to pooling of blood after an operation, both of which need immediate treatment, or be due to other conditions such as poor circulation or heart trouble.

The aim of treatment for lymphoedema is to try to shift fluid from a swollen area to another part where the lymph system is not damaged, so it can drain away the fluid as normal. A number of hospitals do now have specialist lymphoedema clinics but, alas, not enough.

You can obtain a directory of treatment centres from the British Lymphology Interest Group or the Lymphoedema Support Group may know which is the nearest to you. Also the Support Group stocks a very simple instruction booklet which you can buy (*Lymphoedema: advice on treatment*) that describes all the treatment methods mentioned below. Beneficial treatments for lymphoedema are good skin care (see page 103), compression sleeves, exercise and massage.

Compression sleeves These are designed to stop the build-up of fluid and provide support but they can only do the job if they fit properly and provide sufficient pressure in the right places. For example, the pressure needs to be greatest (that is, the sleeve tightest) at the part nearest the hand, so that the fluid is pushed upwards. Any wrinkling in the sleeve will just make fluid build up below the wrinkle.

If possible, you should be fitted for a sleeve by someone who is experienced in treating lymphoedema. In some hospitals they may be made to measure but ready-made ones can be just as effective, as long as they fit correctly. It is important that the sleeve is changed regularly. After a few months, much of the elasticity is lost. Also, as swelling reduces, a differently fitting sleeve will be required.

For severe swelling, bandaging can be a great help but specialist knowledge of where to apply most pressure is required and this will probably only be found in a specialist treatment centre.

Exercise   This is essential to prevent stiffness in the swollen arm and to help fluid drain. Experts recommend doing a simple sequence of arm exercises twice a day.

Massage   Encourages the lymph system to work better and can help ease the discomfort of the swelling. It does not have to be done by a professional to be of benefit. You can do it for yourself but may need the help of a partner, because you need to work on both your front and on your back. If you prefer, you can use one of the commercially available electric body massagers but some are better than others for this purpose, so take advice.

Experts recommend a 15-minute session twice a day, aiming for strokes firm enough to move fluid but not so firm as to irritate the skin. It is important to follow specific instructions provided by your clinic or by the lymphoedema advice booklet already mentioned, so that you know in which direction to massage the fluid.

A gentle form of massage specially designed to move lymph is manual lymph drainage (MLD). It does need to be done by an expert, however. It was developed in Germany and at present the only place where training is given in the UK is the Clare Maxwell School of Massage in North West London. They may also be able to tell you if there is an MLD therapist practising anywhere near you. You can also contact the organisation MLD UK. See Useful Contacts.

Compression pumps   These are small pumps attached by tubing to an inflatable sleeve. When air is pumped into the sleeve, the sleeve inflates, pushing fluid up the arm to relieve congestion at the bottom. After a few moments, the sleeve deflates again. The process is repeated for as long as the pump is switched on. Many doctors tend to recommend these pumps, if nothing else. However, they may not have anything more to offer than the self-help methods described above and are only really worth trying if these have not worked, especially as the pumps may need to be used for hours daily to get any good effect.

In many cases they will be positively counter-productive. This is if the chest or abdomen is congested as well, leaving the fluid in the arm nowhere to drain. The fluid in the chest or abdomen must be cleared by massage first, otherwise using the pump will just cause more discomfort.

42

....

SEX AND SEX-RELATED PROBLEMS

THIS chapter takes a look at the natural process of sexual arousal and how it works for us physically and emotionally. It also tackles the range of common or not-so-common problems that may prevent enjoyment of sex and looks in detail at sexually transmitted diseases. It doesn't set out to explore in any depth the variety and richness of 'normal' sexual practice, nor to define what normal sexual practice is. It assumes, however, that women may be contentedly heterosexual or lesbian, be in monogamous relationships or have more than one partner, be celibate by choice or otherwise and masturbate as well as or instead of having sex with a partner.

· Female sexual arousal ·

The same physiological pattern of sexual arousal is experienced by both women and men, with variations for each decided simply by anatomy. (See page 209 for a description of how the female reproductive organs are organised.) Women are as capable as men of sexual desire, sexual arousal and achieving sexual satisfaction and are also as keen.

The famed sex researchers Masters and Johnson have described the basic pattern of arousal as having four distinct phases. While it is helpful to describe sexual response in this way, the different phases are not rigid and may not be so clear in some people as in others.

· I Excitement ·

The first sign of sexual excitement in a woman is that the vagina becomes more moist with lubrication, as the vaginal walls secrete a clear liquid to prepare the vagina for the friction of sex. As arousal continues the inner part of the vagina lengthens and widens by ballooning out. (Normally the vagina is a collapsed tube, with its walls resting against each other.)

The vagina's colour changes from reddish purple to deep purple, as blood flow to the area increases. The extra blood flow also makes the uterus swell and lift upwards from the pelvic floor muscles, which also helps to make the vagina longer.

The urethral sponge is the name given to a pad of sensitive tissue which lies just inside the vagina, between its upper wall (if you are on your back) and the urethra. It can be felt through the vagina wall and intense, firm stimulation of it during the excitement phase leads it to swell. It is then capable of contributing to the intensity of orgasm. It is this area which has been popularised as the G-spot.

The heart rate and blood pressure increase and the nipples become erect. Then the whole of each breast and the areola (the dark area around the nipples) engorges and swells too. Usually a sexual flush occurs, a reddening of the skin that spreads from the abdomen to the breasts and neck.

Women can become excited as quickly as men but usually need more prolonged and direct physical stimulation whereas men may be sufficiently stimulated by fantasies, looking at something that turns them on or by specific sights and smells. The excitement phase may last for minutes or hours.

• 2 Plateau •

This phase may or may not be very distinct from the excitement phase as it is mainly a continuation of it but at a high level of excitement which is maintained, rather than increased further, until orgasm. During this phase the sex flush is at its most extensive and muscle tension increases considerably throughout the body, often creating involuntary jerking movements. The breasts are at their fullest size and the uterus expands further and lifts further upwards. Breathing is very fast.

The outer third of the vagina becomes congested with blood and this in effect narrows and tightens the passageway into the vagina. Masters and Johnson called this the orgasmic platform. The inner lips of the vagina carry on darkening to a deep red and this is a sign that orgasm is close. This colour change is the most marked in women who have given birth.

When excitement is at its peak, the clitoris retracts under its hood and so cannot be directly stimulated any more. The Bartholin's glands may secrete lubricating fluid at this stage.

• 3 Orgasm •

Orgasm is the culmination of sexual arousal and excitement, when all the tension is released in an intensely pleasurable whoosh. Physiologically, the event is similar for women and men – although only men ejaculate in any real sense – and lasts for only a few moments.

Physiologically what occurs is that the outer third of the vagina, 'the orgasmic platform', starts to contract strongly and rhythmically. The contractions may be less than a second apart at first, then, as they weaken, occur slightly less frequently. A woman may have as many as 15 contractions or as few as three, according to Masters and Johnson's researches. The uterus also contracts at this time but in an irregular fashion and there is tension throughout the rest of the body as well. Breathing is extremely fast and blood pressure and heart rate are even further raised.

The intensity of the experience of these sensations depends upon the degree of sexual excitement attained. Some women may have a 'mild' orgasm after less intense excitement, or more than one orgasm; others may have a deep, perhaps even overwhelming one, after prolonged intense arousal. The experience of orgasm is very variable (see below).

Some women may experience a leakage of fluid at orgasm. This is not urine but fluid secreted by glands which open into the urethra and which correspond to the prostate in men. But these glands are not necessarily well developed in most women and therefore only a minority are likely to experience the 'female ejaculation'. Absence of it – or of multiple orgasm, for that matter – certainly isn't a sign of sexual insufficiency .

• 4 Resolution •

This is the phase when everything starts to return to normal. The orgasmic platform disappears as the outer third of the vagina returns to its previous size, the clitoris re-emerges from under its hood, the inner lips return to their normal colour, the walls of the inner two thirds of the vagina collapse again and the uterus shrinks down and descends to its usual position. The sex flush fades, the breasts gradually return to their usual size and blood pressure, heart rate and breathing quite quickly slow down again and become normal.

For women who may have more than one orgasm if sexually stimulated again, this resolution phase does not occur until all orgasms are over.

• The female orgasm •

There is a lot of confusion about clitoral orgasm and vaginal orgasm, whether they are the same thing and, if not, whether one is better than the other. The clitoris, made up of erectile tissue and similar in everything but size to the penis, is the most sensitive of the female sex organs. Stimulation of the clitoris is usually necessary for orgasm (but not always): depending upon the exact position of the clitoris, the position during sex and maybe the likes and dislikes of individual women. Indirect stimulation of the clitoris during penetrative sex may or may not be sufficient for triggering orgasm. Probably at least half of all women need or prefer direct clitoral stimulation, manual or oral, to bring them towards orgasm.

Although sensations of orgasm start in the clitoris, the intensity of orgasm may be experienced as deeply internal or deep inside the vagina. What happens is that nerves supplying the clitoris send messages of pleasure along a network that serves the whole pelvic area, so that waves of sensation are experienced throughout this region. Contraction of the pelvic floor muscles is essential for orgasm, so orgasm cannot truly be described as occurring in the clitoris although powerful sensations which heighten the process emanate from there.

The experience of orgasm varies from woman to woman and from occasion to occasion. Descriptions in romantic novels often make orgasm appear to be something almost overwhelmingly sudden and ecstatic, an explosion of lights and colour, a transportation for a few seconds out of this world. Some women may feel something so remarkable. For many orgasm is more a warm flooding of feeling. Or it may be like an exquisitely pleasant muscle spasm. Or it may be so powerful that your whole body shakes uncontrollably and pleasure courses through the whole pelvis. You may feel faint. Occasionally, some women do faint. There may be a sense of being on the brink of something big and then experiencing only the briefest of pleasurable moments. Or an enormously pleasant sensation may suddenly almost overwhelm you.

Some women can only have an orgasm when they masturbate. This isn't weird or awful, even if you have a partner. It just means that you know how to stimulate yourself best.

• Not having an orgasm •

Some women think they have never had an orgasm, although they may still find sex pleasurable. The lack of orgasm may be because they are not sufficiently aroused. Others are aroused sufficiently but are left unable to have an orgasm because stimulation isn't maintained around the clitoris for long enough. This can, of course, be very frustrating but may also lead to pelvic congestion, with accompanying abdominal and back pain.

However, many women are just not bothered about whether they have orgasms or not and prefer not to feel that they have to strive for pinnacles but just to let the experience be loving and gentle and come to its own natural conclusion, whatever that may be on any occasion.

The mind, of course, plays an enormous part in the sexual experience. If you do not want to be with whomever you are having sex with, even if sex is not being forced upon you, you are unlikely to allow yourself to feel aroused or to give yourself up to the occasion sufficiently to achieve orgasm. In free and loving sex you are making yourself deeply vulnerable to another person and this can be threatening or frightening, so many women may hold back, which prevents them from experiencing full excitement or orgasm.

Many women may feel frightened of losing control or of being overwhelmed by feelings – or imagine that they might be overwhelmed – and so hold back on sexual arousal and orgasm for this reason.

Being with someone they love and trust deeply may be important or vital for sexual abandonment and full sexual feeling for some women. Others may need to feel passionately excited about their partner or may only be able to experience excitement and orgasm if their partner is relatively unknown and there is the thrill of the new, and limited risk of vulnerability. Problems in relationships affect desire and ability to enjoy sex, of course (see Loss of Desire, page 352.)

• Sexual fantasies •

Many women like to fantasise during sex or masturbation. Many women do not. There is certainly no right or wrong about it. Women who don't fantasise shouldn't feel that they are less sexually mature or adventurous; women who do fantasise shouldn't feel that they must be less naturally sexy for needing to.

Fantasies can heighten the sexual experience for many women and are therefore worth having. Some women feel guilty if they fantasise about someone other than the person they are making love to, or about another person, known or unknown, during masturbation. This is likely to be a problem only if it hides a problem, such as a reluctance to be with your partner. Some women who usually experience orgasm only during masturbation and not during intercourse find that fantasising during sex with their partner helps them get more excited and more able to achieve orgasm, and as a result feel closer to their partner.

Many women have fantasies about rape or about sex that is in some way forced upon them. Or they may fantasise about having sex with a stranger. This doesn't mean that they really do want any of these thing to happen.

Rape fantasies are not really rape fantasies at all. In rape, there is commonly frightening violence, always fear and no pleasure. In fantasy, women are enjoying the idea of sex that is pleasurable but imposed upon them. Often it is women who have to take a lot of control in their daily lives, whether running the family, their jobs or both, who fantasise about 'rape' or domination. Fantasies of being forced into sex may also be a way of abdicating responsibility for what is happening or a way of letting go for women who have guilt feelings about sexual enjoyment. For some women, however, fantasies about rape in any form may be perceived as sick, because of how terrible the experience is in reality, and therefore are pushed firmly out of mind.

• Sexual problems •

There may be a number of reasons for having problems with sex. Fear and ignorance about one's own anatomy or about quite what happens during sex may lead to physical difficulty. Certain illnesses or excessive fatigue may make sex more difficult or more painful. Most commonly, however, unresolved or unvoiced difficulties in relationships, fear of intimacy or some discomfort about sex learned from childhood perceptions of parents' attitudes may cause loss of desire and lack of sexual response.

• Vaginismus •

At least 27,000 women in the UK are estimated, by the Royal College of General Practitioners, to suffer from vaginismus, an involuntary spasm of the muscles surrounding the entrance to the vagina (and sometimes also the muscles of the thighs, stomach, anus and buttocks) when an attempt is made to insert something such as a tampon or penis. The clamping effect means that nothing can be inserted.

• Who may get it? •

Sufferers of vaginismus are most commonly aged between 15 and 24 and they imagine, at least at first, that their problem is physical: that their vagina is the wrong shape or too small. But vaginismus is emotional, not physical. The causes may be superficial or deep but, either way, need confronting as early as possible so that the condition doesn't ruin your relationships and your life. For, as many sufferers have found, the shame experienced is so great that it can devastate self-image and permeate one's whole experience of life, because the world presented to us in magazines, newspapers, adverts and television is a very sexual one.

Women with vaginismus are not asexual. Many may enjoy oral sex, masturbation and mutual masturbation but just not be able to allow penetration. Others may have previously enjoyed sex but have developed vaginismus later.

While there may be many causes of vaginismus, it is not always necessary to root them out. A number of young women do not realise, for example, that they themselves are in control of their pelvic floor muscles which, among other things, govern entry to the vagina. If women are shown that they can grip and let go of a finger with those muscles and that the muscles are the same ones used to stop a flow of urine, this may be sufficient to help them over the fear that causes them to clamp their muscles.

• Causes •

Anything which causes physical pain during sex may, in some women, lead from a natural reluctance to have sex to an inability to have sex. Certain sexual infections which make the vagina sore, dryness of the vagina caused by hormonal abnormalities, or allergic reaction to rubber in the condom or diaphragm may all be such causes.

For some women a bad previous experience of sex, perhaps with an insensitive or brutal partner or as a result of child abuse or rape, can cause vaginismus. Unresolved feelings or guilt about having had an abortion can sometimes play havoc with women's sexual responses. Vaginismus that occurs only with one particular partner may be an indication of problems within that relationship rather than a sexual problem in the woman.

It may not be easy to pinpoint the cause of vaginismus which, for some, may stem from parental unease with or distaste of sex which is unconsciously passed on. Or there may be unconscious fears about what penetration means (perhaps hurt or damage or annihilation), fear of intimacy, lack of self-esteem and self-love or an unconscious need to fight against being too dependent and vulnerable.

• Getting help •

With an understanding partner and when the causes of vaginismus are not deep, it is often possible to overcome it gradually without having to resort to professional help.

Treatment, if sought, may be physical or psychological. One simple method often used by sex therapists involves objects called vaginal trainers which are made in graduated sizes and are smaller than a penis. The therapist encourages the woman to relax (a medically qualified therapist may give intravenous valium to help someone relax if she is extremely tense) and then gently inserts the smallest trainer or helps her to do it. The aim is to work up in size herself and then for her partner to do it, so that the woman gradually overcomes both the fear of penetrating herself and of being penetrated.

A different behavioural technique which may help is desensitisation, where the therapist teaches a woman to relax and then asks her to imagine aspects of making love which she fears, beginning with the one that causes least fear and working up to the most feared: penetration. (For more details on the desensitisation technique, see page 157.)

A third approach is sensate focusing, where couples do not even try to have penetrative sex (enabling the woman to relax) but, with the support of therapists, to work up to it slowly from kissing, stroking and massaging. For details of organisations to contact in order to find these kinds of help, see Useful Contacts.

Brief psychotherapy may be appropriate for some: in up to four sessions a woman is helped to explore her anxiety and how it is affecting the way her body performs. If this is not sufficient and problems are deeper and more complex, lengthier psychotherapy may be the best way to try to unravel them while being supported through the emotional pain or fear this may uncover. This process might take months or years.

Vaginismus is only a problem if you want penetrative sex and can't have it. Not everyone does want penetrative sex. But not wanting it because you can't allow yourself to have it is a different matter and warrants seeking help, if your life is being made less happy than it might be.

There is a very helpful book about vaginismus: see Further Reading.

• Pain during sex •

The medical term for this is dyspareunia and it can have many causes, including vaginal infections, vaginal dryness or problems such as endometriosis or pelvic inflammatory disease. It can certainly also be painful if you start to have penetrative sex before you are sufficiently aroused when your vagina may be too dry. The discomfort may then cause you to tense up, increasing the pain.

If you experience pain every time you have sex, and particularly if you have any other symptoms such as abnormal vaginal discharge or heavier than normal periods or cramps, you should see your doctor. However, pain during sex can often have a psychological cause: if you are emotionally uncomfortable about having sex for any reason, such as problems within a relationship or feelings of guilt.

• Difficulty reaching orgasm •

Some women have never had an orgasm, either through masturbation or during sex with someone else. Sometimes this is because of fear or embarrassment about their own bodies which prevents them from feeling comfortable about exploring their own genitals, and so they are not able to learn what makes them feel good. It is perfectly possible to experience orgasms with a partner when you have never masturbated, but if you are fearful about sexual feelings and frightened to masturbate, it is unlikely that you relax sufficiently during sex with a partner to reach orgasm.

• Getting to know your body •

It is good to feel comfortable with your own body. If you know how it works and can see how your genitals look, there is less room left for fear. If you have never masturbated, it may be a good idea to take some time for yourself when you will not be disturbed, undress completely and look at your body.

Get a hand mirror and sit with your knees raised and apart so that you can look at your external genitalia. Explore with your fingers what gentle touching feels like, around and inside the vagina. Try to find the clitoris (see page 210) and see how stimulation of it feels good. See how touching your breasts, your nipples and the skin of other parts of your body (such as light stroking of the stomach and thighs) feels to you. Experiment with finding positions that feel good, such as on your back, on your stomach, on your hands and knees, and try to pleasure yourself.

Just aim to enjoy the sensations, not to have an orgasm, but respond to your body's excitement in whatever way feels good, such as more and faster stimulation or slower sensual stroking, and let your feelings lead you. The more you know of your own body and what feels good, the more easily you can guide a partner. Some women find it pleasurable to use a vibrator or to fantasise while they are masturbating.

• The role of emotions •

Even if a woman knows she is capable of orgasm, emotions can get in the way of sexual fulfilment in all sorts of ways. We may be so anxious to have an orgasm, for ourselves or to please a partner, that we try too hard instead of just letting go and experiencing our feelings. If with a new partner, we may be worrying about whether we are being sexy enough or exciting enough and how our bodies look, or we may be anxious about what our partner is going to do next. Worry makes it hard to stay in the moment and enjoy it.

We may not find what a partner does sexually satisfying but be too embarrassed to ask for what we want in case we sound critical and hurtful. Or we may feel that if a partner spends too long on our pleasure, he or she will be annoyed or aggrieved if we still don't reach orgasm. We may even be so used to 'faking it', to prevent this, that it feels too late to speak up.

If a woman feels any guilt about having sex, for any reason, she is less likely to relax sufficiently to achieve orgasm. Feeling aggrieved by one's partner or angry about something going on within the relationship, especially if these feelings have not been expressed, may make it hard to give oneself fully to sexual arousal, excitement and orgasm. These kind of feelings or issues need to be acknowledged and addressed in order for our sexual experience to change.

• Loss of desire •

Loss of desire is common in both women and men and certainly isn't instant proof that your partner has lost interest in you, or vice versa. Various factors such as stress, undiagnosed illnesses, unresolved guilt and pain about a childhood trauma can all take their toll on once-lively libidos. The cause of losing desire is rarely related to sex itself.

• Causes •

There are so very many pressures on relationships and on individuals within relationships that it is not surprising if the total abandonment and absorption in sex that may have thrilled both partners at the start quite quickly disappears. Financial worries, worries about work, the responsibility of looking after young children or dependent parents or both, the sheer exhaustion of caring for others and running both a home and full-time job inevitably push sex into second – or sixth or seventh – place. Depression or lack of fulfilment in other areas can also affect your libido.

Loss of desire is also, however, often a symptom of an underlying breakdown in communication within a relationship. Unfortunately, women and men tend to view the loss of interest in sex in different ways: men are more likely to think the problems in the relationship stem from the lack of sex whereas women feel the sexual problems are secondary to the relationship problems. (The women are right, say the sex therapists.)

Sexual problems escalate if a couple cannot share their feelings, particularly the negative ones like anger, upsets, irritations and hurts. The accumulation of anger and bitterness that can stem from not clearing the air every single time a problem occurs is a powerful inhibitor of a woman's sexual feelings. Women, particularly, may not realise that they feel angry (the emotion they are conscious of may be anxiety) but the effects on sexual interest are the same.

When a woman is assertive within a relationship, there may be problems if her partner doesn't know how to handle that. Men who don't like a scene or who simply try to pacify a woman when she is angry may well suffer from a loss of sexual desire themselves, and this can only change if they are given help to be more open – and angry, where appropriate – within their relationships.

Fear of intimacy can also play a part in loss of desire. It may be easier to feel strong desire in more casual relationships where you are not called upon to expose vulnerability in a way which is vital for real emotional intimacy in a long-term relationship. It is not uncommon for couples to feel desire right up until the moment of commitment and then lose it. Sometimes this results from a power struggle – usually an unconscious one – between two partners. If you are fighting to keep control of both the relationship and your emotions, it is hard or impossible to 'let go' and give up control of sexual feelings either.

It may be important to realise whether you or your partner 'use' sex to assuage needs other than desire. Some women want a lot of sex because it provides reassurance that they are still desirable/loved/wanted. Or they may be seeking intimacy through sex and might really be more satisfied with a cuddle. Sex may be a means of releasing tension or anger. It may be a means of escape from feeling low, bored or miserable about some other aspect of life. Using sex in this way may be fine but it may also make it harder for you to recognise your real needs, both emotionally and sexually.

• A difference in desire •

Often, a loss of sexual desire isn't so much a loss as a change in desire. The heightened desire that comes from the novelty and tension of sex within a new relationship is impossible to maintain for any real length of time. Desire that is experienced within a familiar and safe relationship is different, although it can be just as strong. It may not have urgency but it can be a powerful medium for the expression of deep mature feeling.

Different levels of desire or differences in when you and your partner feel desire may also be more the problem than actual loss of desire. Research shows that in most long-term relationships men tend to become aroused more quickly and more often than women. Men's desire for sex tends to be dictated more by biological urges which express themselves in terms of time (for example, requiring sex every day or every three days or whatever) whereas women's desire is more oriented towards the state of the relationship.

If there is an underlying problem in the relationship that is causing differences in desire, this has to be sorted out before any changes in sex habits can be of any use. It can be helpful, while this is going on, with or without professional help, if the heat is taken out of the conflict of one person wanting sex, and the other person not. A useful way to do this is to agree not to have sex on, say, six particular days rather than to agree to have sex on one particular day a week (or whatever arrangement is appropriate). The partner who wants more then knows what to expect and isn't so frustrated; the partner who wants less feels freed from pressure and guilt.

• Unrealistic expectations •

Expert in human sexuality Dr Elizabeth Stanley believes couples may want unrealistic things from sex, that is, parallel arousal and simultaneous orgasm with anything less signifying sexual failure. She suggests, where the problem is differing desire not caused by underlying conflict, creating a 'his and hers' ladder. Rung one represents being in a romantic cuddling mood and rung six is orgasm. In between lies a range of mild to quite strong sexual feelings and arousal.

She thinks it is unrealistic to expect both partners always to be on the same rung of the ladder at the same time but that both can still share pleasure. If the man feels sexy and the woman doesn't, she can derive pleasure from his satisfaction without needing her own. If it is the other way about, he can bring her to orgasm without needing to have an erection. If couples can learn not to mind if the intensity of pleasure isn't equal on every occasion, sex ceases to be associated with pressure to perform.

There are no norms about how often couples ought to have sex; some couples even choose to have periods of celibacy. If the frequency or infrequency truly suits both partners, you need have no anxiety.

• Physical illness and effects on sex •

A number of illnesses or conditions may affect one's feelings about oneself sexually (and therefore enjoyment of sex) or reduce one's ability to enjoy sex in the ways we might have been used to.

Naturally, the loss of a limb or body part can severely affect body image and self-confidence. A woman who has had a breast removed for cancer very often feels her sexuality has been partly taken from her. Radiotherapy to the vagina and cervix for cervical cancer may make sex painful at first and scarring may narrow the vagina, which doesn't help when trying to come to terms with the impact of the cancer on one's life. Drug treatments for any cancer may result in loss of hair while the cancer itself may cause very severe loss of weight, all of which makes it unsurprising if a woman ceases to feel in any way attractive for a while.

It can also be very hard indeed to come to terms with cancers or other problems of the intestines which require part of the bowel to be cut away and the creation of an ostomy (an opening on the abdomen). A bag or pouch needs to be fitted over the ostomy for the removal of faeces and is permanently in place, even when making love.

The difficulties that these devastating consequences of illness may bring cannot be over-estimated. But with love and support from caring others, and particularly from a sexual partner to help build back confidence and belief in one's own attractiveness, all can be successfully overcome – and indeed have been, by countless women.

Angina and a history of heart disease may not necessarily need to alter one's sex life, although many people fear the consequences of exertion at the start. But chest pain during sex, or pain, breathlessness and palpitations that go on for more than 15 minutes afterwards could be warning signs.

Chronic respiratory diseases such as bronchitis and emphysema may, in their later stages, make sex more difficult because of difficulty in breathing during any exertion. For conditions such as asthma, fear of attacks during sex is usually greater than the likelihood and risks can be reduced by avoiding making love anywhere that allergens may be most problematic (for example, on feather pillows or on grass) or, as a last resort, using an inhaler before sex.

Some illnesses, such as epilepsy, multiple sclerosis, depression and an underactive thyroid can cause a loss of interest in sex. Conventional methods of sex when a woman has rheumatoid arthritis may be extremely painful, particularly if the arthritis is in the hips. Sex may be extremely uncomfortable with a prolapse. Fortunately, in most cases, there are ways to get around particular disabilities.

Medical specialists or voluntary organisations concerned with particular illnesses should have useful advice to offer if you think a sexual problem may be linked to a physical illness. You can contact the Patients Association (see Useful Contacts) to find out if there is an association or self-help group for any particular condition you are interested in.

• Sex therapy •

Sex therapists are specially trained to help with sexual problems that are psychological rather than physical. Sometimes you may see someone on your own but more usually you attend as a couple. Different therapists use different methods but most will offer counselling or psychotherapy, use behavioural techniques or a combination of both. The therapist will talk with you about how you see your problem and will usually explore possible causes. You may need to look at general difficulties you have in relating to your partner, not just at the sexual aspects. Obviously you both need to be willing to work on these, as well as the sex side. If the relationship has irretrievably broken down, no amount of sex therapy will work and you may choose to separate, as an outcome.

Besides looking at your relationship and depending upon the nature of your particular problem, you may be given help to relax sexually and to rediscover your natural sexual responses by going back to basics and enjoying touch and closeness without full sex (a behavioural technique called sensate focus, in which you gradually build up confidence to enjoy sex fully). You may be given a specific programme to follow to achieve this and/or exercises to do, such as pelvic-floor muscle strengthening. Women who have never reached orgasm may be helped to learn to masturbate.

Some organisations to contact for help are the Institute of Psychosexual Medicine, the Association of Sexual and Marital Therapists, The Family Planning Association, or Relate (formerly the National Marriage Guidance Council): see Useful Contacts.

• Rape •

Most of us now know that rape is not about sex or lust, but about power. There are many different types of men who rape; few are actually psychopathic, most live normal lives and more are known to their victims than are strangers. There are also many different reasons given for why they have done or do it, either by the men themselves or by therapists who try to understand them. Nevertheless, the effects on women are the same.

• Emotional reactions •

Rape is always a violation of oneself and may often be utterly terrifying, with death feared as the final outcome. After a rape a woman may feel so shocked that she is numb and appears calm, or she may be extremely fearful and irrational. Some women are too ashamed to admit what has happened, as if it were their own fault. They may feel filthy, polluted, disgusted, despairing and emotionally as well as physically violated.

It is best not to try to suppress feelings about rape but to find support from loving family and friends or trained helpers to express as fully as possible the wide range of emotions which may be experienced for some time afterwards. Women who can do this may manage to lessen the impact of this dreadful trauma on their lives. However, the aftermath of rape can be devastating, even with support, and it may take a long time to learn to trust again and not to feel fear in circumstances others find ordinary. Much will depend upon a woman's sense of self and on the reactions and supportiveness or otherwise of partners, family and friends. Relationships may be strengthened; equally they may crack under the strain of different and difficult emotions.

• Practicalities •

Many women prefer not to press charges for rape, feeling this may prolong the whole horrifying experience and make it even more difficult to get back into their ordinary lives. They may also fear callous treatment or being disbelieved by a court. Others feel very strongly that they want to see justice done. A woman who is raped and might later consider pressing charges shouldn't bath or shower before contacting the police: however much she may feel the need to get rid of contamination, this will destroy important evidence that could pinpoint the attacker. Someone who has been raped has to be medically examined if she contacts the police (a woman can ask for her own GP to be called) and clothes are likely to have to be taken away for forensic examination.

Emergency contraception may have to be thought about. The morning-after pill is preferable to the emergency fitting of an IUD, in case the rapist passed on a sexually transmissible infection which could then ascend to the uterus. Even if a woman doesn't think she has been injured, she should see a doctor, preferably a genito-urinary specialist, for tests to check that she has not been given any sexually transmitted disease.

• Getting help •

There are now a number of rape crisis centres, and women who work there are enormously sympathetic, helpful and knowledgeable. The central Rape Crisis Centre in London can supply details of local centres and phone helplines. Your local Samaritans should also know of relevant telephone numbers. See Useful Contacts.

43

VAGINAL AND SEXUALLY TRANSMITTED DISEASES

NOT ALL infections described in this section are necessarily caught sexually but they can be.

If you have any symptoms of vaginal or vulval itching, discomfort or vaginal discharge, it is best to go directly to a genito-urinary clinic (GU clinic) at a hospital for diagnosis, rather than to your GP. Doctors who are specialists in genito-urinary medicine are experts in a whole range of problems from sexually transmitted diseases, vaginal or bladder infections through to problems with sex and contraception. They have access to the widest range of tests and checks, and are the best people to ensure you receive the right diagnosis.

GU clinics are a far cry from the old 'special' clinics or VD clinics, which have long gone, and the ambience is very different too. It is extremely unlikely that you will find any of the staff making assumptions or judgments about your moral character or sexual proclivities as a result of your visit there. Attending a GU clinic is not a statement about your sexuality either.

Most women are likely to suffer from some kind of genito-urinary infection at some time in their lives, even if they don't have sex. Cystitis, thrush and even trichomoniasis can all be self-generated. Herpes can be transferred to the genitals from a cold sore. Scabies and lice are caught by close contact with another person, but not necessarily by having sex with them. Even the diseases which are only sexually transmitted may be the result of your current partner's present or past sexual encounters rather than your own.

If you do have a lifestyle which includes more than one sex partner, it is a good idea to have occasional checks at a GU clinic, even if you have no symptoms. Some of the diseases with the worst consequences for women may not have any symptoms until the damage is done (see chlamydia, page 373 and gonorrhea, page 377).

Most large hospitals should have a GU clinic. Ring to check and to find out whether you need to make an appointment or just come along and wait in a queue. You do not need referral from your GP and your visit to the clinic remains confidential unless you wish your GP to be informed of the outcome.

• Thrush •

This is the colloquial name for a yeast-like fungus caused by an organism called *Candida albicans*. It may also be termed monilia or monilial vaginitis. Its

natural home is in the intestines and it lives there without causing any problem but it can also migrate to the vagina, because the anus and the vagina are
so close. Even in the vagina, however, it should not cause a problem if there
isn't too much of it there. Usually this is the case, as the healthy vagina is too
acidic for the liking of this fungus and so it cannot proliferate. But if the
acidity of the vagina drops (see how below), the thrush may become more
profuse and give rise to a vaginal infection.

• Symptoms •

You usually become aware of a vaginal discharge that is greater than normal.
It is thick and whitish and may even look like cottage cheese. You may be
aware of a strongish, but not foul, smell. Your vagina may feel extremely
sore because the discharge, however copious, acts as an irritant that dries and
cracks the skin. If there are cracks in the skin around the vaginal opening,
you may find it a bit painful when you urinate.

A very common symptom is itchiness, which is an allergic reaction to the
infection and so may be experienced as a severe symptom even if the thrush
attack itself is mild. Not all women have itch with thrush.

Thrush usually arises non-sexually but once you have got it you can pass it
to your partner who can then pass it back to you. Men rarely have visible
symptoms of thrush however, although occasionally they may have a little
pain on urinating and a light clear discharge from the penis. More commonly,
they may notice a slight reddening of the penis under the foreskin which is
usually an allergic reaction to the presence of the fungus. (Uncircumcised
men are more prone to catch thrush, as it likes to settle under the foreskin.)

• How you develop thrush •

Thrush likes it warm, moist and not too acidic. The acidity of the vagina is
usually higher than thrush can thrive in but various factors can cause it to fall.
Broad spectrum antibiotics are a major cause of lowered vaginal acidity as they
kill off bacteria in general, rather than just the type for which they have been
prescribed. Amongst those which succumb are bacteria called lactobacilli
which live in the vagina and perform the necessary function of converting
glycogen, a sugar-like substance found in vaginal secretions, into lactic acid. It
is lactic acid which creates the normally acidic environment of the vagina.
After a course of antibiotics, it takes time for the lactobacilli to re-establish
themselves. In this intervening period, thrush may take its chance to proliferate, slowing down even more the return of adequate numbers of lactobacilli.

Be aware of this risk particularly if taking antibiotics for cystitis. The drugs
may clear up the attack but in the process precipitate thrush which may then
be transferred the very short distance to the urethra and irritate it enough to
cause another bout of cystitis. A vicious cycle is then set up.

You may find you suffer more from thrush if you take the contraceptive
pill. The oestrogen content of the combined contraceptive pill helps increase

the amount of glycogen in vaginal secretions. (The same effect occurs during pregnancy when oestrogen levels are raised.) Progestogen-only pills may also be a problem as they work by thickening cervical mucus so that it is hostile to sperm. Thrush may find a chance to thrive in this extra moisture.

The IUD is also associated with increased risk of thrush because thrush is often a secondary infection that takes hold when another micro-organism has already altered the vaginal environment. The IUD is associated with an increase in virtually every genital infection, as the thread that hangs down from the cervix can act as a ladder for micro-organisms to climb. The IUD may also irritate the uterus, causing tiny tears through which infection can enter.

Many women find themselves especially prone to thrush before and during a period, when vaginal acidity falls. Blood is alkaline. (So too is the semen of some men, which means a sexual partner might be part of the problem.) Using tampons during a period can be painful if you have thrush because tampons, as well as the thrush, have a drying effect on the vagina.

Tight jeans and nylon pants are popular with thrush, as both prevent air from circulating and absorbing moisture. Also, anything that is tight around the crotch causes friction, heat and irritation. Even pads which some women like to wear inside pants, to prevent any vaginal discharge or stress incontinence staining underwear, can help precipitate an attack of thrush by rubbing relentlessly against the top of the legs as you move. Sex can trigger thrush for the same reasons, if you are low on lubrication.

Some chemicals found in medicated soaps, bubble baths, vaginal deodorants and antiseptics and any harsh detergents in which underwear is washed can irritate the vagina in some women and alter the balance of vaginal secretions in thrush's favour.

If thrush is something you are prone to, you are particularly likely to suffer an attack if you are under stress, feeling run down and/or not eating properly. At these times the immune system can't function at its best and is less than usually able to fight infection.

You also need to watch what you eat. Thrush likes sugar and unrefined carbohydrates, which increase the amount of glycogen in vaginal secretions to levels higher than lactobacilli can cope with. Diabetic women tend to suffer more than average from thrush because of raised blood sugar and also the increased sugar in their urine. As the urethral and vaginal openings are so close, this sugar may provide fine fare for thrush.

• Effects if untreated •

The main effect of thrush is discomfort. However, it can live in other places besides the vagina and generally affect your whole sense of well-being. Some complementary health practitioners, and some orthodox ones, believe that it can be implicated in some long-term problems such as headaches, heartburn, gastrointestinal disorders and sore throats if it takes firm hold, so it is wise to get it treated or take steps to prevent it, or seek further investigations if it recurs as frequently as every month.

Thrush may even cause temporary infertility. In one study of 40 women who had no sperm or inactive sperm in their cervical mucus after post-coital tests, 35 were found to have thrush instead, which had acted on the mucus to make it inhospitable to sperm. Treatment corrected the problem.

• Treatment •

If you see your GP rather than a genito-urinary specialist for diagnosis, do insist on an internal examination and vaginal swabs being taken, as vaginal discharge caused by other infections may mimic thrush. Many GPs do not routinely take swabs. This is unfortunate as GPs diagnose 80 per cent of the vaginal discharge they see as thrush, when in fact the majority of cases of vaginal discharge is caused by a different micro-organism that needs different treatment (see Bacterial Vaginosis, page 362).

The conventional treatment for thrush is with an antifungal agent that may come as a tablet, pessary or cream. The most usual treatment is with one-dose, three-dose or six-dose pessaries. The one-dose pessary is obviously the most convenient and generally viewed as sufficiently effective, as there is only a little less overall amount of the drug in the one-dose than the three-dose regimen. However, in intractable or severe cases, some doctors like to pre-scribe six doses to be sure.

Do tell the doctor if you are pregnant or trying to get pregnant, as certain antifungal agents are not suitable in pregnancy.

Antifungal creams may be prescribed as well to ease itching or soreness of the skin around the vagina and anus. It is important that a regular sex partner is given antifungal cream too because, although it is often thought thrush can't survive long enough on the penis to cause a problem, there are very many cases of re-infection through a partner.

It is now possible to buy a one-dose treatment for thrush: Canesten 10% VC, sold in pharmacies with an applicator and enough cream for just one dose. This is fine as long as you are absolutely sure you have thrush, or if you are prepared to pay to find out and then see a doctor within a few days if your symptoms haven't cleared. Various genital infections can cause discharge and need different treatment.

Do not self-diagnose or buy an over-the-counter thrush treatment if you are pregnant or have additional symptoms such as abnormal vaginal bleeding, blood-stained or foul-smelling discharge, blistering of the vagina, pain when urinating or fever or chills. See a doctor for investigation and correct diagnosis.

If you suffer from regular attacks of thrush that are related to the menstrual cycle, a low-dose oral antifungal drug taken at the high-risk time (such as flu-conazole 50mg for the last two days of your period) might be useful to try for six months, if your doctor recommends it.

If you suffer from highly recurrent thrush not related to the menstrual cycle ask your GP for a blood test to check that you do not have undiagnosed diabetes.

• Prevention and self-help •

1 Don't wear clothes that fit too tightly around the crotch or which don't let air through.

2 Avoid harsh chemicals whether they are packaged as bath salts, scented soaps or detergent, etc. Stick to pure soaps or avoid using them at all around the vagina if you can bring yourself to. The vagina cleans itself and wiping around it with cotton wool soaked in tepid water is all you need to do. Wiping yourself with cotton wool soaked in olive oil may help recurrent itching.

3 During an attack of thrush, dry yourself with a hair dryer that is not too hot, rather than a towel. It is less painful and more hygienic.

4 It probably isn't a good idea to take long soaks in the bath if you are prone to thrush, and certainly never when you have an attack. However, at least one expert has found that nine out of ten women with abnormal vaginal discharge only shower and never bath, which may mean showers don't always flush everything undesirable out. A quick bath at least once a week might be advisable.

5 Always wipe from front to back after using the toilet to avoid transfer of any organisms, including thrush, from the anus to vagina. If you like your anus to be stimulated during sex or masturbation, ensure that the same finger isn't used for vaginal stimulation afterwards. Avoid having anal sex followed by vaginal sex if your partner doesn't wash his penis in between. (But anal sex brings its own risk factors: see HIV, page 361.)

6 If you are particularly prone to thrush before or during a period, try increasing the acidity of the vagina by inserting spoonfuls of natural live yoghurt (which contains lactic acid) or a tampon soaked in the yoghurt in the vagina for a few days before your period starts. It can be a difficult messy business, however. Easier, if more costly, is to buy from a pharmacy a tube of the vaginal jelly Aci-gel, which has the same effect and comes with its own applicator. Another option is to fill a large washing-up bowel with warm water and a little vinegar and to sit in it for a few minutes.

7 If you use tampons during a period, don't use a size that is larger than necessary, thinking you can leave it in longer. Large tampons are even more drying than ones which are the right size for your flow. Change your tampon at least every four to six hours.

8 Never have sex when you are not lubricating properly. If you are dry because you don't want sex, don't have it. If you are dry for other reasons but still feel sexy, use a vaginal lubricant (see Vaginal Dryness, page 262) or baby oil (but don't use anything oil-based if you use a condom or diaphragm as the oil will rot the rubber).

9 Consider whether the contraceptive pill or IUD, if you use either, may be contributing to your problems. Are you prepared to try some other form of contraception and see?

10 Avoid any unnecessary courses of antibiotics, such as for bad colds or coughs which antibiotics don't help anyway.

11 Don't neglect to eat regularly and sensibly, with plenty of fresh fruit and vegetables in your diet. Minimise the amount eaten of sugar (also in alcohol) and refined carbohydrates such as white bread and flour.

12 Some women find that they can abort an attack of thrush at the start if they use the yoghurt treatment described above. It doesn't work for everyone, though, so do seek treatment if nothing happens or if symptoms flare up again soon afterwards.

• Bacterial vaginosis •

This is an extremely common vaginal infection which a great many women will probably never have heard of. Unfortunately, a number of GPs are still unfamiliar with it too. Records show, however, that bacterial vaginosis causes more cases of vaginal discharge than thrush, yet GPs diagnose vaginal discharge as thrush 80 per cent of the time (presumably without taking vaginal swabs) and as bacterial vaginosis only 10 per cent of the time. As the treatments are different, it is highly worth ensuring you receive the correct diagnosis. The best way to do this is to go to a genito-urinary clinic.

You may hear bacterial vaginosis referred to by its initials BV. Some doctors may still refer to it as non-specific vaginitis, although this is incorrect and out-dated. (The infection is not non-specific and there is no inflammation, which is what is meant by -itis endings on words.)

BV is thought to be caused by a bacterium called gardnerella (named after the Dr Gardner who first described it) along with mixed anaerobic bacteria. Anaerobic bacteria live without air: gardnerella can live with or without it.

Like thrush, BV can live quietly in the vagina without problem as long as the bacteria are in small numbers. Like thrush it can be sexually transmitted but this isn't the main way women get it. Unlike thrush, it is only found in women who are or have been sexually active.

• Symptoms •

BV doesn't always give rise to symptoms but it usually does. The symptoms are a thin creamy whitish-grey discharge that is often frothy and smells foul and fishy. The smell may be strongest after a period or after sex. There is not usually an itch with BV unless the discharge has been present profusely for some while and has made the vagina sore.

Sometimes women themselves cause an itch by using inappropriate creams or ointments to try to soothe the soreness or by putting perfumes of some description on themselves or in the bath to mask the smell. Obviously this harms rather than helps but is an understandable response by women who have been told by doctors that tests for thrush are negative and therefore there is nothing wrong with them.

BV doesn't cause symptoms in men but they can certainly pass it on or re-infect you.

• How you develop BV •

BV, like thrush, is keen on conditions that are not too acidic, so things that reduce vaginal acidity (see Thrush, page 357) can equally well encourage BV to take hold, but it is very rare for both to occur together.

BV can be caught during sex with a man who is carrying it. It may be triggered in some women after childbirth or gynaecological surgery. The IUD, associated as it is with an increase in genital infection generally, may be a culprit.

BV can often be a secondary infection. About a third of women with gonorrhoea also have BV and it is often found in women with trichomonas or genital warts. This is not to say that most women with BV also have gonorrhoea, trichomonas or warts, because they don't.

• Effects if untreated •

BV can be a risk factor for pre-term labour and late miscarriage because, it is thought, of infection tracking up into the cervix. Research has shown that women in whom BV is detected early in pregnancy (prior to 16 weeks) are at five times the normal risk of going into pre-term labour any time from 24 weeks onwards or of miscarrying between 16 and 24 weeks. Miscarriage is the more likely outcome.

In this research, one in five women attending antenatal clinics was found to be harbouring BV.

Undiagnosed BV is also associated with recurrent urinary tract infections and post-operative infection.

• Treatment •

Conventional treatment is with a week of an antibiotic-like drug called metronidazole, 400mg twice a day, or – preferable as far as the patient is concerned – a single 2g oral dose of metronidazole. Partners should be treated too.

Alcohol reduces the effectiveness of metronidazole and also interacts with the drug in a way that makes some people feel nauseous or violently ill. It should not be given in the first three months of pregnancy and if used later in pregnancy should be given vaginally not orally. There is now also another drug that is gentler and safe to use in pregnant women, called clindamycin, as a vaginal cream daily for a week.

The big trouble with BV is that it has a high recurrence rate, although whether this is because of reinfection from an untreated partner is unknown. Certainly, up to 40 per cent of women with BV get it again.

• Prevention and self-help •

See prevention and self-help section for Thrush (page 361).

• Bartholin's abscess or cyst •

The Bartholin's glands lie one on either side of the entrance to the vagina and produce secretions to lubricate it. If the duct from one of the glands is blocked, the secretions which are produced have nowhere to go and cause the gland to swell and form a cyst. This may feel uncomfortable when walking or having sex but is not usually painful. If infection sets in, however, an abscess may form and this is highly painful indeed. The development of a Bartholin's abscess is not unusual if a woman is suffering from a vaginal infection. It is a common accompaniment to gonorrhoea.

• Treatment •

Antibiotics may help fight the infection and the cyst may need draining or removing surgically. If cysts and abscesses repeatedly form, it may be necessary for the whole gland to be removed.

• Trichomonas •

Trichomonas is a protozoan, a single-celled organism larger than bacteria, which commonly lives in the rectum in both women and men without causing problem. It can also live in the vagina, urethra and bladder in women where it *does* cause problems (and in the urethra and prostrate in men, where often it doesn't). The infection that is caused when problems do occur is called trichomoniasis. It is a very common infection and is usually, but not always, sexually transmitted.

• Symptoms •

Trichomonas usually causes a thin, frothy yellowy-green discharge which has an unpleasant fishy smell. Because the discharge itself is an irritant, it makes the skin around the vagina itchy, sore and inflamed. Urinating can be painful. Trichomonas can spread to the urethra and cause cystitis too, but beware of being diagnosed as having only cystitis by any doctor who doesn't take vaginal swabs.

Trichomonas often occurs with other genital infections (40 per cent of women with gonorrhoea also have trichomonas) and then the discharge may be thick and whitish. You may notice some bleeding after sex but more likely it will be too painful to have sex if you have trichomonas.

Men very often have no symptoms although they can pass it on or pass it back sexually if they are untreated. Those who do get symptoms are likely to have a thin whitish discharge from the urethra and maybe some pain when urinating or the desire to urinate more often than usual. (This last is usually the case if trichomonas has infected the prostate gland.)

• How you develop trichomonas •

The most common way of catching it is via sexual transmission. Trichomonas likes conditions to be warm and wet and is therefore far happier in the vagina than the male urethra but it is still able to hang in there for a week or so before being eliminated in a man's urine. This means that you can certainly catch trichomonas from a man who has sex with you within a week or so of having sex with someone else who has it.

A fair amount of trichomonas can be contracted by self-contamination alone. Trichomonas can easily make its way from the rectum to the vagina, especially if given a helping hand by poor hygiene – wiping from back to front instead of from front to back after using the toilet, using the same finger or device for anal stimulation followed by vaginal stimulation or having anal sex followed by vaginal sex without the penis being washed first. (For the risks of anal sex, see section on HIV, page 382.)

As trichomonas can survive outside of the body for a few hours if it is left somewhere moist and warm, it can be caught by sharing a towel or flannel with someone who has it. Occasionally it can be contracted from a swimming pool, particularly if you stay in your wet swimming things for a while afterwards. Very rarely, it can be caught from upward faecal splashes from the toilet bowel, if the previous user of the toilet was infected.

• Effects if untreated •

Trichomonas harboured during the third term of pregnancy may raise by three or four times your risk of having a premature or low-birthweight baby, which are more generally susceptible to infections. It may sometimes be responsible for pneumonia or respiratory distress in babies when there is no other identified cause, if the mother passed on the infection during pregnancy.

Infection with trichomonas can cause changes in the cells of the cervix similar to precancerous changes but, if trichomonas is the only cause of such changes, they quickly return to normal after treatment.

Trichomonas may cause temporary infertility in men if present in large quantities in semen. Fertility is restored once the infection is treated.

• Treatment •

Trichomonas is treated with the antibiotic-like drug metronidazole, except in early pregnancy when it cannot be used. It may be prescribed in 200mg tablets to be taken three times a day with food for seven days or, preferably for the patient, in a single 2g oral dose. Alcohol should be avoided as it can reduce the drug's effectiveness and also interact with it to cause severe nausea. Sex should be avoided till treatment is complete.

Partners always need treating, even if trichomonas doesn't show up in urethral tests. Although it is detected in only 10 per cent of urethral tests it is found to be present in the prostate fluid and semen of up to 90 per cent of male partners of women with trichomonas.

• Prevention and self-help •

1 If you have sex with more than one partner or your partner has sex with more than one partner, it is wisest not to use an IUD as your form of contraception, as your susceptibility to genital infections is increased.
2 Do all the right hygienic things, such as wiping from front to back and avoiding organisms from the rectum being passed to the vagina by penis, finger, vibrator or any other device.
3 Don't share towels or flannels.
4 Wear clothing loose around the crotch and natural fibres next to the skin, so that air can circulate and you can keep cooler and drier. Trichomonas likes warm damp places best.

• Genital herpes •

Herpes is an extremely common virus. There are four different types but only two of them, HSV (*Herpes simplex* virus) 1 and 2 can give rise to genital herpes. HSV 1 is more familiar to us as cold sores which usually appear on and above the lips and occasionally on the nose and cheeks.

HSV 1 is a part of life: a third of children have caught it by the age of three and virtually everyone by the age of 25. Once infected, we remain carriers of the virus for life because it doesn't go away. It causes infection in the area where it entered the body, then enters the nerve fibres, travels up the nerve and ends up in the nerve root where most often it remains dormant for life. However, it can sometimes cause a recurrence of symptoms in the same place it first infected if we haven't built up enough resistance against it.

It used to be thought that HPV 1 and HPV 2, which causes genital herpes, were rather more distinct from each other than they actually are. A fair proportion of cases of genital herpes (up to 60 per cent in some cultures) are in fact caused by HPV 1 transferred to the genitals via oral sex.

Genital herpes appear most usually on and around the vaginal lips, the clitoris, inside the vagina, on the cervix and around the anus in women (and on the penis and around the anus in men). They can often also be found on the thighs and buttocks, and occasionally on the mouth.

There are likely to be as many as a million sufferers in the UK at any one time, with a great many cases going unreported to doctors or unnoticed by the 'sufferer'. Yet a decade ago, genital herpes was the subject of scare stories, with Americans claiming an epidemic and newspapers announcing huge rises in case numbers here. The alarm was fuelled by the fact that herpes is incurable, and the impression given was that if you had genital herpes your sex life was effectively over.

In fact, this is all wildly out of proportion (although unfortunately the image has to a certain extent stuck). It is only an unfortunate minority of people who suffer recurrent attacks and, as much can be done by sufferers themselves to reduce the likelihood of recurrences, herpes may in fact have far less serious consequences than many other genital infections.

However, for those who do have frequent recurrences, herpes is undoubtedly extremely unpleasant and may severely affect both social and sexual relationships. But the good news is that frequent recurrences can be prevented by drugs.

• Symptoms •

Genital herpes usually appears as clusters of little red spots with white blisters somewhere in the genital region. However, it may sometimes appear as a single tiny spot.

Herpes takes a while to show after contact with a person who has it: usually between two and 20 days with an average incubation period of six. The little blisters burst and form painful open sores. At this stage it can be excruciatingly painful to pee as the acidic urine comes into contact with the sores and causes a burning sensation, often mistaken initially for cystitis. (However, with cystitis there is an increased need to urinate whereas with herpes there is not.)

Sometimes the sores themselves become infected by bacteria and there can be painful swelling in the lymph glands in the groin. You may have an abnormal vaginal discharge too.

The first attack of genital herpes is almost always the worst as it can be accompanied, in some people, by a high fever and sometimes a backache. And yet others have no symptoms that they notice at all, not even the blisters if they are hidden in the folds of the vaginal lips.

The length of time from the appearance of the blisters to when they burst, crust over and heal is usually 16 to 18 days for a first attack and anywhere from three to eight days for any subsequent ones. Genital infections caused by HSV 1 are usually less severe than those caused by HSV 2, and cause fewer recurrences.

Recurrent attacks are much milder, whichever type is the cause, because the body has had a chance to build up some resistance. About half of people who have an attack of herpes never get another one. In others, attacks may range from only a few in a lifetime to a couple a year or, for an unfortunate minority, one almost every month; but recurrences do very often just tend to decrease with time. In recurrent attacks there is normally no fever and usually there are fewer lesions on the genitals.

• Warning signs •

For most people an attack of herpes is heralded a day or two before by some kind of warning sign, known as the prodomal sign. Such signs vary from individual to individual but may include an itch, a tingling sensation, a dull ache in the groin, tenderness, a feeling of pain in the pelvis and/or legs, or just a sensation that something is about to happen. Such signs are not likely to be noticed the first time around but, if you have had herpes once, they can be very useful warnings of another attack.

However, when you have just been diagnosed as having herpes, you are more likely to be aware of all sorts of odd sensations in the genital region because your attention is more focused there than usual. Most of these sensations will not be anything to do with herpes, just false alarms which subside once you start to relax and not worry so much that you are about to have a new attack every day.

Most symptoms in men are the same as those experienced by women. Where women may experience an abnormal vaginal discharge, men may notice a mucous discharge from the penis, if the urethra has been infected.

• How you develop genital herpes •

Genital herpes is most commonly acquired through sex with a person who has herpes during its active stage. The virus is shed just before the blisters erupt and, most profusely, while the sores are open. Some people have asymptomatic herpes, which means that they don't ever develop blisters, although they can still pass on the virus. However very little virus is around to catch in these cases, compared with the amount in circulation when sores are visible, and so the risk of passing on herpes when it is asymptomatic is reckoned to be low.

The virus is normally passed to a partner by entering through any breaks in their skin or through particularly soft parts, called mucous membranes, which line bits of the body including the genitals and the eyes. Although it is infectious, its infectivity is low compared with that of some other genital infections. According to one estimate you have a 15 per cent chance of catching herpes if you have sex with someone who is shedding the genital herpes virus at that time, or if you have oral sex with someone who has a cold sore. If you already have HSV, whether you know it or not, you can't catch it again.

Herpes can live outside of the body for a little while so it is indeed possible to catch it from towels and, according to some evidence, from toilet seats. You can give it to yourself, of course, if you touch a cold sore on your face and then touch your genitals, but this is rare.

When you have had genital herpes once there are a number of trigger factors which may precipitate a subsequent attack. These vary from person to person but most commonly include being over-stressed and run down, having a fever or another infection, tight clothing around the genitals, particularly of synthetic fibres that don't allow the skin to breathe, and nude sunbathing, where the genitals are exposed to sunlight. Some women find that they are most vulnerable to an attack when they are having a period; others that sex in certain positions can sometimes bring on an attack because of heavy friction and bruising.

• Effects if untreated •

Herpes cannot be treated in the sense of being cured, and in fact treatment only helps relieve symptoms rather than have any more lasting benefit. So the risks of herpes are the same, whether you have treatment for an attack or not.

There is some evidence that herpes on the cervix is a risk factor for cervical cancer. However it is not a strong one and not an independent one: other risk factors are necessary too to increase your likelihood of getting it.

Because herpes can be transmitted by the finger there is a risk of transferring it to the eye, causing conjunctivitis and ulceration that can lead, if not checked by antiviral drugs, to impaired or loss of corneal vision and permanent scarring. This is not common, yet HSV is the main cause of corneal blindness in the western world.

Herpes infection of the eye is far more likely to occur through touching a cold sore on the lip and then touching the eye, but it could be the result of the transfer of infection from the genitals, particularly during love-making. In the same way that cold sores and genital herpes can recur, so can herpetic eye infections, with stress, illness, menstruation and ultraviolet light again being the main trigger factors.

If you get an eye infection which you suspect may have been caused by HSV, (symptoms are usually itch, burning sensations and the feeling of grit in the eye, a watering eye and a very severe headache) it is important to tell your doctor, who should refer you to an ophthalmologist for correct diagnosis and treatment.

Herpes is dangerous to a baby during childbirth if there is an active attack at the time of delivery. However it is a first attack which is most dangerous, as a woman who has already had herpes is likely to have passed on her antibodies. A baby born with herpes usually has lesions all over its body and the disease is fatal in 60 per cent of cases. Those who survive are likely to have brain and/or eye damage. Having a delivery by Caesarean section can avoid such terrible consequences.

• Treatment •

There is no cure for genital herpes but the first time you think you have it you should go to a genito-urinary clinic for diagnosis as soon as possible. The virus is usually shed when the blisters have just broken and once that period has passed it may not be possible to make a certain diagnosis.

Antiviral drugs, most usually one called acyclovir, can be given to relieve severe symptoms of a first attack and come as both tablets and cream. The tablets are usually the more effective. There are other antiviral drugs also in use or being developed to treat genital herpes, some of which may be similar to acyclovir but need to be taken less frequently than the five tablets of acyclovir required daily.

Acyclovir can also be taken continuously, at a lower than normal dose, to prevent attacks in those who suffer very frequent recurrences (six or more attacks a year) or unusually severe ones. This is expensive, of course, so not prescribed lightly.

After a first attack, there usually is no need for medication and self-help methods are enough.

• Prevention and self-help •

1 As with all genital infections, the more sexual partners you have, the higher your chances of getting herpes. However, it is worth remembering that genital herpes has as much to do with past lifestyles as with present ones. Even if you are in a totally monogamous relationship, you or your partner may have been infected with the herpes virus years previously without ever realising it, in which case an unrecognised recurrence for one might lead to infection for the other. Any accusations of unfaithfulness from either party are therefore not necessarily justified!

2 The condom helps protect against herpes but not absolutely entirely, if a herpes blister is developing at the point where the condom stops.

3 Never have genital contact if you or your partner has genital herpes, or kiss or have oral sex if you or your partner has a cold sore. The time to keep clear is from the first warning signs, if you have them, through till the sores are completely healed over. If you are careful about herpes, you need never pass it on.

4 Wash hands thoroughly with soap and water after touching any sores.

5 Don't share towels and flannels.

6 Make sure you have regular cervical smears. Ask your doctor, or the specialist at the genito-urinary clinic, whether you need one at shorter than the usual interval or not.

7 Make sure that you don't let the skin around the genitals become too dry and sore or too hot and humid. This means avoiding any irritating chemicals such as perfumed soaps, etc, and wearing cotton underpants and clothes that are not too tight around the crotch.

8 Keep at least bikini bottoms on if sunbathing

9 Make sure you have enough fresh fruit and vegetables in your daily diet. Various vitamins and minerals in these foods help keep our immune systems in proper working order. When your immune defences are down you are more vulnerable to a recurrence of herpes.

10 Try not to have more stress in your life than you can feel OK about. (Some people thrive on stress.) If you feel burdened by stress and defeated and anxious a lot of the time, you are putting yourself at risk. It is stress accompanied by depression that most often precedes a herpes recurrence.

11 One important thing not to get stressed about is herpes itself, hard though that may seem at first. If you find yourself dwelling on the possibility of having a recurrence and anxiously inspecting yourself for signs, you are more likely to get one. If, for instance, you have sometimes had an attack during a period and you start to expect one, you are more likely to be anxious at this time and therefore more vulnerable: a self-fulfilling prophecy rather than anything that was actually inevitable. If you can manage to relax and not expect an attack at any particular time, you should be able to break any pattern that has become established in this way.

12 If you are not in a long-term relationship, do not feel you must announce you have had herpes to any prospective partner that you meet. Get to know him or her first and let them get to know you, so that they can build up a trust that you are someone who is responsible about herpes and won't lightly put them at risk. People who react badly to the news that you have herpes do so through uninformed fear. If you sound confident about it yourself, you are far more likely to be able to dispel others' worries.

13 To relieve or shorten the symptoms of a painful attack, try the following suggestions:
   • Bathe the sores in a tepid solution of salt water: 10ml (1 heaped tsp) to 600ml (1 pint) of water a few times a day.
   • Put a little salt in your bath and keep your bath cooler than usual, if you find hot ones increase the pain.
   • Pass urine in a warm bath or shower, to reduce the acidity of the urine against your skin.
   • Try a cool shower to soothe sores or put ice cubes next to them, wrapped in a clean cotton cloth (and don't reuse the cloth).
   • Keep the genital area as dry as possible; applying a little witchhazel to the sores can help.

14 For someone to talk to who knows what it is like to have herpes, contact the Herpes Association. They also provide information sheets if you send a large SAE: see Useful Contacts.

• Genital warts •

Warts are caused by a group of viruses known as human papilloma virus (HPV). The virus changes skin cells that normally form flat skin into cells that form heaped-up skin, resulting in a wart. There are many different types of HPV, each producing warts of a distinct appearance. HPV 1, for example, causes plantar warts, the type found on the soles of the feet. HPV 6, 11, 16 and 18 are the ones associated with genital warts, also known medically as *Condyloma acuminatum*.

Genital warts can be found anywhere around the external genitalia and the anus in both sexes, and in women also on the walls of the vagina and the cervix. Warts like moisture, which helps them to spread, so they are often found in association with a vaginal discharge caused by another infection. They can sometimes be found in the mouth.

• Symptoms •

The most obvious symptom is the wart itself or a whole group of them scattered around the genital and anal area, which are easy to see. However flat (early stage) warts on the cervix cannot be seen without the aid of a colposcope (see page 220). Some genito-urinary clinics, but not all, have colposcopes, so flat warts on the cervix may be missed in many cases.

The only other symptom in women is that often they have an abnormal vaginal discharge at the same time, not caused by the warts but creating an environment conducive to their proliferation. They may become particularly profuse in pregnancy, when women are more susceptible to these kinds of infection.

In men warts are more common in those who are uncircumcised, as they like to congregate under the foreskin where it is moist and warm. But they can be found anywhere on the penis and around the anus, and in the rectum in men who are homosexual or bisexual. Men can have flat warts on the penis which can only be detected by colposcope.

• How you develop genital warts •

Genital warts are sexually transmitted. If your partner has genital warts, visible or not, you have a 60 per cent chance of catching them during sex. Genital warts can also be passed to the mouth by an infected partner during oral sex.

• Effects if untreated •

Genital warts are believed to be associated with an increased risk of cervical cancer, particularly in younger women. Wart virus has been detected from cervical smears in much cervical precancer and cancer, with HPV 16 and 18 more usually associated with cancerous changes that progress to malignancy, and HPV 6 and 11 associated with lower risk and precancerous changes that are more likely to regress on their own .

An increase in incidence of genital warts over the last ten to twenty years has certainly corresponded with an alarming increase in young women of pre-cancerous cervical lesions (early abnormal changes in cervical cells which may regress spontaneously, or progress to invasive cancer if untreated). Whereas cervical cancer used to be suffered mainly by older women and it took years for abnormal cell changes to become malignant, there seems to be a more aggressive form of the disease which progresses more quickly and which affects mainly younger women. This new, more aggressive form may be associated with wart virus.

This is not to say that having, or having had, genital warts means you are going to get cervical cancer. It is unlikely that genital warts alone are responsible but are one important risk factor which can increase the chances of developing cervical cancer when in conjunction with other risk factors. These are: starting sex early (when the cervix is still immature); numerous sexual partners; having one partner who himself has other partners; a history of sexually transmitted diseases; and smoking. (For more information on cervical smears and cervical cancer, see page 272.)

• Treatment •

There are several methods of removing warts and what you get will depend on the resources or preferences of your local clinic. Warts can be removed by laser. They can be frozen off with liquid nitrogen, a method called cryosurgery.

In very many clinics the first line of approach is still to apply some caustic substance to the warts to burn them off or to apply a podophyllin preparation (containing podophyllum, an extract from a fungus which has the effect of stopping the cell infected with the virus from dividing and growing). This treatment has to be repeated every few days until the warts go away. Some warts can be very persistent and keep coming back, and obviously they are more likely to do so if your partner still has his. Both of you must be treated.

Genital warts can be self-treated with podophyllotoxin 0.5 per cent which can be prescribed by a GP. One self-treatment pack, Warticon Fem, comes complete with a mirror. However, occasionally GPs have prescribed the highly caustic podophyllum for women to use for self-treatment at home and this can be very dangerous, as the slightest inaccuracy in applying it can cause chemical burns of the normal surrounding skin. Podophyllum is not licensed for self-treatment in the UK and should only be used by professionals. Surrounding skin has to be protected with paraffin or petroleum jelly.

• Prevention and self-help •

1 Using a barrier form of contraception reduces your risk of catching genital warts. A condom is best but a diaphragm can be helpful too.
2 If you have had genital warts or get them repeatedly, try and arrange for an annual cervical smear. This isn't an entitlement, but some GPs are willing to do yearly smears in such instances. Family planning clinics and genito-urinary clinics also take smears.
3 If you are prone to genital warts and you smoke, you could, if you choose, instantly eliminate one of these two risk factors for precancerous cervical changes by stopping smoking.
4 Help yourself by eating lots of fruits and vegetables containing beta carotene, which the body stores and uses to form vitamin A when it needs it. Studies have shown a protective effect against cervical cancer, as well as some other cancers. Vegetables rich in beta carotene include carrots (very high), broccoli, green leafy vegetables, sweet potatoes and tomatoes. Fruits include apricots, peaches and prunes.

• Chlamydia •

Chlamydia (full name *Chlamydia trachomatis*) is the most common sexually transmitted disease in the Western world. There are about 170,000 new cases in the UK every year, with some devastating effects in women, yet very many women still haven't even heard of it.

This is not so surprising as it may seem. Chlamydia is a bacterium but an odd one. It contains no living cells and, more like a virus, is dependent on the energy produced by the cells of its host (that is, people) for it to grow and reproduce. It cannot be detected by the usual means for detecting bacteria and so for many years was not detected at all. It is only with today's more sophisticated diagnostic procedures that chlamydia has been realised to be so widespread.

Chlamydia can live in various parts of the body, including the liver, lungs and throat, but in adults it is almost always sexually transmitted and is found mainly in the sexual organs. It is highly infectious, with a 70 per cent chance of catching it from a partner who is carrying it. Women diagnosed with gonorrhoea are especially likely to be harbouring chlamydia.

• Symptoms •

Unfortunately, even tragically, as many as two-thirds of all women with chlamydia experience no symptoms at all. When it does produce symptoms these are likely to be a slight increase in vaginal discharge caused by the cervix becoming inflamed, soreness, and a frequent need to urinate, which is often painful.

These symptoms are, of course, similar to those caused by a combination of other vaginal or genital infections, such as thrush, herpes and cystitis, so the diagnosis may be missed if women are not fully tested. Chlamydia can also infect the rectum, causing painful bowel movements, occasional bleeding and burning sensations. If it is transferred to the eye by hand, you are likely to suffer a nasty conjunctivitis.

If there are no symptoms alerting a woman to the need for investigation, the infection can travel upwards and damage the reproductive organs, in which case the first symptoms are those of pelvic inflammatory disease, such as heavier periods, pain during sex, backache and feverishness.

It is now known that the insidious chlamydia is responsible for about half of what used to be termed non-specific urethritis (NSU) in men, the most common sexually transmitted disease for which men seek treatment. (NSU is still the diagnosis when the infecting organism is some other unidentified one.) Chlamydia is symptomless in one in ten men. Usually it causes a clear but not profuse mucus discharge from the penis and a tingling sensation when urinating. These symptoms tend to occur within two or three (but maybe as long as six) weeks after catching the infection.

• How you develop chlamydia •

In adults chlamydia is almost always acquired via sex with a partner who has it. It can, however, be transferred from the genitals to the eyes and, less certainly, vice versa. Once it has been caught, even if it is symptomless for years, there is no chance of its going away again on its own. It can quietly do damage to the fallopian tubes and this process may be speeded up by gynaecological procedures such as having an IUD fitted, an abortion or a D&C, as the infection can then be introduced to the higher reproductive organs.

• Effects if untreated •

The risks are particularly serious for any woman wishing to have children. Chlamydia causes inflammation of the cervix and, if untreated, may ascend into the womb lining and the fallopian tubes, causing an infection called salpingitis. A high proportion of cases of pelvic inflammatory disease (see page 234) and infertility resulting from blocked fallopian tubes is caused by chlamydia.

Because it so often remains symptomless, many women may only discover they have it when they try and fail to become pregnant and start having infertility investigations.

Women who have chlamydia when pregnant are at higher risk of an ectopic pregnancy, premature birth, stillbirth or of their baby dying shortly after birth, as well as having a greater chance of suffering pelvic infection themselves after delivery.

Babies born to mothers with chlamydia have nearly a 50 per cent risk of being infected with the disease themselves, in the form either of an eye infection (chlamydial conjunctivitis) or pneumonia. The conjunctivitis usually develops when the baby is about a week old; correct and sufficient antibiotics must be given to prevent permanent scarring of the cornea and impaired vision. The pneumonia may not develop for several weeks and again needs correct identification and treatment. Between 10 and 20 per cent of babies born to mothers with chlamydia are likely to get it.

Chlamydia has been found in some cases of early abnormal changes of the cervix but isn't thought a real risk factor for cervical cancer. Treatment for the chlamydia appears to reverse any cervical abnormalities.

• Treatment •

Ironically, for a disease with such potentially horrendous consequences, the treatment is simple and effective once given. The greater problem has always been that chlamydia may not be tested for early enough, especially if a woman has no symptoms. Gynaecologists may not have laboratory facilities available to them for testing for chlamydia, so women with unexplained pelvic pain (that might be caused by chlamydia which has started to do its damage) will do better to go first to a genito-urinary clinic, where usually all the necessary facilities are available.

The usual treatment, for both partners, is three 500mg tablets of oxytetracycline or an equivalent antibiotic for seven days and two 400mg tablets of metronidazole daily for five days. Erythromycin is given instead of oxytetracycline in pregnancy. The wrong or insufficient antibiotic treatment will only damp the infection down for a while but not cure it.

If you have any signs of pelvic infection (for example pelvic pain, some bleeding, fever), there are no testing facilities for chlamydia in your area and you are obliged to rely on your GP, ask for your treatment to cover the possibility of chlamydia: that is, the correct drug regimen, as stated above. Do not settle for being prescribed just ampicillin or metronidazole, if you have not been checked for chlamydia and been found free of it.

• Prevention and self-help •

1 If you have any kind of abnormal vaginal discharge, soreness, unusually frequent need to urinate and pain when you do so, go to a genito-urinary clinic for a check.

2 If you are going to have a gynaecological procedure such as a D&C or an abortion and you have a sexual history which gives you reason to be concerned, it might be worth going to a genito-urinary clinic first and asking to be tested for chlamydia, so that this can be treated if present before you have the surgery with all its attendant risks of giving chlamydia a free ride upwards.

3 It would be wise to avoid the IUD as your main form of contraception if you have a number of sexual partners. The oral contraceptive pill is not a good choice either, as pill users are at two to three times the average risk of getting chlamydia. Barrier methods, such as the condom and diaphragm are best.

• Lice and scabies •

The pubic or 'crab' louse, the body louse and the head louse are all members of the same family of sucking lice. The pubic louse is found mainly in the pubic area and around the anus. Its hind legs have claws which hang on to the pubic hairs and which render it faintly crab-like in appearance, thus its nickname. There are usually more females than males in residence which is unfortunate, as the females lay a prodigious number of eggs. They are very small but possible to see with the naked eye.

Scabies is caused by mites. Mites are smaller than lice and have eight legs, some of them ending in things that look like suckers. Unlike lice, they like to lay their eggs under the skin, so they dig themselves a hole in the outer layer. The genital area is only one of a number of areas of the body which the mite finds attractive.

• Symptoms •

The symptoms for both lice and scabies are the same in women and in men. With lice you are likely to have an itch which comes on mainly at night but some people don't get even that. The itch can be mild or extremely irritating and sometimes there is a rash or tiny spots. However, by the time these symptoms make themselves apparent the lice are likely to have been settled in for a month. In fact, symptoms are thought not to be symptoms as such but an allergic reaction to their established presence. The other sign of lice is a glimpse of the louse itself, but this is rare.

You are even less likely to see the mite but it induces a similar allergic reaction, again about a month after its arrival. In this case itching may occur day and night. It is usually worse at night, and can be absolutely maddening, with buttocks, thighs and armpits particularly affected. If the itch gets scratched, the holes dug by the mites to lay their eggs can become infected with bacteria and cause a rash.

Neither lice nor mites jump.

• How you develop them •

Lice are most commonly sexually transmitted but it is also possible to become infected if you simply share a bed with someone who has got them. However, the possibility of getting lice just from sleeping in a bed previously slept in by someone with lice is extremely remote, unless you are using the bed in shifts, because pubic lice – unlike body lice – cannot survive on their own for more than 24 hours. The likelihood of catching scabies this way is extremely low too. But you don't need to have sex to catch scabies. Close contact is quite sufficient and sharing a bed is the likeliest occasion for transfer.

• Effects if untreated •

Unpleasant as these infestations are, they do not lead to anything worse.

• Treatment •

There are special lotions, benzene derivatives, which kill off both. One application is usually enough. For lice, the lotion is applied to the pubic region only and for scabies it is applied over the whole body, from the neck downward. Special shampoos were used but these are not ideal as they are washed off too quickly to have an effect. Partners need treatment too but there is no need in either case to do anything special to either clothing or bedding.

• Gonorrhoea •

Gonorrhoea is caused by a bacterium known as the gonococcus or *Neisseria gonorrhoeae* which, under the microscope, looks like a coffee bean in shape. In women, the cervix is almost always infected but sometimes the urethra, rectum and occasionally the throat is too. In men it is found in the urethra and sometimes the throat. In homosexual men, but rarely in heterosexual men, it can be found in the rectum.

Gonorrhoea is highly infectious. After one act of sex with a person who has it you have a 90 per cent chance of getting it yourself. You can also infect someone else from the moment you have it: there is no incubation period. It is the most common sexually transmitted disease in the world.

• Symptoms •

Tragically, there can be virtually none for women. About 50 per cent of women have absolutely no symptoms at all; the rest may experience just a slight increase in vaginal discharge but of no very distinct character. A few may have pain on urination. In rare cases, when the rectum is infected, there is a slight discharge from there. Later there are symptoms but these are the symptoms of pelvic inflammatory disease, which untreated gonorrhoea can cause (see page 234).

About a third of women who have gonorrhoea also have bacterial vaginosis and nearly half have trichomonas, so, if they are lucky, they will have sought treatment for the symptoms of these. However, this is where the benefit of going directly to a genito-urinary clinic for tests comes in: whereas a GP may just test for the organism suggested by your symptoms, the GU clinic automatically tests for gonorrhoea and so will not miss it, whatever other infections you might have with it.

Another way to become alert to gonorrhoea early might be through symptoms experienced by your male partner, if he is a regular one. Within ten days of sex with an infected person, men usually get a thick yellowish discharge from the penis and experience intense pain on urination. However, some men do escape symptoms or have less obvious ones.

• How you develop gonorrhoea •

In sexually active adults it is almost always transmitted during sex with a partner who has it. Oral sex is responsible for its being found in the throat. Anal sex is the cause of its presence in the rectum in homosexual men but in a woman involvement of the rectum is far more usually due to the fact that the openings of the vagina and anus are close.

It is theoretically possible to catch gonorrhoea from the much-feared toilet seat but this is less of a likelihood for women than men (for anatomical reasons) and not at all common for them either. However, young girls who have never had sex can catch it from an infected towel or flannel. This is because the make-up of vaginal moisture is different before puberty, such that the gonococcus can survive in it and cause soreness around the vaginal entrance.

• Effects if untreated •

If untreated, gonorrhoea can ascend to cause infection in the fallopian tubes, often blocking them and leading to infertility or ectopic pregnancy because a fertilised egg cannot reach the womb. When the fallopian tubes have been affected, a woman may experience her first symptoms, such as low pelvic pain, heavier and more painful periods, backache and feverishness. In rare cases she may suffer peritonitis, an inflammation of the lining of the abdomen which can be fatal if untreated.

Women with gonorrhoea on the cervix at the time of giving birth can have babies with infected eyes. Within two days of birth, the eyes become red and swollen with a discharge and must be treated quickly with antibiotics to prevent scarring and permanent impairment of vision.

Untreated gonorrhoea can also give rise to arthritis, as it can have an effect on the joints.

• Treatment •

Treatment for both partners is with a single dose of oral penicillin, although more may be needed if there are complications. It is safe to take in pregnancy but there is an alternative for those allergic to penicillin. The gonococcus has the alarming ability to develop strains which are resistant to the penicillins most usually used in treatment. Fortunately, the pharmaceutical industry is just about keeping ahead with the development of different types of penicillin drugs.

• Prevention and self-help •

1 Choose your contraceptive method carefully if you have more than one sexual partner. The pill is actually protective against gonorrhoea but significantly increases the risk of chlamydia (see page 376), so is not ideal at all. The IUD is associated with an increase in all kinds of genital infections. Barrier methods are best.
2 Go for investigation immediately if you or a partner develop symptoms. Be particularly alert if your partner is bisexual.

• Syphilis •

Syphilis is relatively rare in women these days but there are periodic increases in syphilis in homosexual and bisexual men, which may therefore lead to increases in its incidence in women. Also, increases in both sexes are often linked with poverty and drug use.

Syphilis is caused by a bacterium called *Treponema pallidum* and known as the treponeme. The areas of primary infection in women are the lips of the vagina, the clitoris and around the opening to the urethra. Sometimes it can affect the cervix. In men, symptoms usually appear on the penis. In both sexes infection can also occur around the anus, occasionally the mouth and, rarely, the nipples. It is possible for a baby to be born with syphilis if the disease has not been treated in the mother but this is rare these days, as pregnant women are still routinely tested for syphilis.

• Symptoms •

It can take as long as three months after sexual contact with an infected person for the symptoms of primary syphilis to show but more usually something has shown within a month. Because the infection, once in the body, blocks the blood supply to the skin in the area where the bacteria entered, the first sign is a single ulcer (chancre) at that spot. The area may be inflamed and the local lymph glands swollen. The ulcer may be so tiny as to be almost invisible; equally it might extend to about 1cm (⅜in). It is hard to the touch and usually painless.

Nothing further happens during the next six to eight weeks. In the majority of cases the chancre has disappeared by the time that symptoms of secondary syphilis become apparent. Usually a red spotty rash or other sores appear on various parts of the body which may disappear again quickly or stay around for some weeks. There may be flat warty-looking growths on the vagina (these are not of the same family as genital warts). Often people with syphilis get spots on the tongue. As well, there will be fever, aching muscles, bones and joints, fatigue, loss of appetite and even loss of hair, because syphilis attacks the whole body. At this stage it is very common for all the lymph glands and the liver to be enlarged.

These symptoms eventually resolve themselves even if no treatment is given and the infection then becomes latent. In many people it remains latent until the end of their lives and causes no further symptoms: in a few the disease progresses and is then known as tertiary syphilis. It can then affect the skin, the bones, the nervous system (including the brain) and the cardiovascular system and lead to dementia and heart failure. But tertiary syphilis is very very rare indeed today.

• How you develop syphilis •

Syphilis is acquired sexually. It has to find a cut or graze in the skin to enter by, which is why homosexual or bisexual men who have anal intercourse, where tearing of the tissues is common, are at especial risk. The disease can be passed on for two or three years from the time of the appearance of the chancre, if untreated.

• Effects if untreated •

A woman who has syphilis when pregnant can pass the disease on to her baby. If the disease is in its early infectious stage, she is more likely to miscarry; but if it is in its early latent stage – up to two or three years after first symptoms – there is an 80 per cent chance of the baby being born with various defects of the skin, bones, eyes and nervous system. However, congenital syphilis is very rare because in Britain a pregnant woman's blood is routinely tested for syphilis, among other things, when she first attends the antenatal clinic.

• Treatment •

Syphilis is cured quite easily with a course of penicillin injections for 14 days. Penicillin is safe in pregnancy and is always effective because the treponeme, which causes syphilis, has not developed any resistance to it, unlike the organism which causes gonorrhoea. There are alternative drugs available for those allergic to penicillin. You should be advised to have follow-up blood tests to check the treatment has worked, and avoid sex till a month after treatment is complete.

• Prevention and self-help •

1 Be aware that you may be more at risk if you have a partner who is actively bisexual.
2 The condom is protective but not entirely. A woman who has syphilis may still infect a man at the base of his penis, the part that isn't covered by the condom, and he can then pass it to you.

· Hepatitis B ·

Hepatitis B is a viral infection which causes inflammation of the liver and can have potentially serious complications. In this country it is very commonly contracted sexually and is 100 times more infectious than AIDS (that is, 100 times easier to catch if you have sex with an infected person). Even after sufferers have recovered, some of them – usually men – become silent carriers of the disease and can unwittingly pass it on for the rest of their lives. Probably about one person in 1000 in Britain is a silent carrier and is at greater risk of the long-term complications.

· Symptoms ·

The symptoms are the same in women and men. Between one and three months after contact with the virus, you usually experience tiredness, nausea and loss of appetite. These are the only symptoms in about half of people who contract hepatitis B. The rest develop jaundice, fever, tenderness around the liver and there is a tendency for urine to be darker than usual while stools are lighter.

This acute phase of the illness may last for up to a fortnight and be followed by a long period of depression and lethargy which may persist for up to six months.

· How you develop hepatitis B ·

Hepatitis B is commonly acquired by sex with a partner who has it, or with a carrier of the disease. It can be passed not only through cuts and abrasions but in semen, vaginal secretions and saliva; but levels of the virus in blood are by far the highest.

Non-sexual methods of acquiring the disease are mainly by splashes of contaminated blood entering through a cut in the skin or via needle pricks, so medical and nursing staff, dentists and hygienists are at high risk, as well as, of course, intravenous drug-users. More general possible sources of infection are contaminated needles not sterilised properly after use for acupuncture, ear piercing, tattooing and electrolysis.

· Effects if untreated ·

The disease slowly wears off on its own but if high levels of the virus persist in the blood for more than six months, you can become a carrier, with which there are the long-term risks of relapse and increased risks of cirrhosis and liver cancer. About one in ten people becomes a carrier. The risk of later liver cancer is 273 times greater than in a non-carrier.

Babies can acquire hepatitis B from their mothers at or around the time of birth.

• Treatment •

Although possible treatments are being investigated, there is nothing universally available. There are, however, vaccines to protect against contracting hepatitis B altogether. They are recommended for high risk medical professionals and may be given immediately after birth to babies of infected mothers, to reduce their risks. The vaccine is also available to others but not generally on the NHS, and it is expensive.

• Prevention and self-help •

1 If you have a partner who is actively bisexual, you are at greater risk of contracting hepatitis B. It is a good idea to use condoms and avoid anal intercourse and the swallowing of semen.
2 Check when having any commercial procedure that entails a needle prick, such as electrolysis, that the practitioner uses an autoclave for proper sterilisation of needles or, better still, disposable needles.
3 Any woman who has recently had hepatitis B should avoid the contraceptive pill, at least until tested to ensure that liver function is normal.

• HIV and AIDS •

AIDS is the most frightening of sexually transmitted diseases because there is no cure and it can be fatal. At the beginning of 1980 no one had heard of it. Now everyone has heard of it and probably everyone feels fearful of it, but there are still more questions than answers about how it is caused, how it might be treated and how far it affects women.

AIDS stands for acquired immune deficiency syndrome, the name given to a group of normally uncommon infections and cancers which may occur when the body's immune system breaks down. HIV stands for human immunodeficiency virus. It is believed that infection with HIV may lead on to AIDS but certainly not in all cases. About half of those diagnosed with HIV appear to go on to develop AIDS within ten years.

Most scientists believe that if HIV gets into the bloodstream, it attacks certain white blood cells (T4 cells) which are part of the body's immune system and designed to help fight disease. HIV invades the cells and, because of a similarity between the make-up of these cells and HIV, forces them to make more of the virus which eventually kills the T4 cells, leaving the body open to infection it cannot fight.

However, there are differing views. One, for instance, is that HIV doesn't kill T4 cells but tricks the immune system into destroying itself: AIDS thus being an auto-immune disease. This would mean prevention needs to be directed towards damping immune response down rather than building it up.

Some researchers believe that HIV cannot cause immune suppression by itself but needs co-factors, such as other sexually transmitted diseases. A minority of scientists believe that HIV is not the cause of AIDS at all, although it may commonly be present, and that immune suppression is caused by dangerous sexual lifestyles, drug use (the social drug amyl nitrate known as 'poppers', has often been implicated in reducing immune function), poor diet and/or poor hygiene etc.

Some experts claim HIV/AIDS can affect homosexuals and heterosexuals equally (pointing to worldwide figures), others that heterosexuals are at far less risk and only suffer equally in parts of the world where other debilitating diseases (such as tuberculosis) and poverty are rife. There really are as yet no answers to satisfy everyone and many of the disputes surrounding the disease, and the amount of research money that is put into it, are political rather than scientific.

• Symptoms •

HIV causes no symptoms, at least initially, in the majority of people, which is why it is impossible to calculate how many people harbour the virus. Sometimes, however, some people do experience cold-like symptoms shortly after infection, which may include swollen glands, night sweats, a cough that doesn't go away and weight loss. These symptoms are probably dismissed as flu.

Some people develop other symptoms at a later date, such as persistent swelling of the lymph glands in the neck, armpits and groin, intense fatigue, dry cough, diarrhoea, thrush in the mouth, cold sores, night sweats, fever, unexplained bleeding and unexplained weight loss.

Women with HIV may be more prone to persistent vaginal thrush, menstrual disorders, pelvic inflammatory disease and precancerous cervical changes. All of these and the above symptoms are signs that the immune system is not functioning effectively.

A number of women and men with HIV may develop AIDS. This term is used when certain more serious conditions associated with a severely compromised immune system develop, such as a particular form of pneumonia known as PCP (*Pneumocystis carinii pneumonia*) and rare cancers such as lymphoma and Karposi's Sarcoma, along with night sweats, fever and cough.

• How you catch HIV •

HIV can be transmitted sexually and by the use of shared needles and syringes. It can also be passed by a mother to her unborn baby or via breast milk to a newborn baby. There is a 15 per cent chance of a baby being infected.

There is sufficient HIV in an infected person's blood, semen or vaginal fluid to be infectious to someone else. Although it is present in saliva, there is not sufficient virus to be transmitted by this means. A man can infect a woman during penetrative sex without a condom because semen entering her vagina or anus can be absorbed into her bloodstream. A woman can infect a man during penetrative sex without a condom if infected vaginal fluids or menstrual fluid can gain entry to his bloodstream via a cut or tiny tear in the skin of his penis, or through his urethra.

Scientists have calculated from studies that a woman has a one in a 1000 chance of catching HIV from having sex once with an infected man. A man has a one in 2000 chance of catching HIV from having sex once with an infected woman. Studies of hundreds of stable heterosexual couples in which the man has HIV have indicated that, over several years of unprotected penetrative sex, a woman has a one in five chance of having the virus passed on to her by an infected partner.

Lesbian women are not immune from HIV transmission during sex, although the risks are much lower. If a woman has HIV, licking her clitoris or vulva during her period can be risky, as little cuts and sores in the mouth or bleeding gums are common and allow HIV access. Any sex act may be risky, even if there is no penetration of any kind, if as a result infected vaginal fluid or blood enters a cut.

Also, sharing sex toys, such as vibrators, can be a source of infection.

Women who inject drugs are at risk if they share needles and syringes because small amounts of blood remain in syringes which may then be injected into their own bloodstreams. In some undeveloped countries, doctors may reuse needles without sterilising them properly, or at all.

You are unlikely to become infected with HIV from a blood transfusion as all donated blood is tested. You are also extremely unlikely to receive HIV-infected semen via donor insemination, if you are using this method to conceive, as all NHS and private clinics in Britain have to test prospective donors for HIV antibodies (but you may need to take care if making private arrangements).

HIV cannot be caught from kissing, using the same cup or cutlery as someone who has HIV, sitting next to someone with HIV, mosquitoes, swimming pools, damp towels or lavatory seats. There is only a very small risk of catching it by giving first aid to an accident victim who has the HIV virus and there has been no known case of catching HIV from mouth-to-mouth resuscitation.

• Effects and consequences •

There is, tragically, no effective treatment for AIDS, although some of the infections which occur because of it can be treated. Ultimately, someone who has full-blown AIDS is likely to die of it, although this may be many many years after first becoming HIV positive. The best protection currently is prevention.

Effects of a different kind are the powerful psychological and social ones. It is devastating to learn you have a potentially fatal disease, particularly if you feel well and have only discovered you have HIV through a test (see page 386). Despite massive efforts at public education, there is still stigma and fear associated in many people's minds with a diagnosis of HIV, let alone AIDS.

If you have HIV you do not have to tell your employers or even your doctor, and you will need to think very carefully about whom exactly you will tell and how. Partners, family and friends may be wonderfully supportive, or they may be frightened and, in their fear, push you away. Fortunately, there are a number of very helpful and sympathetic support groups which can offer advice or just a listening ear: see Useful Contacts.

It is important to be aware that the shock of the diagnosis may bring on symptoms of stress which you may mistake for symptoms of HIV. The mind is powerful and fear itself may induce, temporarily, symptoms that are similar to those of HIV.

As mentioned above, a possible consequence of HIV is that a baby born to an infected mother has a 15 per cent chance of developing AIDS too, either in the womb or during birth. (It is not possible to know till the baby is 18 months old whether he or she is affected, as all babies are born with the same antibodies as their mothers and the maternal antibodies don't disappear till 18 months after birth.) However, even children who do have the HIV virus may be perfectly healthy and reach adulthood without undergoing any significant health problems.

If you are HIV positive during pregnancy, you do not necessarily need to have a Caesarean birth or any other special measures taken, but at least one study has recently been published which suggests Caesarean delivery can reduce risk of transmission of HIV.

• Treatment •

There is no single established approach to treatment of HIV or AIDS symptoms and expertise in this area is concentrated in a relatively small number of hospitals where the majority of sufferers have been treated. You can get a great deal of information about current treatment approaches and where to go to find out more from the national AIDS charity, the Terence Higgins Trust: see Useful Contacts.

The doctors most experienced in dealing with HIV and HIV-related illnesses are the genito-urinary specialists (see page 357). They can monitor your health on a regular basis and treat symptoms as appropriate. You can have regular blood tests to check on the health of your immune system.

Treatment approaches fall into three main categories.

- There are anti-HIV drugs, which aim to inhibit an enzyme produced by HIV and without which it cannot multiply. However the strong drugs needed (AZT or zidovudine is the most well-known) have significant side-effects and are never altogether effective, if at all. Hopes that AZT might be able to prevent AIDS ever occurring if taken by asymptomatic people with HIV have not been proved. Most doctors would recommend use of one of these drugs, however, if someone has AIDS symptoms and a low count of the crucial white blood cells.
- Fighting infections which may arise because of HIV and AIDS. Many odd infections may occur when the immune system is badly damaged, usually caused by common micro-organisms which a normal immune system effortlessly fights off. There are now a number of treatments which have improved very significantly over the last decade or so. The pneumonia known as PCP used to be fatal, for example, but now can be treated with drugs. Maintenance doses may prevent recurrences.

- Looking for drugs or means to strengthen the immune system or to return it to effective functioning. Vaccines are still being looked at but there have been set-backs over the years in efforts to create one which would prevent anyone who is HIV positive from ever developing AIDS.

Very many people with AIDS have, not surprisingly, turned to complementary medicine for help, whether in conjunction with more orthodox approaches or instead of them. Many of these methods concentrate on natural means of strengthening the immune system, for example through healthy diet and rest, reducing stress, etc. Other therapies which are commonly tried and for which a degree of success has been claimed include acupuncture, healing, aromatherapy, homoeopathy, massage, visualisation and vitamin and mineral supplementation. HIV self-help groups are a good source of information and opinion about these.

• HIV testing •

This test can be used to find out whether a person has HIV by testing for antibodies to HIV. It is not a test for AIDS. You may test positively for HIV (termed HIV positive) and yet feel perfectly well. Having a positive result merely means you have been exposed to the HIV virus: it is no indicator of how well you are or will remain.

There are a number of reasons why some women choose to have an HIV test. They may have met a new partner and both want to be sure of being HIV-free, so that condoms can be dispensed with. Or they may want to get pregnant and be sure of being AIDS-free.

If you are thinking about having an HIV test for these or any other reasons, you need to think very carefully indeed about how you would react to a positive result or to your partner having a positive result. It is not easy to live with a diagnosis of HIV, especially when there are no cures for the condition.

On the other hand, if you are so worried for any reason about your risk of being HIV positive that you feel you would cope better with knowing you did have HIV than with the constant uncertainty of not knowing, a test may be right for you. You may also wish to have the opportunity to have your health regularly monitored and to take all the protective steps you can.

A few employers ask for HIV tests. You will have to weigh up your desire for the job against your feelings about a positive result, should there be one. Insurance companies occasionally ask for an HIV test if they have reason to think you are bisexual or a drug user, although goodness knows quite how they would have reason to suspect. A positive result will mean no insurance and difficulty finding insurance elsewhere: a negative result may still leave you with a higher premium. (The Association of British Insurers claims that you are not penalised for a negative result but that the underlying reason that you were asked to take the test will still be taken into account. This could amount to the same thing.)

If you do decide on a test, you have to wait three months from when you had reason to suspect you contracted HIV (if this applies), as antibodies take three months to show up in the blood. The test can be carried out confidentially at any genito-urinary clinic and counselling should be available for a positive result. If tested by your GP, the result will be put in your medical records.

You are required to give just a small sample of blood for the test and will probably have to wait up to three weeks for your result, although same-day results are available in some places.

An excellent booklet on testing and the issues it raises is produced by the Terence Higgins Trust (see Useful Contacts). It is called *Testing Issues*.

• Prevention and self-help •

1 If you are not in a monogamous relationship with someone you know to be HIV-free, the best advice is to practise safer sex: avoid doing anything during sex which allows blood, vaginal fluids or semen to pass from one of you to the other. This means, if you want to have penetrative sex, using a condom. Used correctly, the condom can provide 98 per cent protection against HIV infection – and other more common sexually transmitted infections too. This is important because the presence of another sexually transmitted disease, particularly one that causes breaks or tears in the skin, increases the risk of catching HIV.

An effective alternative to the condom used by the male is the condom used by the female: the femidom, which is fitted in a similar way to the diaphragm (see page 396). The femidom has the advantage of partially covering the external genital area and the material it is made of is known to be impermeable to HIV. However its efficacy against HIV in practice has not yet been assessed.

The diaphragm is by no means as protective as the condom. It may perhaps reduce risk of HIV transmission by 50 per cent. Nonoxynol-9, the most commonly used spermicide in the UK, is easily capable of inactivating HIV. Alas, however, it appears to irritate the cervix and vagina, causing tiny lesions which might actually provide a port of entry for HIV.

Some studies have found that women on the oral contraceptive pill have some protection from HIV; others that their risks of catching it are increased. The major findings against it are that it thins the vaginal and cervical wall linings, increases the risk of chlamydia and thrush and suppresses the immune system. Studies of the IUD are also conflicting, although the evidence here is stronger that IUD use increases the risk of HIV transmission. In two studies, risks of infected men passing HIV to women with IUDs were treble the usual. Also, the IUD is known to increase risk of other genital infections.

If you borrow or lend a vibrator or any other sex toy, or use one with a female partner, wash it thoroughly between uses.

2 If you are HIV positive, ask for a yearly cervical smear as you will be at higher risk of precancerous cervical changes. It is also advisable not to smoke as this together with HIV can put you significantly more at risk of cervical cancer.

3 If you are HIV positive, make sure you have a healthy balanced diet, with plenty of fresh fruit and vegetables, and avoid the use of recreational drugs.

44

CONTRACEPTION

IF 100 women have sex without contraception for a year, between 80 and 90 of them will end up pregnant. Obviously, chances of getting pregnant are higher the younger you are and the more often you have sex but, if you don't want it to be you, it is vital to use suitable contraception.

Different forms of contraception may suit different women or the same woman at different times in life. So we all need to make very careful choices, taking into account not only preference but lifestyle and any relevant medical history. There are seven main types:

- natural birth control
- barrier methods (diaphragm, cap, male condom, female condom)
- chemical (sponge, spermicides)
- hormonal (pill, injectables, implants, vaginal ring)
- intrauterine device (IUD)
- hormonal IUD
- sterilisation

A GP, not necessarily your own, and experts at family planning clinics can help you make a good choice.

· Where to go ·

You can arrange for your own GP to provide you with contraceptive services, if this is a service he or she offers or, if you would prefer, you can arrange to see a GP in another practice for this service only. You can get a list of the names of GPs who offer contraceptive services from your local library, post office or Family Health Service Authority (address in the phone directory). GPs who offer contraceptive services have a C after their name. Some GPs do not offer the full range of contraceptives available. If this is the case, they should be able to tell you of the family planning clinic nearest to you which does have the full range.

You may prefer to go to a family planning clinic anyway, as the staff there are specialists. Find the address of your nearest one not only from your GP but from the phone directory, from the Family Planning Association, or from the free NHS Helpline: see Useful Contacts.

· Natural birth control ·

This is discussed first, not because it is especially recommended but because, unlike all the following methods, it doesn't involve any artificial device. Natural birth control is a method in which you work out, from bodily clues, the time in the month when you are fertile. You then avoid sex around that time (sperm can live in a woman's body for up to seven days) or use a barrier form of contraception.

Many women may think that natural birth control is practised only by women whose religion bars the use of artificial means of contraception. However, a number of women use the method because it is natural and eco-logically sound and there is no need to take, fit or insert anything alien in order to have pregnancy-free sex.

It isn't a popular method. Only 1 per cent of women opt for it. But with very careful use and commitment – and both are vital – it can have a safety record similar to many artificial forms of contraception. About two women in 100 would fall pregnant in any year of careful use and with less careful use, 20 might become pregnant.

· How do you use it? ·

You need to be taught this method by someone who is professionally trained to do so. In large towns it may be possible to find the method taught at a GP practice or family planning clinic. If not, the Natural Family Planning Service (see Useful Contacts) can provide a list of NFP teachers locally. Whether a teacher comes to your home, works with a small group, charges a small fee or expenses or works on a voluntary basis will depend upon the individual concerned.

The most effective natural birth control method is the sympto-thermal method which combines a number of approaches, as any one method on its own may be far from foolproof. By the sympto-thermal method a woman is taught to keep a record of the length of her menstrual cycles, take her temperature on waking every morning, check her cervical mucus secretions, check the position of the cervix (not strictly necessary) and be aware of other revealing physical and emotional signs.

It is perfectly normal for menstrual cycles to vary in length by as much as a week. According to NFP teachers, having irregular cycles is no barrier to calculating fertile periods and, in fact, teaching women with irregular periods to recognise their fertile time should help them calculate when their next period will start. Although the length of time from the beginning of a period till ovulation occurs may vary considerably, a period almost always starts about 14 days after ovulation.

Taking your temperature every day can be an aid because normal tempera-ture usually drops slightly before ovulation and then rises as the level of progesterone rises. It should stay raised until your period starts. You need to know your own normal temperature at rest (that is, before you get up in the morning or have a hot drink). The norm is 37 °C (98.6 °F) give or take 0.5 to 0.8 °C. After ovulation you will be looking to detect a rise of at least 0.2 °C. However, some women detect such a rise but aren't ovulating and some women have no detectable rise but are ovulating.

Cervical mucus can change markedly during the menstrual cycle. As oestrogen levels rise, the mucus becomes clearer and stretchier and more inviting to sperm. After ovulation, the mucus become thick, white and sticky and inhospitable to sperm. But although it sounds simple to tell the difference, it isn't necessarily easy. Some women do not produce much mucus anyway and other secretions, such as discharge from a vaginal infection or semen in ejaculate, may confuse the issue.

Fluctuating hormonal levels during the cycle affect the cervix so that there are minor changes in both how it feels and where it is lying.

There may also be other signs of the stage in your cycle. At ovulation some women experience pain (a cramping on the side of the ovary that is releasing the egg), some spotting of blood or breast tenderness.

• For whom is it unsuitable? •

Natural birth control is unsuitable for anyone who doesn't want the daily chore of checking temperature first thing before you have done anything active. (You can't leap out of bed to answer the door to the postman and then come back and take it, nor can you have a waking-up love-making session first.) You must also check cervical secretions at night. You really do have to be committed.

• Advantages •

1 It is absolutely natural, so you can't do any harm to your body.
2 It gives women a lot more sense of their own body and how the menstrual cycle works.
3 If you want to become pregnant at any point, you can use the same knowledge to pinpoint the fertile days in your cycle and increase your chances of conceiving.

• Disadvantages •

1 You need to be taught properly, which entails finding a teacher (some areas may not be well served). You will need a few sessions (perhaps adding up to about four hours) over a period of a few or several months before you will be deemed sufficiently and safely practised at the method.
2 You need absolute commitment.
3 Successful usage means periods of avoiding sex, which affects spontaneity, especially if your sexual interest tends to heighten around ovulation. Or it means using barrier contraception during the possible fertile period, which you may feel defeats the whole object.

• The diaphragm or cap •

Although diaphragms are often also called caps, the cap is a slightly different device (see page 391). But both are barrier methods of contraception and act to prevent sperm from entering the cervix and heading for the womb. Both are used with spermicide, chemicals which kill sperm and therefore increase the safety of the method.

The diaphragm and cap can be very effective methods of contraception if used carefully by experienced users. However, two or three women in every hundred users fall accidentally pregnant, so if not used carefully they can be quite risky methods. Studies show that between 4 and 8 per cent of women may fall pregnant in their first year even if they use it carefully and 10 to 18 per cent may fall pregnant if they don't use it carefully. The highest failure rate is with young fertile women who on average tend to have sex more often than older women. It is the chosen contraceptive method of only two per cent of women overall.

• What is it like? •

Diaphragms   These are dome-shaped devices made of soft latex rubber with flexible metal rims. There are three types: the flat-spring, the coil-spring and the arcing-spring. The rim of the flat-spring diaphragm is flat metal and the whole thing folds over flat when you bend it. The rim of the coil-spring diaphragm contains coiled wire which makes it more malleable when you bend it. The arcing-spring version has a rim which is a mixture of both and forms an arc when folded over. All come in a range of sizes. The right size is the one which allows the diaphragm to cover the cervix when opened out and also fit snugly behind the pubic bone.

Cervical caps   These are smaller than the diaphragm and, as the name suggests, they simply fit over the cervix. There are three different styles of cervical cap too, slightly differing in depth, width and general shape. They are made of rubber with no metal rims and also come in different sizes to fit individual women. Cervical caps are less popular than diaphragms.

You need to be fitted for the correct size by a family planning doctor and come back regularly for checks every six to 12 months. You should always be re-measured if you lose or gain any significant amount of weight (over half a pound) or have a baby, miscarriage or abortion.

You shouldn't be aware of a correctly fitting diaphragm once it is in place. If you do feel it, this is a sign that the size isn't right or the type you have doesn't suit you.

• How do you use it? •

Your doctor should show you how to insert the diaphragm or cap. It is important to be confident that you can get it into the right position.

1 Squirt a little spermicidal cream or jelly on both sides of the dome of the diaphragm and put a very little bit on the rim as well. If using the cervical cap, squirt spermicide only on to the inside. If you don't like jellies or creams or find the whole thing gets too messy, you may prefer to use either a foam which you can put into the vagina with an applicator or a spermicidal film which you can either insert with your finger or place inside the dome of the diaphragm. (For more on spermicides, see page 397.)

2 Fold the rim of the diaphragm over with your thumb and index finger. In whichever position you find easiest – lying on your back; sitting squatting; one leg raised, bent at the knee and supported on a chair – slip the folded diaphragm upwards and slightly backwards into the vagina. If using the cervical cap, push it up into the vagina open end first until it covers the cervix like an upturned cup. Suction then takes over to keep it in position.

3 Check that the diaphragm or cap is covering your cervix correctly by inserting a finger into the vagina and feeling for it through the rubber. The cervix has the shape and feel of the tip of the nose, although it is usually a bit bigger and wider once you have had a baby. The other end of the diaphragm should be fitting behind your pubic bone.

4 If you find it hard to feel your cervix because of its position, try pushing down as if you were trying to push the diaphragm out. This should help to bring it within reach. It is also a good thing to do in the early days of diaphragm use as a means of checking you have inserted it correctly. You shouldn't be able to push it out if it is in its proper position.

5 You can insert the diaphragm or cap any time before making love, even much earlier in the day if you choose. However, if more than three hours pass before having sex, you need to add more spermicide.
   If you have sex more than once, you need to use more spermicide before each time. After sex, the diaphragm or cap must be left in place for at least six hours. You shouldn't leave it in for more than 30 hours, however, as this increases risk of infections including, but rarely, the one which causes toxic shock syndrome (see page 488).

6 Take the diaphragm out by hooking your index finger under the rim and pulling. For removal of the cervical cap, push the open end off the cervix with a firm tap to release the suction. Push downwards if you have any difficulty doing this.

7 Wash the diaphragm or cap in warm water and unperfumed soap. Check the state of it every time you wash it, to ensure that there are no holes in the rubber. An easy way of doing this is to fill it with water, or to hold it up to the light. Rinse the diaphragm or cap carefully, dry it (but never put talc on it) and put it away in its container.

8 Make sure that you never allow your diaphragm or cap to come in contact with any oil-based creams, lubricants or bath oils, as these can rot the rubber. If you are not sure whether certain creams, including those for medical use, contain oil, ask your local pharmacist.

• For whom may it be unsuitable? •

Women who are prone to urinary tract infections may not find the diaphragm or cap a good choice as both are associated with increased bouts of these infections (though urinating before and after sex and washing after sex may lessen the risks). Women with a prolapse may find they cannot keep them in place and women with a retroverted (tilted back) uterus may have similar difficulty.

If your cervix is difficult to reach for any reason, you may not trust the method because you can never be sure you have the device in place correctly. A very few women may be allergic to the rubber or to spermicide. Otherwise, it can be used by almost all women, as there are no side-effects. The biggest deterrent to its use, however, may be the need for forethought involved (see below).

• Advantages •

1 The diaphragm or cap can offer some protection against some sexually transmitted infections and cervical cancer.
2 It doesn't have any adverse side-effects on your body.
3 You only need to use it when you are having sex.

• Disadvantages •

1 You have to remember to put it in.
2 Stopping foreplay to insert it affects spontaneity. (Many women with an active sex life choose to put it in every night so that spontaneity is not affected. This may not be so practical or desirable if you are not in a regular relationship.)
3 Many women don't like having to use spermicide, finding it messy or a nuisance both during sex and afterwards, when it gradually drips out. The smell of spermicides may be a turn-off to some during oral sex.
4 Sometimes the diaphragm bothers men if they can feel it during sex.

• Male condom •

The condom is a thin rubber covering for the penis which stops sperm entering the vagina after ejaculation. Used carefully, just two women in every 100 will fall pregnant in a year when relying on this method of contraception. Up to 15 per 100 will get pregnant in a year if condoms are not used so carefully. It is the contraceptive method chosen by one in five women and, as a barrier method, has the added benefit of conferring significant protection against sexually transmitted diseases, including AIDS, and PID and cervical cancer, both of which can often be caused by sexually transmitted organisms.

Condoms can be bought from pharmacies, garages and many shops and supermarkets. Some are also available free from family planning clinics, genito-urinary clinics and from some GPs – but not the most jazzy versions! Wherever you acquire condoms from, always make sure the packet carries the BSI Kitemark, which means the product is tested for quality and is of sufficiently high standard. Before you open a packet, check the expiry date on it – condoms can keep for a few years if unopened – and don't use a condom that feels dried out or overly sticky. Keep unopened packets in a cool place to preserve them at their best.

• What does it look like? •

The condom is a thin latex rubber sheath open at one end with a thin rim. At the other it is closed and either teat-ended, to collect semen, or plain-ended. Some are made of thicker rubber than others; some have ribbing or protruding bits designed to increase sensation during sex; some are flavoured or scented. Ordinarily, condoms are transparent but are made in all different colours as well. Most contain lubricant, usually a spermicide. The one area where there is no variety, however, is in size: at least in the UK, one size fits all.

• How do you use it? •

1 The condom needs to be placed on the man's penis before the penis touches the vagina. Cases of condom failure are often due to sex play in which the penis and vagina are in contact before full sex and when small amounts of semen may leak out during arousal.

2 Open the packet of condoms and unroll one carefully on to your partner's erect penis. (Never unroll it completely first and then try to slip it on.) Although the rubber is surprisingly strong, you could still do damage if you catch it on a ring or a sharp fingernail.

3 Hold the closed tip of the condom tightly with the thumb and forefinger of one hand while you unroll its length with the other. Doing this stops air collecting in the closed end which semen could push upwards on ejaculation and then follow, to emerge out of the other end. Also, if you hold the end, you won't put the condom on so tightly that there is no room for sperm to collect.

4 Condoms that contain spermicide don't contain a lot of it, so you may choose to use additional spermicide (see page 397) but you don't have to. If you want to add to the lubrication of your vagina, use something water-based, such as KY jelly, not oil-based such as baby oil or Vaseline as they will rot the rubber.

5 After ejaculation, it is important that your partner withdraws from the vagina before his erection has completely gone, otherwise the condom will come off and semen will be deposited in the vagina. Either you or he should hold the rim of the condom as he withdraws to ensure it doesn't slip off while he is doing so.

6 After he has withdrawn, your partner can easily slip the condom off. One of you should wrap it in tissue and throw it in a bin. Don't flush it down a toilet as condoms are not biodegradable. And never wash out a condom and keep it to use again, as it may no longer be effective.

• For whom may it be unsuitable? •

Condoms are only likely to be a problem if your partner consistently has difficulty in maintaining a firm erection or cannot achieve one. Some men, and women, are allergic to the spermicide or lubricant used in some condoms but changing brands can usually solve this difficulty.

• Advantages •

1 They are the most protective of all contraceptive methods against sexually transmitted diseases and are useful for this purpose even when not used as a contraceptive.
2 They are easy to keep (or carry) around.
3 You only use them as you need them and, if you haven't had sex for a while, you don't have to worry about whether they still 'fit'.
4 The condom can help a man maintain an erection longer, if this is a difficulty for your partner.
5 If you don't like things wet and messy, the condom helps to ensure that the bed stays dry.
6 You can see if a condom rips or if it slips off before your partner withdraws, giving you time to think about emergency contraceptive cover (see page 417).

• Disadvantages •

1 You have to remember to have condoms handy.
2 You can't be completely spontaneous about having penetrative sex because the condom has got to be put on first. But many couples incorporate the rolling on of a condom into their sex play, so that it is seen as part of sex rather than an interruption of it.
3 Some men, and women, claim sensation is reduced, although certainly modern condoms are very fine and should hardly lessen sensation at all.
4 The condom still has a poor image for some women who associate it, however unjustly, with teenage sex, illicit sex or unadventurous sex.

• The female condom •

The female condom is still relatively new, so there are no figures for its efficacy but according to research so far it is reckoned to equal the male condom. Like the male condom, the female condom is a barrier method of contraception. However, it not only prevents sperm from entering the vagina but from touching the vulva as well and is therefore also extremely protective against sexually transmitted infections and some of the possible sequels, such as pelvic inflammatory infection and cervical cancer.

The female condom can be tricky to put on, so it might be advisable to ask your GP or family planning doctor for guidance. One study found that failure rate could be as high as 15 in 100 women, given only verbal or written instructions on its use. It is also suggested that you continue with another method of contraception until you feel you have properly got the hang of using it, if you like it.

The female condom is available from pharmacies and a variety of shops, but it isn't cheap. It is free from family planning clinics that supply them. Unfortunately there is no BSI Kitemark for it yet.

• What does it look like? •

There is at present only one female condom on the UK market, called the Femidom. It is a soft polyurethane sheath, far larger and wider than a male condom, and covers the vagina and vulva. There is a rim at the wide, open end and a ring inside the closed end. The material is much stronger than that used for male condoms.

• How do you use it? •

1 Unlike with the male condom, you can put on the female condom well before having sex. Make sure it is in place before there is any mutual genital contact between you and your partner, otherwise leakage of semen during arousal could find its way into the vagina.

2 As with the male condom, you need to make sure you do not snag the material when putting it in place.

3 Squeeze the sides of the ring inside the closed end together and use this to help you insert it, like a tampon, into the vagina, far enough so that it is past the pubic bone but not so far that the external genitalia aren't covered. The rim at the open end should lie flattened against the vulva. You need to ensure a snug fit here. One of the common reported problems with new users is that the penis somehow slips between the condom and the vaginal wall. Another is that the condom may slide in and out of the vagina during sex if it isn't in place correctly.

4 Use any vaginal lubricant you like, if you want one. You don't need to avoid oil-based ones because Femidom isn't made of rubber. However, there are likely to be other versions of the female condom on the market soon, if not on it already, and some may be made of latex rubber.

5 After your partner has ejaculated, hold the open end of the condom, twist it over on itself to make it leak-proof and remove. Throw away in a bin; don't flush down the toilet, as it isn't biodegradable.

6 Never wash and reuse a female condom, no matter in how good condition it looks. It is not safe.

• For whom may it be unsuitable? •

Women with weak vaginal muscle control may find it difficult to use.

• Advantages •

1 It provides excellent protection against sexually transmitted diseases.
2 It is only used when you are having sex and has no side-effects.
3 It can be put in place before penetrative sex, so need not adversely affect spontaneity.
4 Unlike the male condom, your partner doesn't have to withdraw his penis soon after he has ejaculated, as the female condom stays exactly where it is regardless of how soft or hard he is.
5 As with the male condom, it can serve to keep you and the surface you have had sex on relatively dry, if this is something you want.
6 You can see after use if it has developed a rip and so have time to consider emergency contraceptive cover.
7 If you don't have sex very regularly, you can choose just to keep a few handy in case, instead of opting for a form of contraception that gives daily protection, or for which you have to be fitted.

• Disadvantages •

1 You have to remember to have one around and to have it close by when you start sex play.
2 Some women don't like the fact that their partners can see part of it outside the vagina.
3 It is expensive, if you have to buy it.
4 If you want your partner to have direct manual or oral contact with your genitals, the advantage of being able to put the female condom on beforehand is lost.
5 Some people are put off because its loose fit often makes it sound squelchy or rustly.

• Spermicides •

Spermicides are chemical preparations that help prevent pregnancy by killing sperm or making them unable to swim properly. They also form a physical barrier of jelly, cream, foam, etc, which makes it hard for sperm to penetrate the cervix. Although a small proportion of women do rely on them for contraception, they should really be seen as an adjunct to barrier methods such as the diaphragm or condom. Using them for a year without another method could leave up to 25 users out of every 100 pregnant. Spermicide is available free from family planning clinics and can be bought from pharmacies and many shops, supermarkets and garages.

• What do they look like? •

Spermicide comes in several forms. There are jellies, creams, foams that you put into the vagina with an applicator, foaming suppositories, tablets that melt in the vagina or soluble squares of thin film which melt in the vagina.

There will be an expiry date on the packet, which you need to keep a check on if you store them for occasional use.

• How do you use them? •

Spermicides need to be inserted high into the vagina, either with a finger, an applicator or on the back and front of the diaphragm. You need to read the instruction leaflets to see how much you are supposed to use and how long you need to leave before they are effective. Foams are effective straight away; tablets need some minutes to melt. If more than three hours pass after insertion but before you have sex, you need to add more. The same applies if you have sex more than once, with more spermicide needed before each time.

Unopened packets of spermicide should be kept in a cool dark place to preserve them properly.

• For whom may they be unsuitable? •

Anyone can use spermicide.

• Advantages •

1 Spermicide is easy to obtain and easy to use.
2 It only needs to be used when having sex.
3 Most spermicides contain the active ingredient nonoxynol-9, which may protect against many sexually transmitted diseases including AIDS. (But there is a downside to this too: see Disadvantages.)
4 If you tend to be dry, spermicide is an effective lubricant.

• Disadvantages •

1 Spermicides are not reliably effective against pregnancy when used alone, only in addition to the condom, diaphragm or cap.
2 Some women find them messy both at the time of use and afterwards, as they may drip out slowly over some hours.
3 You have to remember to have some handy and to stop and insert it, so spontaneity of sex is affected.
4 Some women and their partners find that the skin on the vulva, in the vagina or on the penis becomes red and irritated by certain spermicides.
5 Nonoxynol-9, the active ingredient in most British spermicides, may irritate the cervix, causing tiny abrasions which may allow entry to any micro-organisms, including HIV.

• Sponge •

This could have been a lovely contraceptive method but alas, didn't live up to expectations. Even with careful use, ten women in every 100 using it for a year will get pregnant. With less care, up to 25 could fall pregnant. It has now been withdrawn from the market.

• Combined pill •

The combined oral contraceptive pill contains oestrogen and progestogen, a synthetic form of progesterone. Oestrogen and progesterone are the two female hormones made by the ovaries which govern the events of the menstrual cycle. The pill works by preventing ovulation from taking place, by altering the action of the fallopian tubes so that the movement of the sperm and egg are impeded, and by preventing the lining of the womb from thickening sufficiently to nourish any embryo.

First developed in the 1960s and much refined since, it is still the most popular form of contraception with one in three women users of contraception in the UK opting for it, and one in two of those aged under 24.

There is now a large range of combined contraceptive pills available, with varying amounts of oestrogen and progestogen in each. Oestrogen-dominant pills can help sufferers from acne, excessively greasy skin and hirsutism. Progestogen-dominant pills can be of benefit to sufferers from benign breast disease, dysmenorrhoea, fibroids and endometriosis. The newer progestogens – desorgestrel, gestodene and norgestimate – even have a slightly beneficial effect on blood cholesterol. If, however, the UK government limits GP prescribing of oral contraceptives to certain brands only, it is feared that only older, cheaper brands with more side-effects (weight gain, breast tenderness and nausea) will be available on the NHS.

Theoretically, the combined pill is 99.8 per cent effective as a contraceptive. However its practical efficacy level is put at 97 per cent because it has to be taken daily (and can therefore be forgotten) and because certain drugs interfere with its effectiveness. Alarmingly, however, one in five pill users regularly forgets a pill, according to one large recent survey of 10,000 women, and doesn't use another form of contraception as a back-up afterwards. The result is that, although the pill provides nearly 100 per cent safety, 18 per cent of all unplanned pregnancies are in pill users. It is essential therefore, if the pill is to live up to its potential, for instructions in its use to be followed precisely.

• What is it? •

The pill is just a very small tablet, its exact appearance varying from manufacturer to manufacturer. They are usually provided in blister packs, so that you can see all of the pills in the packet through one side and press them out individually through the other. Each pill has a day of the week printed under it and an arrow and the idea is that you follow the arrows and days of the week around until you finish the packet. Usually there are 21 pills in the pack. Some contain 28.

There are three types of combined pill. Monophasic are the conventional type, in which all of the pills in the pack are the same. Biphasic and triphasic pills are special formulations where the content of the pill alters at different stages of the month in an attempt to mimic the levels of nature's own hormones. Biphasic are two-stage pills taken over 21 days and triphasic are three-stage pills. The colour of the pills for each phase is different, to reduce the chances of your taking the wrong one on the wrong day. However, they are not popular with family planning experts as a pill of first choice because of the increased risks for error. They are more likely to be prescribed when a monophasic one doesn't suit you.

• How do you use it? •

If you are a new user, you should take your very first pill on the first day of your period and this will give you immediate contraceptive cover. If you want to start the pill after giving birth and you are not breast feeding, you need to wait 21 days after the birth until increased risk of thrombosis has reduced. After a suction termination (a method of abortion used before 12 weeks) or a D&C for a spontaneous miscarriage, the pill can be started immediately.

Whatever the day that you take your first pill, this will be the day that you start each new pack of pills, because you take the pill for three weeks and then have seven pill-free days before starting a new pack. (Some pill brands contain 28 pills, seven of which have no active ingredient and are taken on the pill-free days if women think they would find it hard to remember to start taking the pill again on the right day after a seven-day break. These are called Everyday combined pills or ED pills.)

During the pill-free days (or the inactive pill days with ED pills) you will have a bleed, although this is not a real period. You do not need to use additional contraceptive cover during the seven pill-free days because the formulation of the pill is such that you are covered at this time.

It makes sense to aim to take your pill at the same time each day, to ease the problem of remembering to take it, but it doesn't matter exactly when you take it as long as it isn't more than 36 hours after you took your last one. (Or, more simply, if you usually take your pill at 11pm at night, you can be up to 12 hours late in taking it without losing contraceptive cover.) New users are advised to start by taking the pill at night just in case of mild side-effects such as nausea which may pass unnoticed if asleep.

It is vitally important to do the right thing if you accidentally do miss taking a pill. You also need to follow the procedures below if you are pre-scribed antibiotics, if you have extremely severe diarrhoea or if you are ill and vomiting frequently.

• What to do if you miss a pill •

1 If you are more than 12 hours late in taking your pill, take it as soon as you remember it and carry on taking the rest as normal but you need to use an additional form of contraception for the next seven days.
2 If you have fewer than seven pills left in your pack to take, don't take the pill-free break. Start your next pack immediately you reach the end of the old one. If you are using the ED pill and the seven days would take you into the inactive pills, miss these out and start a new pack.

3 Take the pill for the appropriate day, if you are using the monophasic pill. If you use biphasic or triphasic ones, stay with the same dosage pill as you were taking before. You are likely to experience some breakthrough bleeding, even while taking these pills from the new pack. Look at the packet insert for specific instructions.

4 Don't be tempted to forget all about these procedures if the pill you have forgotten is the first or second of a new pack. You may think that, because you have just had a 'period', you are unlikely to be fertile. In fact these are the most dangerous pills to miss because, after seven pill-free days as well, it is possible an egg could have had time to mature and you could ovulate. If you do miss these crucial pills and then have unprotected sex, you should investigate emergency contraception.

5 If you have been prescribed antibiotics, you only need to use additional contraception for the first seven days, however long your course of antibiotics is, because the gut gradually develops resistance.

6 If you have a period of vomiting that lasts over some days, take additional precautions from when the vomiting started and then for seven days from when the illness was over. If you vomit just once, more than three hours after taking the pill, you do not need to take any extra precautions. If you vomit just once within three hours of taking the pill, you are covered if you take another pill straight away afterwards.

7 Remember that, if you have had to go straight from the end of one pack of pills to another without a break, your pill-taking day will probably have changed, so you will have to start remembering a new start date for each pack.

• For whom may it be unsuitable? •

If you suffer from any of a number of conditions or smoke more than 40 cigarettes a day you will be advised against the pill. Before anyone is prescribed the pill, a doctor should take a detailed medical history and family history and measure blood pressure.

Conditions which may be worsened by the pill (and therefore it is not prescribed) include heart or circulation disorders, stroke, liver disease, any cancer that is oestrogen-dependent, such as breast or ovarian cancer, certain gynaecological conditions, diabetes with complications, certain types of migraine (focal or crescendo), gallstones and some others.

If a close relative developed heart disease before the age of 45, you have high blood pressure, are overweight, smoke up to 40 cigarettes a day or have uncomplicated diabetes or migraine, you will be considered at higher risk but not necessarily denied the pill if you are prepared to be sensible. Certain types of pill suit certain conditions better than others. Smokers, if they can't give up, and those severely overweight will probably be advised to stop the pill and change to some other method at age 35. It used to be thought that increasing age was itself a reason for stopping taking the pill at 35. However, women who are not at risk for any other reason can safely carry on taking the pill into their forties.

• Advantages •

1 The pill when correctly used is extremely safe, and therefore guarantees peace of mind.
2 It has a number of benefits aside from its contraceptive effects including:
   • less risk of iron deficiency anaemia
   • less painful periods
   • less risk of fibroids
   • less risk of ovarian cysts
   • less risk of benign breast disease
   • less risk of pelvic inflammatory disease
   • less risk of ovarian and endometrial cancer
   • possible reduction in rheumatoid arthritis and thyroid disease.
3 There is no mess.
4 Sex can always be spontaneous.

• Disadvantages •

1 Forgetting the pill leaves you at high risk of pregnancy.
2 There may be a range of side-effects. Some are usually temporary, such as mild nausea or slight weight gain after first starting the pill. Others may persist if the pill doesn't suit you. Side-effects associated with oestrogen-dominant pills are nausea, breakthrough bleeding, breast tenderness, fluid retention, increased vaginal discharge, headaches, dizziness. Progestogen-dominant pills may cause lethargy, loss of periods, loss of desire for sex, acne, depression, oily hair, weight gain and dry vagina. Report any such side-effects which bother you to your GP because a different brand of pill might suit you better.
3 You are at slightly higher risk of heart disease and stroke, thromboembolism (blood clot in a vein) and high blood pressure.
4 There is 70-per-cent increase in the incidence of breast cancer under the age of 36 in women who have taken the pill for eight to ten years, according to studies. However, although an increase of 70 per cent sounds vast, it actually amounts to three and a half women instead of two per 1000, developing breast cancer before the age of 36, as fewer than 2 per cent of all new cases occur in women under this age.

   According to an analysis made and reported by the Imperial Cancer Research Fund, there is no evidence of an increase in breast cancer in middle-aged women who took the pill when young (although not all other experts are so confident that an increase would yet have shown up). An American study found a small increase in the risk of breast cancer if the pill was started within five years of starting periods. Studies over a longer term are needed to confirm or disprove this.

   Most pill enthusiasts believe that women need to be given full information so that they can weigh up the costs and benefits for themselves. Those who fear that the full, adverse effects of pill use over many years may not yet be known, would probably prefer to opt for a different method. Those who like the method and for whom safety from pregnancy is paramount may prefer to take their chances, especially as the pill confers benefits as far as some other cancers are concerned.

5   Pill use does not affect fertility. However, for some women, it may take a few months or even years before they have a period after stopping the pill. This is probably because of infertility or sub-fertility problems which existed previously but were masked by the pill.

6   Some women develop dark brown patches on their face and neck, particularly if they have been in the sun. These patches are known as cloasma and occur in some women during pregnancy too. They may fade after stopping the pill but not always entirely.

7   Women who take the pill are more susceptible to the effects of alcohol.

8   Women who like to take mega doses of vitamin C periodically, for example to try to ward off colds or to enhance their immune systems, need to beware: a 1g tablet of vitamin C interacts with the oestrogen in the pill to increase its potency, effectively making a low-dose combined pill into a high-dose one, with all the associated risks of heart disease and thrombosis.

• Progestogen-only pill •

This is sometimes known as the mini-pill or POP and, as its name suggests, contains no oestrogen. It does quite often have the effect of suppressing ovulation but its main mode of action is to thicken the cervical mucus, making it inhospitable to sperm. It also stops the fallopian tubes from helping the egg or sperm along, making it more difficult for either to make progress, and thins the lining of the endometrium, leaving it less able to support a pregnancy.

It is used less often than the combined pill, with only one in ten pill users opting for it. Yet some experts believe that progestogens will increasingly be the contraception of the future, although not necessarily via the pill. As with the combined pill, used correctly it can provide more than 99 per cent protection but incorrect use greatly increases risk of pregnancy (four in 100 women), especially as you cannot safely take a progestogen-only pill more than three hours late.

• What is it like? •

See Combined Pill, page 399.

• How do you use it? •

You use it exactly as described for the combined pill except – and it is a vital except – you must not let more than 27 hours pass between pills. In other words, you should establish a set time of day or evening when you routinely take your pill and never let yourself be more than three hours late in taking it. If you are more than three hours late or have severe vomiting or diarrhoea, you must follow the procedure for missing the Combined Pill, described on pages 400–1.

Taking antibiotics does not affect the efficacy of the progestogen-only pill. However, some other drugs for various conditions do affect it, so always remind your doctor you are taking it if you are prescribed any other drug.

• For whom is it unsuitable? •

You should have your medical and family history taken before you are prescribed any form of contraceptive pill. Certain conditions, such as some cancers, severe present or past arterial disease and some rare diseases may be worsened by the progestogen-only pill. As it also slightly increases risk of ectopic pregnancy, you will not be prescribed it if you have had an ectopic pregnancy in the past.

• Advantages •

1 As with the combined pill, used properly it can provide great peace of mind that you do not risk accidental pregnancy.
2 Many of the conditions that rule out use of the combined pill, such as a history of heart or circulation problems, severe diabetes and smoking, are not a problem with the progestogen-only pill.
3 Breast-feeding mothers can take it. It should be started not less than four weeks after giving birth.
4 There is less progestogen in this pill than in the combined pill, which reduces any adverse effects.
5 Women who have infrequent periods are more likely to find their fertility returns more quickly after stopping it than if they used the combined pill.
6 Period problems, such as pain or premenstrual syndrome, may be lessened while using this pill.

• Disadvantages •

1 Irregular bleeding is quite common. This could range from spotting or complete cessation of periods, which might bother some women.
2 Some women suffer headaches, weight gain or loss of desire when they first take this pill but the effects don't usually last. You might have some breast tenderness and some women experience depression. Other possible side-effects include hair growth, acne, oilier skin and loss of interest in sex temporarily. See also the list of side-effects on page 402 under progestogen-dominant pills.
3 There is an increased risk of suffering ovarian cysts, although a lot of these just disappear by themselves after a cycle or two.
4 There is a slightly increased risk of ectopic pregnancy.
5 There is a slight reduction in efficacy if you weigh over 70kg (11 stone) (that is, a higher risk of pregnancy).

· Injectable contraception ·

There are two injectable hormonal contraceptives currently licensed for use in the UK: Noristerat, which provides contraceptive protection for two months and Depo-Provera, which provides protection for three months. Both are injections of progestogen, so they work to prevent pregnancy in the same way as for the progestogen-only pill (see page 403).

Injectables are a very effective form of contraception, with less than one in every 100 women using it falling pregnant in a year; but they do have distinct drawbacks (see below).

· How do you use it? ·

If you are considered suitable for it, you have to visit a doctor or nurse at your GP surgery or family planning clinic for an injection in the buttock or top of the arm every two or three months. There is an initial high dose of progestogen delivered into the body and then it carries on slowly being released. It stops ovulation, but also thickens cervical mucus making it hostile to sperm, and thins the endometrial lining.

· For whom is it unsuitable? ·

It may be unsuitable in a number of conditions such as arterial disease, stroke, hormone-dependent cancers such as ovarian or breast cancer and liver disease.

· Advantages ·

1 Sex remains spontaneous.
2 You have to remember an appointment once every couple of months rather than to take something every day.
3 You can't see it.
4 Period pains and premenstrual tension may be lessened.
5 It may be protective against endometrial cancer.
6 The usual reduction in efficacy of progestogen-only contraception associated with weighing over 70kg (11 stone) does not seem to apply, or only slightly, to injectable contraception.

· Disadvantages ·

1 Although the injection is reversible in the long term, you won't necessarily be able to reverse its effects for quite some time after having it. Not only will it give you contraceptive cover for two or three months but for many women it may take over a year before regular periods and fertility return. This could be a very big minus indeed.
2 While having the injections, periods may become irregular or, more usually, stop altogether, which might bother some women.

3 The usual possible side-effects of progestogen such as weight gain, acne, increased hairiness, tiredness, headaches, stomach cramps, depression and loss of interest in sex may occur. These are usually temporary.

4 Not an appealing method to those who are nervous of injections.

• Implants •

These are devices which are implanted under the skin and slowly release progestogen at a controlled rate for five years. At time of publication there is only one implant available in the UK, Norplant, which came on to the market in October 1993, but different varieties will be coming on to the market in the future, one of which may be biodegradable and therefore not need removal.

Family planning experts thought this method might appeal to older women who had had their families. In fact it has been greeted with great enthusiasm by young women. A Mori survey of women found that 44 per cent of those who said they would be interested in trying it were under 24; 38 per cent between 25 and 34 and only 18 per cent over 35.

The implant suppresses ovulation in about 50 per cent of women. It also thickens mucus so that it is not sperm-friendly and prevents the endometrium from thickening properly and being able to support a pregnancy. It has a failure rate of one per cent over the first year and two per cent over the whole five year period.

• What is it like? •

The implant consists of six tiny flexible plastic rods, each containing a set amount of the progestogen, levonorgestrel.

• How do you use it? •

A doctor gives you an injection of local anaesthetic and then inserts the rods in a fan shape just under the skin on the inside of the upper arm. An experienced doctor should be able to insert it in less than 15 minutes. There is likely to be some bruising and swelling for a day or two. Although most women say they can feel the implant, it can't usually be seen. Removal, also carried out under local anaesthetic and with the aid of curved forceps, may take up to 20 minutes but can be considerably less if a doctor is experienced. Sometimes it may require a second attempt, if for example, a lot of scar tissue has formed around the implant.

Doctors are not obliged to be trained in the procedure but the manufacturer has offered training sessions all over the country and well over 5000 GPs and family planning doctors have either taken or applied for it. It is important to be sure that any doctor who inserts it for you has been properly trained as there have been some complaints of problems and pain on removal.

Norplant releases 85mcg of levonorgestrel daily, decreasing by nine months to 50mcg daily and by 18 months to 35mcg, then settles at 30mcg daily for the rest of the five-year period. It is effective as a contraceptive almost at once and, if the device is removed for any reason, fertility returns within days. If the implant is only removed when the progestogen is used up and another one is desired, a second implant can be inserted in the same place.

Ideally it should be implanted on the first day of a period but, if this is not practical to arrange, it can be implanted any time between days two and five, with additional non-hormonal contraception then being used for the first seven days.

• For whom is it not suitable? •

Women for whom progestogen-only contraception is not suitable (see Progestogen-only Pill, page 404 and Injectable Contraception, page 405) may not be right for this one either. For women who weigh over 70kg (11 stone), the failure rate may rise to 7.6 per 100 women over five years.

• Advantages •

1 Once the implant is in place you can forget about contraception for the next five years.
2 If you do decide you want to become pregnant, the implant can be removed and fertility will return almost immediately, unlike with injectable contraception.
3 After a three-month follow-up with your doctor, you need only attend annually for a check.
4 You can breast feed with an implant.

• Disadvantages •

1 Between 60 and 80 per cent of users experience menstrual irregularities in the first year, severe enough that almost one in ten asks for the implants to be removed in the first year, although overall blood loss is usually less than normal. The menstrual irregularities are unpredictable but include pro-longed bleeding, spotting, loss of periods altogether or a combination of all three. However they tend to lessen as time goes on.
2 A quarter to half of women using Norplant experience headaches, although very few choose to have the implants removed for this reason.
3 Some women experience irritation around the implant site. Sometimes the implant is visible when the arm is raised and sometimes the skin over the area darkens. Scar tissue that builds up round the implant may be felt for some time after the implant has been removed and sometimes scarring is visible. A small proportion of women opt for removal because of arm pain.
4 There may be progestogen side-effects, such as weight gain, breast tenderness, acne, nausea, hair growth, hair loss, dizziness and mood change, in up to one in ten women.

5 There may be an increase in incidence of ovarian cysts, if ovulation is suppressed. But many may resolve themselves without treatment.

6 A method which releases a hormone for five years may be of concern as, according to some doctors, it is impossible to be sure at this stage that it is totally safe.

• Vaginal ring •

There are two types of vaginal ring currently being developed and neither, at time of publication, is yet available. One contains progestogen which is slowly released once the ring is in place in the vagina, and works for three months. The other contains both oestrogen and progestogen and will work for four months, but needs to be removed for one week out of each four, during which you have a period.

The progestogen ring was expected to be available by now but met a hitch when in trials red patches were discovered on some women's vaginas. This could indicate thinning of the vaginal walls and have implications for susceptibility to sexually transmitted diseases and vaginal infections. So trials have continued while this is investigated. Also, studies so far show that it is less effective than the progestogen-only pill; up to five women in every 100 using it have fallen pregnant per year.

The oestrogen and progestogen version is still some years away from availability here, at time of publication, so the following refers only to the progestogen ring, which works, as does other progestogen contraception, by thickening cervical mucus to make it inhospitable to sperm, thinning the endometrial lining so it cannot nourish an embryo and, in many cases, stopping ovulation.

• What does it look like? •

It is a small flexible plastic ring, which looks like a washer and is roughly the size of a biscuit.

• How do you use it? •

After squeezing the sides of the ring together you slide it up into the vagina. You don't have to cover the cervix or hook it behind the pubic bone. It can stay anywhere within the vagina and should be kept there automatically by your vaginal muscles. Once you have inserted this ring, you leave it there for the full three months, including through your period and during sex. It is effective immediately if you insert it on the first day of your period. You can still use tampons, although some women find the ring falls out when they remove tampons. Still, no matter, you just reinsert it after rinsing it in water. After the three months is up, you remove it and insert another.

• For whom is it not suitable? •

It will not suit women who have had an ectopic pregnancy, as the chances of another are slightly increased. It shouldn't be used if you have had pelvic inflammatory disease and if you are prone to vaginal infections, as it may increase risk of infections. If you have a prolapse or weak vaginal muscles, you may not be able to keep the ring in position.

• Advantages •

1 The ring doesn't interfere with sex and once in place you can just forget about it.
2 The ring uses a lower dose of hormones than is needed with the oral contraceptive pill.
3 You can take it out if you are not happy with it. If you take it out to become pregnant, fertility is restored immediately.

• Disadvantages •

1 There is the usual progestogen-only side-effect of irregular bleeding and spotting, which bothers a number of women.
2 Some women report irritation of the vagina and increased discharge.
3 The ring may come out when taking out a tampon or if straining on the toilet.
4 The ring may become discoloured which some women may not like, although it actually doesn't matter as far as its efficiency goes.
5 There is a very slightly increased risk of an ectopic pregnancy.
6 There is an increased risk of suffering ovarian cysts, although after a cycle or two these are likely to disappear on their own.

• Intrauterine device (IUD) •

The IUD is a small plastic and copper device which is inserted into the uterus where it can be left for a minimum of five years and where it affects the lining of the uterus so that it cannot support an embryo that tries to implant. The copper in the IUD also helps destroy or immobilise sperm. The IUD is the third most popular form of contraception after the pill and the condom and is used by 7 to 8 per cent of women in the UK. At most one or two women in every 100 will get pregnant during a year of its use. The highest risk time for pregnancy is in the first three to six months after insertion, particularly as this is the time when the IUD might be pushed out by the body if it is going to reject it.

• What does it look like? •

The type of IUD used nowadays is made of a rubbery material called poly-ethylene or polypropylene and copper wire. It comes in various shapes; the most describable ones are those that look a bit like a T or a 7. There are two threads attached to one end which hang down a little way into the vagina. (Under trial at present and looking promising is a threadless IUD.) The IUD can be used by women who have had children and by women who haven't (unlike the older types which were different for each group).

• How do you use it? •

An IUD has to be inserted by a doctor. If it is inserted correctly it can be a very satisfactory method of contraception but if it is not put in correctly you can get all sorts of problems. So it is really worth ensuring that the doctor who puts in yours has a lot of experience of inserting them. Many GPs may just put them in occasionally whereas family planning doctors do it all the time.

Before having an IUD fitted it is wise to go to a genito-urinary clinic to check that you do not have any symptomless sexually transmitted infection, particularly chlamydia or gonorrhoea. If you have an infection present at the time of IUD insertion, the procedure can help the infection ascend to the higher reproductive organs where it can quietly wreak havoc and cause infertility. You would not know until you started to experience the symptoms of pelvic inflammatory disease or found perhaps that, after removal of the IUD, you failed to become pregnant.

The best time to have an IUD fitted is in the last few days of your period. At this time insertion is easier and less painful, because the cervix is softer, and there is less risk of immediate expulsion, which is more likely to happen during the strong uterine contractions that may be experienced at the start of a period. Although doctors would be less keen, it is perfectly possible to fit the IUD at other times in the cycle, up till day 19.

To have an IUD inserted, you need to lie on you back with your knees raised and apart and your feet flat. You may be offered local anaesthetic. A speculum is put into the vagina to push the walls apart and a rod inserted through the cervix to measure the length of the womb. This can be a bit uncomfortable or even painful for some women. Then the IUD is inserted in a flattened form through a hollow tube that is passed through the speculum. The tube is pushed through the opened cervix. When the tube is withdrawn, the IUD stays in place, opening out into its normal shape. It becomes effective immediately.

The threads are then cut so that a short length hangs down into the vagina, long enough for you to feel for to check every so often that the IUD is still in place. (Your partner may feel the threads during sex but this isn't normally a bother.) The threads are also used by the doctor to aid removal. In some cases the threads are cut too short, in which case it may be necessary to go for an ultrasound check to ensure that the IUD is in the right place and able to function. The threadless IUD, on trial, is removed with a special hook.

It may only take a few moments for the IUD to be inserted but any fiddling around with the cervix makes many women feel a bit faint or hot and uncomfortable. Give yourself a minute or two to regain your composure if you do feel a bit odd, rather than heroically swinging your legs off the couch and instantly getting on with your day.

You may be aware of some stomach cramps or vague pain and you may notice a little bleeding for a day or two. If any problems persist or you feel feverish and unwell, go back to your doctor in case you have developed an infection. Quick treatment is essential to prevent potential long term problems such as pelvic inflammatory disease.

You will be asked to return for a check up about six weeks after insertion and then once a year. For the first three months it is wise to check after each period that your IUD is still with you and perhaps a couple of times during the month as well. If all remains fine, you need only make occasional checks, preferably at the end of a period.

• For whom is it unsuitable? •

You definitely should not consider an IUD if you have a number of sexual partners or if your partner does. The more sex with the more people, the higher the risks of catching sexually transmitted diseases which can be especially problematic with an IUD in place, as infecting micro-organisms can literally climb the threads to make their way into the uterus.

Women who have already had pelvic inflammatory disease or who have had an ectopic pregnancy should avoid the IUD. However, the threadless IUD reduces the risk of PID. In early trials, none of the 99 women studied over 22 months developed it despite an expected incidence of 3 to 10 per cent. So should those with an abnormally shaped uterus, scars on the uterus and uterine fibroids. With some kinds of heart disease the IUD may not be advised by your doctor because of increased risks of infection. Also, if you have to take immunosuppressive drugs, you will be more open to IUD-related infections.

If you have heavy periods normally, you may not want to risk the IUD making them even heavier.

• Advantages •

1 Once the IUD is in place and if you have no problems, you don't have to think about contraception for at least five years.
2 Sex can be totally spontaneous.
3 Fertility is not adversely affected after removal.

• Disadvantages •

1 Insertion may be painful, but because it is brief is often considered worth it.
2 Periods are likely to be heavier, with more pain and cramps. There may also be some spotting between periods.
3 The IUD increases the damage which can be done by the sexually transmitted infections chlamydia and gonorrhoea, with particularly high risk of pelvic inflammatory disease. (See Pelvic Inflammatory Disease, page 234, for symptoms.)

4 The IUD can come out, an event most likely to occur, if it is going to occur at all, in the first few months after insertion.You are then obviously at high risk of pregnancy. Check tampons and pads during periods for the first few months. If you can feel the IUD itself and not just the threads it is not correctly in place. Use another form of contraception and see your doctor as soon as possible.

5 In rare cases an IUD, most usually if it is fitted badly, may perforate the uterus and be carried off elsewhere into the abdomen. In such an event you will probably feel pain in the abdomen, maybe experience some bleeding and you will not be able to feel the threads, so this is a signal to go instantly to your doctor to arrange an ultrasound check. Once located, the IUD will need surgical removal.

6 Sometimes the lining of the uterus can start to grow around the IUD, embedding it and making its removal more difficult. Laparoscopy may be necessary.

7 If you do fall pregnant with an IUD in place, there is a slightly greater than usual chance of the pregnancy being ectopic, developing in the fallopian tube instead of the uterus. This is a medical emergency. If the pregnancy is in the right place and you decide to go ahead with it, there is an increased risk of miscarriage or premature delivery if the IUD is left in place, although the baby itself will not be harmed because the IUD is outside the amniotic sac that surrounds the foetus. If the pregnancy has progressed for less than 12 weeks, you will probably be advised to have the IUD removed, if it will come out easily.

8 If threads are cut too short and can't be felt, removal when the time comes is less straightforward than normal. In these circumstances women used to have to go into hospital for removal under a general anaesthetic. This is now not necessary as doctors who are specially trained and have the right imple- ments can retrieve the IUD through the vagina, either with or without local anaesthetic. In the event of difficulty locally, you can ask your doctor to refer you to the Margaret Pyke Centre in London. This is an NHS family planning service and research centre which runs a missing threads clinic and takes referrals from all over the country: see Useful Contacts.

• Levonorgestrel-releasing • intrauterine system

Newon the market, under the brand name Mirena, is the IUD that slowly releases progestogen and which, from studies so far, appears to be almost a completely different animal from the conventional IUD. (It is becoming known as an intrauterine system rather than an intrauterine device in order to distance it from the conventional IUD.) With an annual pregnancy rate of 0.2 per cent, it is as effective as the combined pill properly used and, in effect, more so because there can be no user error.

This method works as an IUD and as a progestogen-only hormonal contraceptive, making cervical mucus scanty and thick and inhospitable to sperm, thinning the endometrial lining, so that the womb is less receptive to any embryo trying to implant, and sometimes suppressing ovulation. However, because it is able to release the lowest effective dose of progestogen, associated side-effects are minimised and there are a number of distinct side-benefits: see page 224.

• What does it look like? •

It looks similar to a T-shaped IUD but has a plastic frame and a silicone capsule on its stem that contains the progestogen, levonorgestrel.

• How do you use it? •

It has to be inserted in the same way as an ordinary IUD, but because the capsule containing the progestogen makes it thicker than the copper IUDs, it may be more difficult to insert. Therefore it will be important to ensure that any doctor who inserts it for you has been properly trained to do so. There have as yet been no studies looking at the ease or otherwise of insertion in women who haven't been pregnant.

The silicone membrane allows slow, steady release of levonorgestrel: 20mcg over each 24-hour period (just 13 per cent of the dose in a standard oral contraceptive) for five years. Some studies have shown the device can work for up to seven years.

• For whom may it be unsuitable? •

It is early days yet but, in the light of information so far, this question should be put the other way around. Many women for whom the conventional IUD is unsuitable would not be excluded from use of the levonorgestrel-releasing intrauterine system. It does not increase risk of pelvic inflammatory disease, instead being protective because the progestogen component works by thickening cervical mucus to keep out sperm, and this also keeps out undesirable micro-organisms.

It does not appear to affect blood pressure, cholesterol levels or carbohydrate metabolism. There does not appear to be any increased risk of ectopic pregnancy. And very few women actually experience the possible side-effects.

• Advantages •

1 Once in place, it works without your having to remember anything and spontaneity of sex is not affected.
2 It appears to offer some protection against pelvic inflammatory disease, with significantly lower rates in under-twenty-fives using this method rather than the conventional IUD.

3 It significantly reduces menstrual blood loss, by around 85 per cent after three months, making it a potential treatment for menorrhagia (see page 223). (It is licensed as a treatment for menorrhagia as well as as a contraceptive in Finland and Sweden.) Women with very heavy flow are usually losing only an eighth of their former amount by six months.

4 It may have a role as a means of progestogen delivery in hormone replacement therapy. (This is under evaluation.)

5 It appears to be able to shrink fibroids, relieve premenstrual pain and may have a role in treating endometriosis.

6 Very few undesirable side-effects are experienced.

• Disadvantages •

1 Some women do not want their periods to become extremely light.

2 Other possible side-effects include increased risk of ovarian cysts, nausea, fluid retention, breast tenderness, acne and depression, but in fact are relatively rare.

3 It may be expelled by uterine contractions shortly after insertion; the uterus may be perforated if it is fitted badly or it may become embedded if the lining of the uterus grows around it (see Disadvantages for IUD, page 411).

4 Insertion may be painful and removal may be more difficult than with the conventional IUD. For removal if threads are cut too short, see Disadvantages for IUD, page 411.)

• Female sterilisation •

This (and the male version, vasectomy) is the most permanent form of contraception, with one in three couples world-wide opting for one or the other. The effect is that you are no longer physically able to conceive.

The failure rate with this method is extremely low indeed: one to three women in every 1000 may still fall pregnant. However, to say this is a surprise to them is putting it mildly indeed. Unlike with other methods of contraception, women who have been sterilised imagine the method is utterly foolproof and tend not even to consider the possibility of pregnancy, for some time, if they miss periods or have other signs usually associated with pregnancy. So, even though the risk of becoming pregnant is tiny, it is important to accept that this risk does exist if you opt for sterilisation.

Sterilisation is not common under the age of 25 or in women who have not had children, although some young women who have made a firm case that they never want to have them have been allowed the operation.

When considering whether sterilisation is a method for you, if you are in a permanent relationship, you and your partner will need to consider whether it is you who should have the operation or he. Vasectomy is simpler: a woman needs a day in hospital whereas a man can go home half an hour after a minor operation in which the tubes that carry sperm to the penis from the testes are cut or sealed. Vasectomy is also more effective: a maximum of one man in 1000 finds the operation leads to a pregnancy in his partner.

• How is it done? •

Female sterilisation is achieved by blocking the fallopian tubes, either by cutting and then sealing them or by putting a clip or ring on to each which effectively holds them closed and stops the passage of an egg to the uterus. The clip or ring method is thought to offer a higher chance of the operation being reversed later, although you should only opt for a sterilisation if you are convinced you want no more children, or none ever.

Whichever method is used, it involves either an overnight hospital stay or day surgery, both with light general anaesthetic, although very occasionally local anaesthetic can be used.

Your GP will need to refer you to a hospital for the operation. You need to be very sure that you are not pregnant at the time that the procedure is carried out, so use contraception very carefully up until that date. Afterwards, the method is effective immediately.

The surgeon usually carries out a female sterilisation via laparoscopy (see page 218). In some cases, for example if a woman is extremely overweight, sterilisation cannot be performed by laparoscopy and a larger incision is required across the abdomen. However it is not that large, about 3cm (1¼in) in length, and the procedure is known as a mini-laparotomy, rather than a laparotomy, which is the operation performed for other more complex pelvic surgery and in which the cut is more extensive.

Very occasionally the operation may be carried out through a cut made high in the vagina, with the benefit that there is no scar to see, but this method significantly increases the risk of infection.

After the operation you should expect to experience some discomfort. If the clip or ring method has been used, there is likely to be some cramping and period-type pain for up to a week. The laparoscopy itself may leave you feeling tired, tender and sore for some days, and often with pain experienced in the shoulders from the carbon dioxide gas that was pumped into the abdomen.

• For whom may it be unsuitable? •

Sterilisation is not generally offered to women under the age of 25 and who have never had children unless they put up an extremely compelling case for it. It is, however, very hard to be adamant at a young age that you will definitely not want children in ten or even 20 years' time. Feelings change not only with time and experience but with experiences within relationships. A single woman who has had no desire to stop her career for a moment to have a baby may feel differently if she meets someone and falls deeply in love.

Sterilisation is not just risky emotionally for those who have never had children. If you have had your family, you still have to think very carefully about every aspect of what losing your fertility permanently means. It is often said that we can never replace a child who dies by having another one but there may be a desire for another child, even if not a replacement, in such a tragic circumstance.

A modern reality to think about is that relationships in which children were conceived all too commonly break down and new ones begin, which may bring the desire to start a new family with a new partner. Although some sterilisation procedures may be reversible and microsurgery techniques are increasing the chances all the time, this should not be considered a norm. If there is the slightest creeping doubt about whether you really want your potential child-bearing days to be over irrevocably, do not choose sterilisation.

You certainly need to feel positively about female sterilisation yourself if you do go ahead. If you are having the operation because your partner is reluctant or downright unwilling to have a vasectomy, think about how this might affect you and your relationship. Will you resent him? How will you feel if your relationship breaks down and he meets someone else and starts a new family, while you have no such opportunity?

Although the peace of mind that comes with sterilisation may be enormous, it is a very big step to take. Talk to someone you trust or whose advice you will respect, whether a friend, your GP or a counsellor at your GP surgery or family planning clinic.

• Advantages •

1 You don't have to think about contraception ever again.
2 Many women find their sex lives more enjoyable or more active, presumably because a continual fear of pregnancy has been removed.
3 The ovaries are not affected by this method. You carry on producing eggs as usual every month and so don't risk premature menopause. The eggs, only the size of a dot, are harmlessly reabsorbed by the body.

• Disadvantages •

1 Every surgical operation carries a small risk. There is always a tiny risk with general anaesthetic plus a small risk of complications arising from the surgery itself, such as damage to surrounding tissues or adjacent organs and infection.
2 Some women find that their periods are heavier and more painful after sterilisation. In some cases this might be because a woman previously used the contraceptive pill and was therefore used to unusually light bleeds. However, it is also thought that sterilisation may affect blood vessels and blood flow, particularly in methods which involve cutting the tubes.
3 The operation may be difficult to come by. Although it is available on the NHS not all areas offer it, as sterilisation tends to be organised on a regional basis. Different regions place different priorities on it, so waiting times can range from a couple of months to well over a year. (Getting a vasectomy is likely to be a little quicker.) If you are able and prepared to pay, you could contact non-profit making clinics, such as the two charities, the British Pregnancy Advisory Service and the Pregnancy Advisory Service: see Useful Contacts. Alternatively, you could have the operation carried out privately.

4 About one in every 100 women who is sterilised regrets her decision later, most commonly because of a later wish to have another child.

5 There is a higher risk of an ectopic pregnancy where sterilisation does fail (failures may most often occur if cut tubes join up again of their own accord, if clips or rings aren't positioned properly or because of other surgeon error). The risk of ectopic pregnancy is also slightly higher when sterilisation is successfully reversed, because of the considerable scarring of the fallopian tubes which may stop an egg getting through.

• Emergency contraception •

Emergency contraception is short-term contraception used after the event: that is, after unprotected sex. It is therefore also known as post-coital contraception. There are two methods: a special dose of the combined contraceptive pill or the fitting of an IUD. The aim is to prevent any embryo that might have been fertilised from being able to implant itself in the womb. Neither method is 100 per cent effective but the IUD is significantly more so, with less than one in every 100 women users of it as an emergency contraception becoming pregnant, compared with up to seven in every 100 women taking the emergency dose of the pill.

Alarmingly, a lot of women don't know emergency contraception exists or how they would go about getting it. According to a 1990 National Opinion Poll survey of over 1000 women, nearly half had never heard of it or didn't know how to get it, and only 10 per cent who had heard of the emergency pill didn't know it could be taken up to 72 hours after unprotected sex, probably largely because of the inaccurate colloquial name of 'morning-after pill' which is often used to describe it.

• How do you use it? •

First you must see a doctor, explain the circumstances and take his or her advice on whether you need emergency contraception and which should be prescribed for you. You may choose to see your GP or a family planning doctor, if this is practical within the timescale. But some women may be embarrassed to see a doctor they know to ask for emergency contraception and may prefer the option of going to a genito-urinary clinic, if possible. There are genito-urinary clinics in most large hospitals and many offer contraceptive advice. Some may be open in late evenings or on Saturday mornings but, if not, there should be a genito-urinary specialist on call.

The pill is taken in two doses of two pills. These are special formulations and are not the same as the ordinary combined pill, so there is no point in doubling up on your own or borrowing someone else's if you usually take the progestogen-only pill. The first dose must be taken within 72 hours of having unprotected sex and the second exactly 12 hours afterwards, whatever inconvenient hour of day or night it might be. Make sure you don't take either dose on an empty stomach, as this increases the risk of being sick.

The IUD must be inserted within five days of unprotected sex, but you need to have seen the doctor first and then make an emergency appointment for the IUD fitting. If you wish, the IUD can remain in place and become your regular form of contraception. Alternatively, if you are bothered about the complications that often come with the IUD or just don't get on with it, you can have it removed at the start of your next period.

• For whom may it be unsuitable? •

Because the special dose pill is – and the IUD can be – of short term effect, there are relatively few conditions that preclude their use. There is really nothing that would prevent use of the emergency IUD as it can be removed so quickly. The emergency pill cannot be used where there is a history of thromboembolism (blood clot in a vein) or a history of focal migraine. However, it can be used by women who would not normally be prescribed the combined pill, such as those who smoke heavily, are overweight, have diabetic complications or high blood pressure.

• After effects •

After taking the emergency pill, you may feel some nausea or actually be sick, particularly after the second dose and particularly if you haven't eaten any food recently. If this happens within three hours of taking the pill, you need to contact your doctor because you may need to take a replacement dose. Some doctors may prescribe an anti-sickness pill to prevent the pills being lost this way.

After the fitting of an IUD, you may experience cramps or pain for a day or two and some spotting of blood. Your next period may be heavier than usual.

The most hoped for after-effect, of course, is that you will not find yourself pregnant. However, if you opt for the pill method but it doesn't work and you become pregnant, there is no evidence that the baby will be adversely affected if you continue the pregnancy. A register kept by the National Association of Family Planning Doctors of pregnancies continued to term following failed emergency contraception has so far not recorded any abnormalities.

The risks of pregnancy with the emergency IUD are as per those described for the IUD on page 409. Women need to understand clearly, however, that in all pregnancies overall there is a 2 per cent risk of major congenital abnormality.

• Future methods of contraception •

We certainly don't yet have the perfect form of contraception, so no doubt research into new methods will go on until we do. Current research is directed towards:

• The development of a contraceptive vaccine which would make the body treat sperm or egg as foreign material and destroy it.

- Reversible sterilisation for either or both women and men.
- A hormonal contraceptive patch.
- A male pill.
- New versions of existing methods, such as new formulations of pills containing smaller and smaller amounts of hormones and differently styled female condoms.

As the Family Planning Association says, however, a successful advance in contraception is not just something that prevents pregnancy efficiently. It has to be a method that women (or men) find comfortable to use, fits in with their lifestyle and that they can trust.

WHEN TO THINK AGAIN

One type of contraception may suit you for a while but changing circumstances in your life may mean it is time for a reassessment. It is good to think again about your chosen method if:

1 Your sexual lifestyle changes. If an old relationship breaks up and you start having sex with one or more new partners, you may find a form of contraception which is protective against sexually transmitted diseases is particularly suitable for a while. If, on the other hand, you are newly settling down for monogamy with one partner, you may wish to consider other forms of contraception which provide good protection against pregnancy but not against infections.

2 You want to get pregnant. You will not want a method which compromises your fertility for some time, such as injectable contraception. Periods may not return quickly after stopping the combined oral contraceptive pill if you had irregular cycles before you went on the pill in the first place.

3 You want to breast feed. The combined contraceptive pill would not suit you. However, progestogen-only pills can be taken.

4 You develop a medical condition. Certain forms of contraception are not advisable for sufferers from certain illnesses or conditions. Look at the 'unsuitable' section for each form of contraception described here.

5 You start experiencing problems or dissatisfaction with your present method. Obviously this is the time to consider whether something else would suit you better.

6 A new method becomes available. Be open to thinking about trying something new that might suit you better, even if you are not dissatisfied with your present method. There may be advantages you haven't considered.

7 You are no longer as fertile as you were. A woman in her forties is a lot less fertile than a woman in her twenties and may feel this is the time when a less reliable but more comfortable method would be safe to try.

8 You don't want any more children. You may decide to consider sterilisation if the idea of never having to think about contraception again appeals to you.

45

WANTED AND UNWANTED PREGNANCY

IF YOU have been using contraception carefully, or your method is one that has taken all the care for you, you will have to make a conscious decision about when to stop and try for a baby, if you want one. This can be extremely hard because the time is probably never perfect. You may be trying to make headway in your career or be consolidating your position. You may have taken on large financial commitments and worry about how you will manage with a loss of earnings, however temporary.

Then there are the huge emotional questions. Although most women think they want a child at some time in their life, there are probably few who do not fear how starting a family will affect their sense of self, their lives, their relationships and their careers. Having a child is an enormous responsibility. In the end, whenever you do decide the time is right or that time is ticking too relentlessly onward to leave it any longer, you have to be prepared to handle whatever happens and accept that you can never really plan fully for how you'll feel and cope.

• Biological facts •

A woman's chances of conceiving become significantly lower as she ages, although, from today's marked increase in older mothers, it is clear that lots of women in their late thirties and early forties do not have too much difficulty doing it. A survey by the Central Statistical Office showed that five in every 1000 40-year-old women had a baby in 1991. Between 1980 and 1991 the birth rate rose by a quarter in 30 to 34-year-old women, but by a half in 35 to 39-year-old women.

Biologically, however, it is easiest to conceive before the age of 25. After the age of 31, fertility is on a definite downward slope and by 40 about half a woman's menstrual cycles are likely to be anovulatory (that is, ovulation does not occur).

Even if a woman who is older does conceive she may sometimes have more difficulty holding on to the pregnancy because she is more prone to conditions such as fibroids in the uterus which may prevent an embryo implanting, and because she has a higher risk of miscarriage (twice as high in women over 34 as in women under 30). Much of this increased risk may be due to the greater likelihood of genetic defects in the foetus.

If an older woman's partner is not young either, his fertility will be declining as well, and his sperm will be more defective.

• Getting ready for pregnancy •

Rubella Your first step may not necessarily be to stop contraception. If, for example, you are not in a rush, you may choose first to have your immunity against rubella checked by going to your GP for a simple blood test. In the event that you are not protected, you can have the rubella vaccination but you then have to use contraception for three months while the vaccine is still circulating in your body. After that it is safe to try and conceive.

Stopping the pill If you are on the contraceptive pill, it is a good idea to stop taking it a few months before planning to try for pregnancy and to use a barrier form of contraception instead. The pill depletes your vitamin and mineral stores, so it may be helpful to have a few months when you can make a point of eating well and getting yourself more back to normal.

Some women find their periods don't return for a few months after stopping the pill, which is another good reason for coming off a while before you would like to conceive. The pill doesn't lower your fertility, however. If your periods don't return for over a year, it is likely that you have an underlying fertility problem which use of the pill simply masked. Alternatively, some women find the pill heightens their fertility and they conceive instantly if not using back-up contraception.

Getting in the best of health Before getting pregnant is the time to try to stop smoking, if you are a smoker, and to lose or gain weight as necessary. If you are overweight when you conceive, you are more likely to have problems during pregnancy. If you are underweight, you are more likely to have an underweight baby.

Many authorities recommend giving up drinking before trying to conceive. One study showed an increase in risks to the foetus when women had been drinking alcohol around ovulation. However, if giving up entirely seems excessively cautious, you might try restricting alcohol in the mid to latter part of each cycle before you conceive.

As folic acid supplements are now recommended from the beginning of pregnancy to reduce risk of having a baby with spina bifida, you might wish to start taking them when you first plan to try for pregnancy. Ask your doctor for advice.

• Making love •

It is best to try to be as relaxed as possible about trying to have a baby. Stress is one of the biggest inhibitors of fertility and trying to plan for sex at the exact moment when you think you are most fertile can be stressful in the extreme. It would be unnatural, of course, if you are actively wanting a baby, not to try to have sex around the right sort of time but you don't have to get any more technical than that.

The fertile period   You are in your fertile period for up to a week before ovulation and until a day afterwards, as sperm can live inside you for up to seven days and an egg lives for 24 hours after ovulation. The more often you make love in this period, the better your chances. It is not true that sperm is weakened if you have sex too often.

If you have regular menstrual cycles or if you have ovulation pain, you will have a clearer idea of when you may be ovulating than if you have irregular cycles. However, as sperm can live for so long, making love several times in a month is likely to lead to pregnancy within a few months, if you are both fertile. Nationally, it takes on average four months to conceive or, put another way, you have a 25 per cent chance of success in any one month.

Pinpointing ovulation   Some women may choose to take their temperature or check their cervical mucus in order to pinpoint their fertile period more accurately. Some may even wish to take instruction in natural family planning by these means (see Natural Birth Control, page 389). However, these methods are not foolproof, and if they add stress, they are not really desirable. You have to remember that planning a pregnancy has to fit in with life's normal demands. You may have a busy job, other children to look after, a partner with an equally hectic lifestyle. The last thing you both want to feel is a dreadful pressure to have sex at all the right biological but wrong psychological moments. Try to keep it light if you can.

Boy or girl   You might be keen to pinpoint ovulation, however, if you are hoping for a child of a particular sex. It is a fact that 'female' sperm swim more slowly and stay alive longer than 'male' sperm, so you would need to have sex at the beginning of your fertile period and then not again till after ovulation if you want to increase your chances of having a girl. But you are only increasing chances, not creating a certainty. And the fewer times you make love, the less your chance of conceiving.

Ovulation kits   If you are having difficulty conceiving or you are just desperate to speed things up if possible, you may be tempted to buy one of the ovulation kits available from a pharmacy. These rather expensive kits detect the surge of a hormone known as LH which is the message to the ovary to ovulate. The LH surge tends to happen within 36 hours of ovulation. You have to keep testing, so that you don't miss it, and sometimes even if the surge does occur ovulation doesn't follow if the ovary doesn't act on the message for some reason. So using these kits might not always have the desired effect.

Getting help   If you have been trying unsuccessfully for a year to become pregnant, this is when to ask your doctor to refer you for fertility investigations if you wish to have them. But you are likely to have to wait, unless you go privately.

• Pregnancy tests •

If you do think you have become pregnant, you can find out as early as the day of your missed period, if you are normally regular. You might prefer to wait a little longer, however, to be on the safe side. Pharmacies sell a number of pregnancy tests. Ask for advice on which are the simplest to use and clearest to read. If you prefer, you can pay for the pharmacy to do a test for you. Find out whether you need to supply early-morning urine or whether a sample taken from any time of day will suffice.

Knowing so early that you are pregnant is not always all good. In the past, women often thought their period was just delayed if it came late one month, whereas in fact they might have conceived but the pregnancy didn't 'take'. Nowadays there is more likely the joy of discovering you are pregnant via an early pregnancy test only for this to be followed by enormous disappointment if a period follows a week or so later.

If, as is to be hoped, you find yourself with a wanted pregnancy, there are a number of good pregnancy books to choose from. Take your pick from a browse through a good-sized bookshop.

• Unplanned pregnancy •

If you find you are accidentally pregnant you have some hard and almost certainly painful decisions ahead of you. You may decide to have your baby and bring him or her up yourself. You may plan to have your baby and then offer him or her for adoption. Or you may decide to terminate the pregnancy by having an abortion.

Unplanned pregnancy is inevitably a shock. You will not have been thinking about making space in your life for a baby. You will not have been thinking through all that this means in terms of changing the way you live your own life. You may not be in a stable relationship or your relationship may be going through a rocky patch. You may feel sure your career will suffer if you have a child now. On the other hand, creating a life is an incredible and awesome achievement and you may feel you want to put your mind to how you could best cope.

It is impossible to think through all of these issues coherently on your own so, if you discover you are accidentally pregnant, it is important to share your thoughts and feelings, rational or not, with someone you can trust. If you have a friend who will listen and support you for as long as you need, make full use of her willing help. If you don't have anyone you feel close enough to, you could try to find a counsellor who can listen to you. There may be someone who does sessions at your GP surgery. Or you may prefer to contact your nearest branch of one of the big pregnancy counselling charities (see Useful Contacts) and arrange to talk to someone there who is especially expert in helping women face this situation.

If you decide to have and keep your baby, clearly you will need to see your doctor and arrange to receive antenatal care. If you want to offer your baby for adoption, this can be set in motion for you by your GP or the hospital social worker or health visitor. You can also contact any local or national adoption agencies directly yourself: see Useful Contacts.

If you want to consider abortion, see below.

• Abortion •

Abortion is a surgical or medical procedure, known by doctors less emotively as termination of pregnancy. It is, however, a huge and deep emotional issue. Women's feelings about ending the life of an unborn child are informed by their culture, their religion, their upbringing, their peers and their personal values.

Many unplanned pregnancies occur because of contraceptive failures, some because of rape, some because of taking a risk and willing it to be all right. Even if you were taking a risk and might have expected it to happen, much of that 'knowledge' may be unconscious or pushed below consciousness, so that unplanned pregnancy always comes as a shock. Having to face its consequences inevitably brings up a whole host of conflicting feelings, even if you are almost 100 per cent certain early on that abortion is the right solution for you.

Many women may have abortions not because of unplanned pregnancy but because of an abnormality detected in a foetus in a much wanted pregnancy. Going for a termination in these circumstances, at what is often a relatively late stage (16 to 20 weeks), is enormously hard emotionally. Even if a foetus is found to be grossly handicapped and even if you have always been adamant that you would opt for abortion in such circumstances, there are likely to be very strong, conflicting emotions, as well as grief and probably feelings of guilt.

Counsellors experienced in working with women seeking abortions or who have had abortions are firm in pointing out that it is important to allow yourself to have those conflicting feelings. Your decision to go for an abortion is not invalid if you allow yourself to acknowledge doubts and even regrets.

The slogan of the pro-choice movement, which has always rallied to fight attempts to tighten the abortion laws, is 'a woman's right to choose'. But having choice was never meant to deny that choice is painful. One of the problems of having a service where abortion is not on demand is that women may feel obliged to make a strong unequivocal case for why they need and want an abortion, fearing otherwise they will be turned down. This doesn't allow them to explore what they are fully feeling.

Not allowing yourself your real feelings about the dilemma of an unplanned pregnancy means not allowing yourself time to grieve and then time to heal. Many women who have had to deny their feelings, or felt they had to because of fears of disapproval from family or society, have found that the suppressed pain and grief arising from abortion did in the end surface, even as long as 20 years afterwards. In some cases, unexpressed grief or guilt about an earlier abortion has prevented women from becoming pregnant later when they did want to, and only when those feelings were brought to the surface through hypnotherapy, psychotherapy or counselling did they then go on to conceive.

There is more about handling emotional after-effects of abortion at the end of this section.

• Who can have an abortion? •

In Britain at present a woman may be allowed to have an abortion if two doctors agree that continuing the pregnancy would put her life or her physical or mental health at risk, or would put at risk the physical or mental health of any children already in her family. It is also allowed if there is a substantial risk that the baby would be born with severe physical or mental handicaps.

An abortion has to be carried out before the foetus is 24 weeks (calculating this date by starting from the day of the woman's last period) as this is when a foetus is now viewed as 'viable': able to survive outside the womb, albeit in intensive care. If the mother's life is at risk or the foetus is discovered late to be grossly handicapped, an abortion may, if necessary, be carried out later.

However, very many NHS hospitals refuse to carry out abortions after 12 weeks of pregnancy, except where a foetus is found in antenatal testing to be abnormal. Even in private clinics 20 weeks is the effective cut-off date, as doctors are concerned to cover themselves in case a woman has inadvertently got her dates wrong (making it possible she could be more than 24 weeks pregnant at the time of termination if they operated right up to the limit).

Notwithstanding, in practice very few abortions ever need to be carried out anywhere near the upper limit allowed by the law. A third of all legal terminations in Britain (nearly 200,000 every year) are carried out before nine weeks' gestation.

• Organising an abortion •

It is possible to have an abortion on the NHS. However about half of all women who have one each year go privately because of greater choice, a wish for secrecy or because of unsympathetic attitudes and unwillingness, or inability on the part of some NHS professionals, to act quickly enough. However, an NHS abortion should be offered routinely and quickly after the discovery of abnormality in a foetus.

Seeing your GP If you are comfortable with your own GP, you should go to him or her as soon as possible. Your GP may be the person with whom you are happiest pouring out your feelings and discussing options. Even if not, they should know where to refer you – a hospital where, it is to be hoped, staff are reasonably sympathetic – and should make the appointment for you.

Don't leave it longer than a week to receive an appointment from the hospital. You should receive a card with a date and time. Ring your doctor or hospital to try to hurry things up. If this isn't possible, because of pressure of patients to see or pure professional intransigence, and you feel too much time is passing, you may need to consider a private abortion. You will need to think private if you are turned down for an NHS abortion, of course. Or you may prefer the private route from the start.

Genito-urinary clinics   Some of these clinics offer abortion counselling and arrange NHS abortions. Ring the genito-urinary department of your nearest large hospital to enquire. You do not need referral by a GP.

Pregnancy advisory services   The two big pregnancy advisory services which are charities, the British Pregnancy Advisory Service (BPAS) and the Pregnancy Advisory Service (PAS), can be contacted directly, although they prefer your GP to make the referral or be aware of what you are doing but they would not press you. They make a charge but cost much less than going completely privately.

The charity Women's Health (see Useful Contacts) may also be able to provide details of any other services available to you locally.

Private clinics   If you go to a private clinic that is not a run by a charity, make sure that it is licensed and what for. Not all licences cover day abortions, for example, and very few are licensed to carry out abortions over 20 weeks.

Pre-abortion counselling   Hospitals and private clinics may employ counsellors. However, much of pre-abortion counselling may concentrate on medical aspects of the abortion rather than on exploring any feelings you have, and may last for only 15 minutes. BPAS and PAS, however, have good counselling services.

You may decide after counselling, or even without counselling, that you want to change your mind about going ahead with an abortion. This is your right, of course, right up till the operation itself. However inconvenient others may claim it is for them or however inconsistent and indecisive you fear you may appear, you need to do whatever is right for you.

Getting informed   If you do go ahead, it can be very helpful to find out all you can about the procedure itself, how it all happens and what things will feel like. Research has shown that the more you know, the less fearful you are and the quicker you heal.

Negative feelings   Accept at this stage, if you can, that you may feel weepy, angry, sad, depressed or guilty, etc, for a while after the abortion. This way you are giving yourself permission to have these feelings if they come up instead of unconsciously trying to suppress them. You may hope you will feel relief after the operation and certainly it is likely to be a relief that the whole agony of decision is over, but you may also feel other more negative feelings that could shock you if you are not prepared for them.

Unfortunately, many women feel that, by choosing abortion, they have forfeited the right to have regretful or sad feelings or to express any good feelings they might have had when they first discovered they were pregnant.

Feelings such as, 'I did feel good to be pregnant when I first knew; I felt so important and powerful; I was grateful to know I was fertile even though I was horrified to be pregnant', etc, are perfectly valid.

• Methods of abortion •

There are a number of methods of carrying out abortion. Prior to 12 weeks, abortions can be carried out by the surgical methods of vacuum aspiration or by dilatation and curettage (D&C). Prior to nine weeks, a medical method involving anti-progestogens can also be used. After 12 weeks, dilatation and evacuation (D&E) may be the method used. More commonly, labour may be induced by prostaglandins given by injection. These methods are described more fully below. A last resort in late abortions is hysterotomy, where the foetus is removed via an incision made in the abdomen.

• Vacuum aspiration •

This is the method used for 99 per cent of early abortions, that is, prior to 12 weeks. It is usually carried out under a light general anaesthetic although you can ask for a local if you like (but not all surgeons may be willing to provide one). A pessary may be inserted into the vagina to soften the cervix so that it is easier to pass a tube through it and a local anaesthetic, if you opt for this, is injected into the cervix.

When the local or general anaesthetic has taken effect, the cervical opening is gently dilated and a thin plastic tube is passed through into the womb. The contents are then sucked into the tube by an electric pump attached to the tube. The abortion is completed in a few minutes.

Afterwards, you are likely to feel cramps as the uterus contracts down to its original size. You may also feel a bit tearful if you have had the abortion under general anaesthetic.

You will be able to go home a few hours later if you have had a local anaesthetic. You can also go home the same day if you have had a general one as long as you have someone to collect you and be at home with you. Some hospitals or clinics may want you to stay overnight.

Some bleeding is likely to occur for about ten days after the operation and you should use sanitary pads, not tampons, during this time. You should also avoid sex until you are certain all bleeding has stopped, so as not to increase risk of infection.

• Dilatation and curettage (D&C)•

This method has been almost entirely superseded by vacuum aspiration for abortions performed prior to 12 weeks. It is usually carried out under general anaesthetic. The cervix is dilated and the contents of the womb are scooped out with a spoon-shaped curette. (See page 219.)

• The 'abortion pill' •

This is a medical as opposed to surgical method of abortion which can be used up till the end of the ninth week of pregnancy (a maximum of 63 days after the first day of your last period). However, for health reasons, it is not a method that is suitable for all women, so you will need to give a full medical history before you may be prescribed it.

You are given three small 200mg tablets of an anti-progestogen called mifepristone to take at one go, in the presence of the hospital or clinic doctor. You need to stay at the hospital or clinic for a couple of hours in case the drug makes you sick, in which case it won't, of course, work. After that you make an appointment to return in two days and then you can go home.

In the next 48 hours the drug works to soften the cervix and act against the hormone progesterone which is needed to help build up the lining of the womb to support the pregnancy. You may experience some bleeding or cramps but are unlikely to suffer a miscarriage at this stage and you can carry on your normal daily routines. If you do have very heavy bleeding, however, you should get in touch with the hospital or clinic at once.

When you go back, a prostaglandin pessary is inserted into the vagina with the aim of inducing contractions and miscarriage within six hours. You stay at the hospital or clinic and will be given something for pain if you want it. If no miscarriage occurs or it is not complete, you will need to have a D&C at this point.

You can go home the same day (unless you needed a D&C) and will experience some bleeding for up to a fortnight, during which time you should use sanitary pads and avoid sex. You should be given an appointment to come back a week later for doctors to check that the method has worked. The abortion pill has a 95 per cent success rate.

This method, although there is no surgery involved, can only at present be given at hospitals or licensed abortion clinics. Even there it is not used as widely as it could be. Eventually it may become possible for GPs to prescribe it but there will have to be a change in the law first.

Some researchers have found that one 200mg dose of mifepristone is as effective as 600mg, at least in pregnancies of up to 56 days, but the larger dose is the only one approved by the regulating authorities in countries that use the method because it minimises the risk of on-going pregnancy in any women who inadvisedly fail to return for the prostaglandin pessary.

A study of the acceptability of both vacuum aspiration and medical abortion by pill carried out in Aberdeen found that 26 per cent of women had a definite preference for the idea of vacuum aspiration and 20 per cent preferred the pill. Those who preferred vacuum aspiration most commonly gave as reasons the desire to be unconscious and the fact that the pill method dragged the whole business out too long.

Those who preferred to take the pill most commonly expressed a fear of anaesthetic or surgery or felt the pill method was more natural. Of women allocated to either method at random and asked their opinion afterward, none who had been less than 50 days pregnant expressed a preference about which method they would want if they ever had to have an abortion in the future. But of those who were between 50 and 63 days pregnant, most found the idea of vacuum aspiration more acceptable. The pill method is more painful the more pregnant you are but this was not, it appeared, a major factor in why they came to this view.

• Dilatation and evacuation (D&E) •

This is a method which may be used for pregnancies beyond 12 weeks and is carried out under general anaesthetic. Larger instruments are needed to remove the contents of the womb the longer the pregnancy has gone on, which in turn means that the cervix needs to be dilated further for these to be passed through.

Prostaglandin gel may be used to soften the cervix (this may take a couple of days in pregnancies of more than 20 weeks) and then dilators are used to widen the opening of the cervix. The instruments required are a forceps and a curette and vacuum suction is used to withdraw the loosened contents of the womb. The procedure may take as little as ten minutes or over half an hour.

Afterwards you may need to stay in hospital for a day. You should avoid using tampons or having sex while the bleeding lasts. Although risks of complications are fewer than with the method described below, you should be alert to signs of infection such as fever, foul-smelling vaginal discharge, vomiting and excessive bleeding.

In clinics licensed to carry out abortions, over half of all 16-week abortions are carried out by D&E. However, there are far fewer doctors able or willing to use this method after 16 weeks, as it requires a lot of skill and is difficult psychologically for many doctors to handle. The method is only used in a small minority of NHS hospitals at any stage.

• Induction •

This is the method most commonly used for 12 to 20-week abortions. Prostaglandins or prostaglandin combinations are injected into the amniotic sac via the abdomen or given as an intravenous drip via a vein. Sometimes prostaglandin pessaries are used but these are often less successful. A woman may feel nausea and have some diarrhoea at this stage.

After a number of hours contractions should start. (If not they may be encouraged by an injection of a drug called syntocinon.) As in a full-term labour, the contractions may start out as mildly painful and then become increasingly severe. You can have pain relief if you want it. However, the contractions do not reach the full severity of those experienced in full-term labour.

After the foetus comes out, the placenta should follow. You may be given a D&C afterwards to ensure the abortion was complete and you will need to stay in hospital for a day or so. While the bleeding lasts you should use a sanitary pad not a tampon and avoid sex. Risks of infection are greater than in earlier abortions, so you should be alert to any signs such as fever, being sick, unpleasant vaginal discharge and excessive bleeding.

No abortion is easy emotionally but induction is particularly hard as you are required physically to go through labour, the process more usually associated with a live birth. There are likely to be many hours of waiting for contractions to start and then there may be several hours of labour.

You may feel particularly upset the later the abortion is taking place, as you may have felt the foetus move and have started to think of him/her as a living being. Afterwards, although you may still feel relief that an unwanted pregnancy is over, it may be harder to come to terms with how it happened. It may be particularly important to seek some kind of counselling help.

• Risks of abortion •

Failure   This is the biggest risk with the abortion pill: it may not work.

Anaesthetic   With the surgical methods, as with any surgery, there are always slight risks of complications and slight risks associated with general anaesthetic.

Infections   One worry with surgical methods is that if you have a symptomless, sexually transmitted infection such as chlamydia or gonorrhoea, the organisms may be helped during the operation to ascend to the higher reproductive organs, where they can do damage and even cause infertility. If you have time on your side and if there is a possibility that you could be harbouring such an infection from a previous or current relationship (that is, if you have had a number of partners or your partner has or has had a number of partners), it might be worth going to a genito-urinary clinic for a check and getting treated first, if your tests are positive.

Future fertility   The biggest worry for many women after abortion is that it could compromise future fertility itself. Two recent large studies which compared women who had abortions and women who went ahead with a pregnancy have found no reduction in fertility in women who have had an abortion and no significant difference in time taken to become pregnant again, when desired.

• Contraception •

It is important that you organise contraception for yourself as soon as possible after an abortion. (See pages 388–419.) You shouldn't, however, agree to sterilisation or the insertion of an IUD at the time of the abortion, even if this is suggested by a doctor. If the IUD is to be your choice, you need to leave time to be sure your body has recovered from the abortion first and that you are infection-free. Sterilisation always needs to be thought about carefully and unless there are very good reasons for opting for it at this time, the upheaval of emotions associated with abortion is unlikely to leave you in the most rational frame of mind to make this most important decision.

• Emotional after effects •

The effect of an abortion is not necessarily over once the operation has been carried out. It carries emotional connotations to do with life and death, with fertility and womanhood, sexuality and identity. For some women, unconscious conflicts in these or other areas may have led to pregnancy in the first place. For others, they can cause conscious or unconscious conflict afterwards. Abortion can have a decisive impact on relationships with partners, with parents and on a woman's whole direction in life.

It is common for women to have a range of reactions to the experience of abortion, some that are experienced immediately, and/or some that may not manifest themselves until years later. It is also not unusual for a woman to adjust, absorb and make sense quickly of what has happened to her and carry straight on with her life. Some women are even able to draw something clear and positive from their experience, however difficult at the time, to carry into their futures. Having an abortion may have been the first decision they have ever made and carried out alone or they may feel powerful to know they are fertile.

As suggested several times so far, it is harder to come to terms and heal if feelings are suppressed, consciously or otherwise. Anxieties or negative feelings that remain locked inside can easily get out of proportion. Not every woman experiences strong and difficult feelings that she needs to express but some are taken unawares by the power of their emotions. If an unresolved and often unrecognised conflict led to the pregnancy in the first place, this is likely to seethe on under the surface at a time when a woman is more emotionally vulnerable than usual.

In some areas of the UK post-abortion groups are run by women who have had abortions, or by therapists (the charity Women's Health should have details: see Useful Contacts.)

Therapy groups may place some emphasis on not only expressing feelings about and describing the experience of abortion but looking at any unconscious issues that may have led to pregnancy and abortion. This is not to induce guilt but to enhance understanding, because sometimes pregnancy and abortion are an indirect way of dealing with conflicting emotional needs (for example, the need to be free and the need to nurture, a desire for and fear of sexuality, a wish to go out into the world of work after bringing up children coupled with the fear of failing). However, there are not necessarily any unconscious issues which need dredging to the surface. A woman's need may simply be to have her feelings, to grieve, to accept and then to move on.

46

INFERTILITY

INFERTILITY affects between one in six and one in ten couples. For those desperate to have a child or those who just naturally expected to be able to conceive when they wanted to, the realisation that it is not going to be easy and perhaps not possible at all is shattering. For most, the enormous emotional investment involved in going through infertility investigations and treatments plus the psychological impact of months or years of anxiety coupled with fervent hope cannot be underestimated.

• How do I know if I have a problem? •

On average, younger couples take about four months to conceive if they are having sex without contraception. If you have been trying to conceive for between a year and 18 months without success, you might want to seek some advice about whether you might have a problem, particularly if you are in your thirties when your fertility is naturally declining.

You might have a problem if your periods are infrequent and certainly if they don't occur at all. If you experience pain after sex, one explanation might be a gynaecological condition which could compromise your fertility (for example, pelvic infection or endometriosis).

You may be surprised to have difficulty conceiving if you already have a child. However, secondary infertility is not uncommon and may be caused by infections, sometimes suffered unwittingly within weeks of a previous delivery when your reproductive organs were most vulnerable, or some hormone imbalance which has developed since your last pregnancy.

Of course, you might not have a problem at all. On average just under 40 per cent of infertility is caused by problems in the male, just over 40 per cent by problems in the female and the rest a mixture of the two.

• Most common causes of infertility in women •

Failure to ovulate This accounts for about a third of all cases of infertility and has the highest treatment success rate (over 90 per cent). It can be caused by hormonal or chemical problems that prevent an egg from developing; a malfunction in the hypothalamus, which controls the pituitary gland, or in the pituitary gland itself, which triggers the production of hormones to start the menstrual cycle; failure of the egg follicle to release the matured egg; cysts on the ovary (polycystic ovarian syndrome); the ovaries failing prematurely (sometimes this spontaneously reverses); damage to the ovaries; or a very very severe shock.

Damaged fallopian tubes This accounts for about a third of female infertility. It can be caused by pelvic inflammatory disease where an untreated infection has scarred (and therefore narrowed) or blocked one but usually both tubes. Many kinds of infection can be responsible, not just the sexually transmitted ones chlamydia and gonorrhoea. Infections from the abdomen, after appendicitis for example, can also spread to the fallopian tubes. Other causes of tubal damage are previous ectopic pregnancy, endometriosis (scarring the tubes and causing adhesions, in which pelvic organs stick together and the fallopian tubes are less able to function) and abnormalities or absence of one or both tubes.

Problems with the uterus This is the reason for infertility in less than 10 per cent of women. Causes may be large fibroids or polyps, congenital abnormalities of the uterus, adhesions in the uterus sticking its walls together, and inflammation caused by infection (not sexual). In these cases the problem is usually not a failure to conceive but a failure of the embryo to implant or stay implanted, causing early miscarriages. Another problem may be a dilated cervix, preventing a pregnancy from continuing. (The usual solution is to put in a stitch early in pregnancy to keep it closed.)

Problems with cervical mucus This is probably the reason for infertility in about 5 per cent of women and may be caused by insufficient cervical mucus or too thick mucus being produced, both of which will impede normal sperm movement. There is also a problem if the cervix is producing antibodies against the sperm.

Psychological causes This is a contentious area and there will be doctors who dismiss the idea and others who are sympathetic to it. Severe stress, including the stress of going through infertility investigations, may well exacerbate the problems of getting pregnant and so may unresolved feelings about wanting a child, fears about being a mother or other unexpressed feelings such as grief or guilt about an earlier abortion.

Most common causes of infertility in men

Few or poor sperm This accounts for 90 per cent of male infertility and the reasons for it can be hormonal, variocele (enlarged veins around the testicles, which may over-heat the testes lying inside them), undiagnosed infection, abnormal sperm (plenty of them and maybe moving all right, but incapable of fertilising an egg for other reasons) and environmental: stress, illness, overweight, poor diet, too heavy drinking, smoking, marijuana and the use of certain drugs, such as to treat depression and high blood pressure.

Immunological problems Up to 5 per cent of male infertility may be caused by the man producing antibodies against his own sperm, preventing them from being released.

No sperm in semen This may be caused by blocked tubes, problems with the muscles that propel semen along the penis or failure of the testes to produce sperm at all, due to injury, severe mumps infection, hormonal problems or twisting of the testes.

Sexual problems Impotence and premature ejaculation may occasionally bring couples to infertility clinics but more usually treatment is sought for these problems elsewhere.

Anatomical problems These are rare but may include the tube carrying sperm stopping short, preventing sperm from being ejaculated into the vagina, the absence of the tubes (vas deferens) that carry sperm from the testes, or improperly developed testes.

• Initial tests for infertility •

If you suspect you may have a problem, your GP can carry out initial checks from a blood test to see if you are ovulating, and, if not, to find out why. Some of the causes for failure to ovulate, including the most common – polycystic ovarian disease – can often be treated at the GP surgery too, without need for referral to a specialist centre.

The initial test for male infertility is the sperm count. This ought to happen at roughly the same time and certainly before a woman is referred for further investigation. However, this is not necessarily what happens. Whereas women are likely to be more used to consulting a doctor about gynaecological problems and may have had symptoms anyway which alerted them to something being awry, most men have no inkling that their infertility could be compromised.

Many are horrified by the thought and may even refuse to contemplate the possibility at the outset. It may therefore often be left the woman to go through the battery of testing first, possibly being subjected to unnecessary invasive procedures, with the man only reluctantly coming into the frame once a blank is drawn.

The second problem with the sperm count is that it is not a sophisticated test. It may show that there are the right sort of number of sperm but not whether they are capable of fertilising an egg, so a man may be given the all clear when in fact he does indeed have a problem. According to the specialised male testing service (the Diagnostic Andrology Service, DAS) at the Hallam Medical Centre in London, a quarter of women who go through the tests may end up with a diagnosis of unexplained infertility, and at least a fifth of these cases may be attributed to a previously undetected sperm defect.

Conversely, many men may be devastated to be told they are infertile because of one bad sperm count, when many life events can temporarily lower sperm count, or because they produce few sperm when in fact those sperm are good quality and likely to lead to a pregnancy with perseverance or with help.

• Where to go next •

Your GP can refer you to a hospital for further tests as necessary. Unfortunately, many regional health authorities will pay only for very basic testing and not for treatment.

Your doctor should be able to advise you; or you can obtain a list of all approved infertility clinics, NHS and private, and the services they provide from the Human Fertilisation and Embryology Authority (see Useful Contacts) which gives the licences. This organisation also publishes information leaflets, including one on questions to ask about the clinic. You can also find out about local NHS services and waiting lists from the Health Information Service: see Useful Contacts.

• Further investigations for women •

The following is the range of tests which may be on offer, depending upon where you go.

Hormone tests   These may have been done by your GP already to see if you are ovulating.

Endometrial biopsy   This is another check for ovulation and entails the removal of a tiny piece of the endometrium (womb lining) a few days before your period. This is a very quick test and is done as an out-patient.

Ultrasound   This can be used also to check for ovulation and for uterine problems but is not widely available, requires great skill and sometimes cannot yield a definite answer.

Post-coital test   A common check to see if there are problems with cervical mucus. You attend the clinic a few hours after sex and mucus from the vagina and cervix is collected for examination. There are no problems with cervical mucus if sperm are seen swimming healthily, at the right sort of speed and in the right general direction.

Laparoscopy   An investigative procedure with a laparoscope (see page 218). During a laparoscopy dye may be flushed through the cervix to see if it 'spills' through the fallopian tubes, indicating they are clear.

Hysteroscopy   An investigative procedure with a hysteroscope (see page 219). May be done under general or local anaesthetic.

HSG   This is short for hysterosalpingogram and is an X-ray of the uterus and fallopian tubes. Special dye injected into the vagina passes up into the uterus and tubes and is visible on the X-ray. If there is any blockage, the dye will not get through. Experts say the procedure, which works best if carried out without anaesthetic, should be painless if the dye is injected very slowly. However there is likely to be some discomfort even with the most sensitive operator and many women may find the procedure painful.

• Further investigations for men •

Sperm tests Sophisticated sperm tests beyond the sperm count are not generally available, unfortunately, but they can be arranged for privately through the Diagnostic Andrology Service (see Useful Contacts) which carries out testing for a number of hospitals. Self-referrals are allowed for diagnosis but GP referral is necessary for treatment.

Initial assessment This includes microscopic examination of sperm and computer-aided investigation of sperm movement.

Functioning tests This is a test to see, for example, whether the sperm is capable of penetrating artificial mucus simulating cervical mucus or to see if anti-sperm antibodies are present.

Acrosome reaction test Sperm cannot recognise and fuse with an egg until a bag of enzymes in the head of the sperm is released by a membrane breaking down at the right moment (the acrosome reaction). The test is to trigger this reaction in a test-tube and, if it isn't present, drugs can be used to try to make it happen.

Hamster egg test A complicated test to investigate sperm's ability to penetrate a test egg.

Hormone tests These measure levels of various hormones which may indicate a number of causes of male infertility, such as the testicles not producing sperm or a benign pituitary tumour.

Surgical investigation of the testicle A very small piece of testis is removed for examination under the microscope.

• Feelings about tests and outcomes •

Going to infertility clinics may be very daunting and frustrating. Because the outcome of the tests is so important to you, you may be particularly vulnerable emotionally and extra-sensitive to any seeming insensitivity on the part of clinic staff. A whole range of emotions are natural, regardless or not of whether they are 'reasonable'; feelings of guilt, shame, anger, depression, inferiority and numbness are common.

It may be particularly hard if you are in a place where pregnant women are also waiting for antenatal appointments or women have come to be examined for a termination of pregnancy. It is a good idea to take someone with you to the clinic for support each time you have to attend.

There are likely to be effects on your life and relationship while all of the tests are going on. You may find it hard to give all your usual attention to your normal daily routines. Because chances of conception are stronger the more often couples make love, you may also feel pressured to have sex when you don't want to. This just adds additional unnecessary stress and it may be better to have sex slightly less but enjoy it more

It can be extra hard, as time goes on, if many people know you are trying for a baby and keep asking you each month if anything has happened. Parents may be well meaning but overly intrusive or they may very determinedly go out of their way to avoid the whole issue of children, which can be equally although unintentionally pressuring.

It may be a time when really there is no right way for others to behave. You may find it hard even to talk to someone who has children or to see any in the street without feeling sad. Some friends may try to be helpful by trying to play up how awful children can be and what a tie they are, but this is never what infertile couples feel cheered to hear. Fortunately, there are some excellent support groups where others who have been through the same mill can offer understanding.

When you finally receive a diagnosis, you may find yourself relieved to know something specific is the cause, even if chances of correcting it are not high. Alternatively, you may feel frustrated to find all is technically normal, even though this means you carry on having a chance to get pregnant each month.

Unfortunately, many women are given a diagnosis of unexplained infertility when in fact not all possible investigative tests have been carried out. It is worth trying to ensure that everything that should be checked has been checked before resorting to expensive techniques such as IVF.

• Treatments for female infertility •

There are a variety of treatments to help overcome infertility in women, depending on the possible cause that has been diagnosed.

• For failure to ovulate •

Clomiphene This is the first drug normally tried. It stimulates the pituitary gland which in turn stimulates the ovaries and promotes ovulation. It is given early in the menstrual cycle, between day one and day five. side-effects may include irregular bleeding, weight gain, hot flushes and depression, but the drug is not taken for long. Clomiphene induces ovulation in about 80 per cent of women given it and half of them will become pregnant.

Human chorionic gonadotrophin (HCG) This may be given along with clomiphene. It is is similar to luteinising hormone (LH) which is produced by the pituitary gland around ovulation and which helps the egg mature and erupt from the follicle. It is injected in the middle of the cycle.

Human menopausal gonadotrophin (HMG) If the methods above don't work, HMG may be tried. This is a very strong drug, containing both LH and FSH (follicle stimulating hormone) which are produced copiously by the pituitary at the menopause in an effort to get the failing ovaries to work. It is given for several days by injection, in the first half of the cycle, and encourages several eggs to be produced, increasing the risk of twins or multiple births. It has to be very carefully monitored; and the risks of multiple births can be significantly reduced with the correct tests at the correct time on blood and urine, plus ultrasound checks.

Pure follicle stimulating hormone (FSH) This contains, as its name implies, FSH and not LH, which isn't always needed and may in fact adversely affect the chances of conception in some women. Women used to have to attend their GP or clinic daily for 14 days for intramuscular injections of FSH but now a high-purity genetically engineered version has replaced the old formulation, and it can be injected under the skin by women themselves at home. It is more expensive than other gonadotrophins but can be particularly useful for women with polycystic ovarian syndrome.

LHRH This is LH-releasing hormone which is produced by the hypothalamus in the brain to stimulate the pituitary to produce LH. This hormone is naturally produced in short bursts every 15 minutes and this can be mimicked in treatment by delivery via a square pump small enough to be worn on the upper arm. A tube from the pump goes into a vein and delivers the correct amount of the drug at the correct times for a period of days. This can often help women with polycystic ovarian syndrome.

• For under-production of progesterone •

If you are ovulating but not producing enough progesterone to build up the endometrium to support a pregnancy, progesterone injections or pessaries may be tried. side-effects may include weight gain, tender breasts and acne.

• For excess prolactin •

If you are producing too much prolactin, the milk-producing hormone, you may be given bromocryptine which slows down the pituitary's production of this hormone. You may have to take it for some months and may experience dizziness, nausea and tiredness.

• For damaged fallopian tubes •

Surgery may be suggested for scarred or blocked fallopian tubes or for adhesions around the tubes. However, this does not have a high success rate and depends upon the nature of the problem (surgery for adhesions caused by endometriosis is more likely to work than for adhesions caused by infection); the degree of the problem (partial block or total block); and the surgeon's skill.

• Trends in treatment •

The National Infertility Awareness Campaign is trying to persuade government to encourage district health authorities to allocate their scarce resources for infertility to more modern options such as IVF and GIFT (test-tube

MONITORING

Women using any of the treatments for failure to ovulate must be very carefully investigated before treatment and closely monitored during it, because of possible links with ovarian cancer. Women should not be given clomiphene if they are already ovulating, in the hope of increasing the number of eggs, and if conception has not occurred after three cycles with clomiphene, they should be checked to ensure the drug is leading to ovulation. Women should not be prescribed gonadotrophins or LHRH without first having had a laparoscopy (see page 218) to confirm all is normal and there there is no disease in the tubes or ovaries.

techniques, see page 440) rather than tubal surgery. However, renowned infertility expert Professor Robert Winston of the Hammersmith Hospital, London, believes that, where both are options, tubal surgery is the better choice if the damage is not too serious. This is because, if the treatment is successful, you can get pregnant in the normal way and get pregnant for a second or more times without further intervention needed. Much of the severe emotional stress commonly associated with IVF may be eliminated as well.

• Treatments for male infertility •

Making lifestyle changes such as giving up smoking, drinking less, eating a healthier diet, getting more exercise (a sedentary lifestyle may lead to prolonged heating of the scrotum), losing excess weight, etc, may improve poor sperm count after a few months.

Certain drug treatment may be effective in some other cases but the success rate isn't high. Although little can be done to improve sperm medically, it may still be worth knowing the exact problem because if, for example, there is no acrosome reaction or inability to penetrate an egg, both artificial insemination with a partner's semen and IVF treatments, with all their emotional trauma and expense, will never work either.

Surgery may be successful for correcting a varicocoele or unblocking tubes (by microsurgical techniques).

• Assisted conception •

There are a number of ways that a woman can be helped to have a baby if the infertility treatments so far described do not work.

Artificial insemination Insemination with a partner's semen may work sometimes when sperm count is low. Sperm may be inserted directly into the vagina via a plastic tube shortly after it is produced. In the few places in the UK where there are sufficiently sophisticated laboratory facilities, sperm may be 'washed' before it is inserted. It is mixed with a special fluid and by one of a number of means the healthy sperm are collected and the dead or inactive sperm are left behind.

'Washed' sperm may sometimes be inserted directly into the uterus via a thin tube which is passed through the cervix. This can be painful.

If the partner's sperm is not viable a couple may opt for artificial insemination by donor. Clinics claim to try as far as possible to match the anonymous donor's characteristics to the 'father'. All potential donors must be tested for HIV before being allowed to give sperm.

• In vitro fertilisation (IVF) •

This is the so-called test-tube baby technique in which egg or eggs are removed from a woman's ovary and mixed with her partner's cleaned sperm in the laboratory. If fertilisation takes place, the embryo or embryos are put into the uterus (embryo transfer).

It has a low success rate. A one-in-three chance of success is the absolute best which the most experienced clinics can offer, and women of 30 and under are much more likely to be successful than women of 40. Chances are also higher if two embryos can be implanted rather than one. If you haven't conceived after four attempts with IVF, your chances are pretty low and most clinics would suggest you have no more tries.

In addition, IVF doesn't suit everyone. It should be recommended mainly when tubal damage is extensive or when there is a problem with cervical mucus but you still need to be ovulating and have an efficiently functioning uterus. Sometimes it is recommended as a try-it-and-see for men with possible sperm problems. This is a rather expensive and emotionally demanding method of investigation, not really to be recommended. Better to get sperm problems fully investigated first (see page 436), at a cost of little over £100 rather than over £1000 for IVF.

A woman needs to take drugs for some weeks before IVF treatment is carried out and these may involve attending for daily injections for a period of time. Ultrasound checks and/or hormone tests are carried out to detect when ovulation is about to occur.

Ultrasound is usually used to assist in the collection of eggs. After a general or local anaesthetic a suction needle is inserted through the vagina and the egg or eggs sucked out. Sometimes this is done by laparoscopy, under general anaesthetic. (Occasionally ovulation has already occurred by the time the process for egg collection is carried out and the whole business has to be rescheduled for another month.) When the eggs are being collected, your partner needs to produce a sample of sperm. Then the laboratory begins its work.

Two to four days later an embryo, if there is one, should be ready to be put into the uterus. This is done via a plastic tube inserted through the cervix and you have to stay on your back for at least 30 minutes afterwards. Doctors usually advise taking it easy for a couple of days and avoiding sex for a week or two. Some clinics follow up the embryo transfer with hormone treatment for a few days.

• Gamete intra-fallopian transfer (GIFT) •

In this procedure, egg and sperm are collected in the same way as for IVF, and with all the preliminaries described for IVF, but are just mixed together and put straight into a fallopian tube, without having been fertilised first. Obviously this technique can only be used if you have at least one tube in good working order, and male sperm needs to be good too.

It isn't very successful, although some centres which use it claim equivalent success to IVF.

• Sub-zonal insemination (SUZI) •

In this very sophisticated technique, still very new, several sperm are injected directly into the egg, underneath the egg's covering that is called the zona pellucida. This gives a greater chance to sperm which don't move very well. However, if more than one sperm fertilises the egg, it cannot develop and has to be thrown away.

Variations on this include PZD (partial zonal dissection), in which the egg cell covering is ruptured to allow sperm easier entry, and DISCO (direct injection of sperm into cytoplasm of the oocyte) or ICSI (intracytoplasmic sperm injection) in which just one sperm is injected actually into the jelly-like substance (cytoplasm) inside the egg (oocyte), avoiding altogether the risk of more than one sperm fertilising the egg.

These techniques are still largely experimental, however, although a few hundred pregnancies across the world have been achieved by them.

• Egg donation •

For women who go through a premature menopause or who do not produce healthy eggs, egg donation from another woman may be an option. However, the egg donor has to be a young woman prepared to go through the kind of procedures which precede IVF treatment. Although the emotional investment is not the same, the whole business is extremely inconvenient, so not many women are prepared to do it.

Once eggs have been collected, they are inserted into the vagina of the woman who wants a baby and chances of pregnancy can be very high in experienced hands: up to 50 per cent.

• Could you cope? •

You may have to be very resilient and determined to handle all the physical and emotional demands of IVF treatment and others similar to it. It can be hard to carry on a normal life because you may have to attend the clinic so often for monitoring or hormone injections. It is also difficult to forget, because of all the preparations, what you are building up towards.

The week to ten days before sophisticated tests can reveal likelihood of pregnancy after embryo transfer or, if there is no test, the 14 days before a period might be expected can be excruciating. Women describe feeling pregnant because they know they are carrying a fertilised embryo and yet they find themselves anxiously watching for all possible signs of an impending period. The disappointment when a period comes can be crushingly strong.

Partners may not always fully understand how draining and demoralising the whole process is for a woman. While they are enormously disappointed, they may want to get on quickly with trying again, whereas a woman may need some months to recover or to think about whether she can even bear to go through it all again.

Some women may prefer to think about other options such as adoption or surrogacy, where another woman bears the partner's child. Yet others choose instead to learn to come to terms with not having children.

The organisations listed under Useful Contacts and books in the Further Reading section should be able to provide you with much helpful information for making your own decisions. You can also be put in touch, via the support groups, with others who know what you are going through and who will gladly listen to all you need to say about your feelings.

47

···

THE MENOPAUSE

THE MENOPAUSE is often called the change of life. It is the time when the ovaries stop functioning and the levels of the hormones produced by them, oestrogen and progesterone, fall. As a result a woman stops having periods.

The word menopause is usually used to refer to the whole time from which the pattern of your monthly periods first starts to change (as less and less oestrogen and progesterone are produced) through to when they cease entirely; although strictly speaking this is termed the perimenopause.

During this time your periods may become irregular and the heaviness of the blood flow may vary from one period to the next. Fluctuating levels of oestrogen may also cause uncomfortable symptoms (see below). This is a process which, for some women, occurs quite quickly (sometimes periods may just stop without there having been any alteration in their nature previously) while for others it may last for years. Most commonly it occurs between the ages of 45 and 55, but it can occur as early as 40 (or even in the thirties in cases of what is known as premature menopause).

Instant menopause is created if you have your uterus and ovaries surgically removed. Even if you have your uterus removed but your ovaries are left in place there is a strong chance that you will enter the menopause early as, in a sizeable proportion of women, the ovaries start to fail within a couple of years of the operation.

The long-term effects of the menopause are a significant increase in the risk of osteoporosis (thinning of the bones), heart attack and stroke.

• Symptoms •

One in five women may notice nothing except the stopping of their periods. Most, however, experience other symptoms as a result of hormonal changes. These include any or all of the following: hot flushes; night sweats; thinning and drying of the skin; breast changes; bloating; psychological effects.

Hot flushes These are caused by falls in oestrogen levels. They are a sensation of heat which can extend over the whole body or spread upwards from the chest or neck to the face, and may be accompanied by sweating.

A flush lasts usually for about three minutes but may sometimes persist for half an hour and can be highly uncomfortable. You may have only one a week or you may have over ten a day. Many women are embarrassed because they think they are turning visibly red while it happens, although in fact the colour change is very minor and the event is probably not noticed by anyone other than yourself.

Flushes may start while you still have your periods and occur only during your period. After periods stop they are likely to become more frequent, continuing to occur in most cases for two or three years but for five years in 25 per cent of women, and throughout life unfortunately for about one in 20 women.

Night sweats   These may be another early menopausal symptom. The sweats can be quite drenching and severe enough to wake you up. After the sweats you may feel shivery and cold.

Changes in skin   Skin may become thinner, drier and more wrinkly after the menopause because of hormonal changes and loss of a protein (collagen) which normally helps to keep skin elastic. The skin of the vagina may become dry and sore. A third of women experience a loss of sexual desire, due to hormonal changes and effects such as vaginal dryness.

Changes in breasts   Breasts may lose a little of their size and firmness. Without oestrogen and progesterone, some women find that their breasts shrink in size, although in very many women breast size stays exactly the same as before. Breasts may tend to drop, because the fibrous ligaments are less elastic.

Bloating   A feeling of bloating in the abdomen, similar to that which may previously have been experienced as a premenstrual symptom may be suffered by some women.

Psychological symptoms   These include mood swings, loss of concentration, forgetfulness, difficulty sleeping and depression. However, although these are symptoms which can all definitely be associated with the menopause, it is important not to attribute all emotional problems to it. Usually the menopause occurs at a time when other changes are going on in women's lives: children may have grown up and just left home; elderly parents may have become more dependent; some women may be contemplating, with equal degrees of fear and excitement, the prospect of going out to work for the first time; others may be thinking about retirement or coping with a partner's impending retirement.

• Long-term effects of the menopause •

Osteoporosis   A thinning of the bones, particularly those in the spine, wrists and hips, severe enough to cause them to fracture even when minimal injury is suffered. One in three women is likely to suffer an osteoporotic fracture in her lifetime, unless taking preventive treatment (see page 479).

Bone density declines after the mid-thirties in both women and men but in women it occurs more quickly, at a rate of 2 to 3 per cent of bone mass per year after the menopause. Women who smoke, drink heavily, take little exercise and have had and continue to have a low calcium diet are the most at risk.

Heart disease and stroke   After the menopause, women are at the same risk of heart disease as men and it becomes a major killer of women. Women appear to be protected earlier in their lives because of the beneficial effects of oestrogen on certain blood fats. This protection is lost once oestrogen stops being produced. For similar reasons, women's risk of stroke is increased after the menopause as well.

· Self-help ·

For hot flushes

1 Avoid wearing clothes made from synthetic materials that prevent air from circulating freely to help you cool down. Wear cotton clothing, preferably in light layers, so that you can remove a layer occasionally if you need to.
2 Avoid alcohol, coffee and spicy foods and stop or cut down on cigarettes, as all these increase the likelihood of flushing.
3 Be aware that drugs for high blood pressure can cause flushing, so if you are on medication for this condition, talk to your doctor about it.
4 Consider evening primrose oil capsules. Some women find that taking them helps improve hot flushes but trials have found them no better than a placebo (a dummy medicine that has no effect).
5 Try showering if you don't already. You may find showering more comfortable than taking hot baths.
6 Try, if you can, putting your arms under cold running water when you are having a hot flush. It can help cool you down more quickly.

For night sweats   Try placing a large towel on the sheet and lie on that, so that you can remove it easily if you have a sweat and still be comfortable in your bed.

For dry skin   Be generous to your skin with moisturising cream, but in the vagina only ever use creams or preparations specifically designed for vaginal lubrication.

Eat well and healthily   Avoid too much in the way of saturated fats, to keep your heart risk low. As constipation can sometimes be a problem, make sure your diet is plentiful in carbohydrate and fibre. Drink plenty of fluids. You may want to consider a vitamin and mineral supplement. There are some that are targeted specifically at post-menopausal women.

Exercise regularly   Do whatever form you may enjoy. Walking briskly is fine. Exercise helps protect against both heart disease and osteoporosis.

Contraception   Carry on using contraception for a while as it is still possible to conceive even during and immediately after the menopause. Keep using it for a year after your last period if you were over 50 when you had it, or for two years if you are under 50 when you have your last period.

Seek support   Talk to friends or family close to you about your feelings on going through the menopause. You may have strong feelings about ceasing to be able to have a child, even though the last thing you actually want is to have a baby. Bound up with this may be a fear that you are no longer as feminine or womanly as you were. Just acknowledging what is happening by sharing your thoughts and feelings (or expressing them on paper for your eyes only) can be sufficient to deal with any sadness, uncertainty or sense of loss you may experience. For many women, the menopause is a liberation and they are able to feel more free and more sexy because all risk of possible pregnancy is past.

Keep up the screenings   Passing the menopause does not mean that you cannot now contract breast or cervical cancer. It is important to maintain regular checks, with breast screening every three years between the ages of 50 and 64 and cervical smears at least every five years till the age of 64.

· Hormone replacement therapy · (HRT)

Most experts now claim that the single most important thing women can do to treat any unpleasant symptoms of the menopause and to protect against its long-term effects is to take hormone replacement therapy (HRT). However, you may have to mention it to your doctor if you are interested as surveys have shown that large numbers of women are still not offered it or even informed about it by their GPs.

HRT is exactly what its name says it is: a replacement of hormones that have been lost. It consists of natural oestrogen and so is not like the contraceptive pill, in which synthetic oestrogen has to be used in order to provide sufficient amounts to prevent ovulation.

Women who have had a hysterectomy need only take the natural oestrogen component of HRT. Women whose uterus is intact must also take progestogen, a synthetic progesterone, for at least part of the month, to prevent oestrogen from acting unopposed on the endometrium, the lining of the uterus. Without progestogen there is a slightly increased risk of cancer of the endometrium, with about eight women in every 1000 likely to develop it. With progestogen the increased risk disappears.

· How do you take it? ·

HRT comes in a number of forms:

- Tablets. Some brands contain the oestrogen and progestogen in one tablet; others require the two to be taken separately.

- Implants, which are tiny pellets inserted under the skin and left there for six to nine months, slowly releasing hormones into the blood. There are distinct drawbacks with this method if you still have a uterus. Because the action of the implant goes on long after it has been removed, progestogen has to carry on being taken for two years after removal of the pellets.
- Patches, which are impregnated with gel and stuck on to the abdomen, a new one being applied every three or four days. The hormones are absorbed through the skin. Some women find patches irritate their skin.
- Creams, which are inserted into the vagina and absorbed through the vaginal wall. Some women find this method fails to relieve menopausal symptoms, as insufficient oestrogen may be absorbed.

As different methods suit different women, it may be important to experiment with different brands of pill or different approaches until you find one that works well for you. If you are keen to have HRT, don't accept unpleasant side-effects or just stop HRT altogether without giving all its versions a reasonable trial.

• Side-effects •

The biggest problem with most current HRT methods is that the progestogen component (if needed) causes a bleed and also may cause premenstrual-type symptoms such as bloating, breast tenderness, abdominal cramps, headaches, irritability and irregular bleeding. The duration of the progestogen therapy may be able to be manipulated on an individual basis by a gynaecologist, but while this may reduce most of the unwanted side-effects, it can increase the heaviness or irregularity of bleeding.

Women who dislike the idea of HRT are usually most put off by the thought of having periods again and possibly premenstrual symptoms. However, there are now new types of HRT being manufactured, in which there is continuous oestrogen and progestogen therapy and no bleed at all. These are obviously proving more popular, although there inevitably have to be some question marks over long-term safety as they are so new: the first came on to the UK market in 1994. No-bleed HRT is most suitable for use with women who have not had a period for at least a year as the low dose of progestogen it contains may not be sufficient to prevent breakthrough bleeding immediately post-menopause.

Also currently being evaluated is the combination of having a progesterone-releasing intrauterine system fitted (see levonorgestrel-releasing intrauterine system, page 412) and taking oral oestrogen alone. With the progesterone-releasing IUD, periods either stop or become very light. Because the progesterone is released directly into the uterus, the amount needed is a fraction of the dose that must be taken orally and therefore side-effects are likely to be fewer.

Any woman who experiences heavy prolonged bleeding should arrange an investigation with her GP, whatever kind of HRT she is using.

Some HRT contains a little testosterone, the male sex hormone, as well as oestrogen and progestogen. This can dramatically improve a woman's sex life.

• How long should HRT be used? •

Some women only take HRT while they have overt menopausal symptoms: perhaps for less than two years. However HRT needs to be taken for at least five years for the effects on bone to become apparent. After five years, risk of hip fracture is halved. Many doctors now recommend that HRT is taken for ten years and some even suggest that it should be taken for life.

• For whom is HRT not suitable? •

HRT should not be prescribed for women who have had breast cancer or endometrial cancer or who have any undiagnosed vaginal bleeding. Some doctors may be reluctant to prescribe HRT if a woman has had a heart attack, previous stroke or blood clots or has high blood pressure, although many experts think this is unnecessarily cautious. Women with diabetes should be monitored carefully if they are prescribed HRT. Endometriosis may recur in previous sufferers even if treatment is started several years after the menopause. Existing fibroids and gallstone may be exacerbated by HRT. There is no evidence that HRT should not be given to a woman with varicose veins.

• Benefits of HRT •

1 HRT, when given correctly, can remove unpleasant menopausal symptoms and protect against osteoporosis, heart disease and various cancers such as those of the ovary, cervix and even the endometrium. It may also reduce incidence of stroke.
2 It can help women keep their pre-menopause figures by preventing the tendency towards central distribution of fat (fat around the abdomen) that tends to occur after the menopause. Also, distribution of fat around the abdomen increases risk of heart disease.
3 Women who had bad menopausal symptoms find that their confidence and zest for life returns because they feel so much better.

• Disadvantages of HRT •

1 The side-effects and return of monthly bleeds associated with some methods may put many women off.
2 There is a very slight increase in the risk of breast cancer. (However, breast cancers discovered in HRT users appear to be less advanced and more amenable to treatments, although there might be a variety of explanations for this.)
3 It may worsen fibroids, endometriosis and gallstones.
4 Some women feel that using HRT is unnatural, although originally, we probably weren't designed to be post-menopausal for very long so the menopause and post-menopause may not be particularly natural either.

Part IV

A–Z OF WOMEN'S HEALTH PROBLEMS

THERE are many conditions and illnesses which, for one reason or another, or reasons unknown, more commonly affect women than men, even though they have nothing specifically to do with a woman's reproductive organs. In this section you will find – described in alphabetical order – all the main physical ailments which are particularly pertinent to women and which have not been covered anywhere else in this book.

48

WOMEN'S HEALTH PROBLEMS

• Anaemia •

ANAEMIA is a deficiency of haemoglobin, the pigment in red blood cells which carries oxygen. It can be caused by insufficient intake of iron, folic acid or vitamin B_{12} in the diet, all of which are essential for forming haemoglobin. It can also be caused by faulty haemoglobin itself. Some inherited diseases, such as sickle cell anaemia, cause faulty haemoglobin. Diseases such as leukaemia and bone cancer also affect its production.

It is the iron- and folic acid-deficiency anaemias to which women are especially susceptible for a number of reasons. About one in ten women has mild anaemia caused by iron deficiency and about a third of all women are borderline for it. Folic-acid deficiency only affects about one in 2000 people but those at extra risk are pregnant women. Although these kinds of anaemia are not themselves serious, they weaken the body's ability to defend itself against illnesses or to recover from injuries or accidents where a lot of blood may be lost. If you are pregnant, healthy development of the foetus may be adversely affected.

Vitamin B_{12} deficiency (known as pernicious anaemia) is not common and usually arises from a problem with absorption rather than a lack of intake, although vegetarians and vegans may be more at risk as B_{12} is most plentifully supplied by meat and dairy products. If ability to absorb B_{12} has been lost, treatment in the form of injections is necessary for life. Without prompt treatment there may be damage to the nervous system.

• Symptoms •

General symptoms of anaemia are tiredness, breathlessness, paleness, fainting, feeling weak and experiencing palpitations. People tend to associate anaemia with looking pale and wan but this may in fact be only a very late sign. With folic-acid and vitamin-B_{12} deficiency, soreness of the mouth and tongue is also common and skin may appear yellowed. If vitamin-B_{12} deficiency is prolonged, you may experience tingling in the fingers and toes and problems with balance.

• Women at especial risk •

I Women who are dieting, especially if restricting their intake of certain foods altogether or just skimping on their own meals, are unlikely to be taking sufficient iron and folic acid in their diet.

2 Women who have heavy periods suffer an excessive loss of haemoglobin which they may not have a chance to make up before their next period. Adequate iron in the diet is essential in these cases.

3 Pregnant women have to make more blood and therefore need to make more haemoglobin than normal. Also, iron and folic acid are needed by the foetus for its healthy development. If normal diet is sufficient in iron, no supplements are needed and absorption of iron improves as the pregnancy progresses. Folic acid supplements, however, are now routinely recommended as insufficient folic acid may increase the risk of neural spine defects (spina bifida).

4 Women who have just given birth are also at increased risk of anaemia for a while. In these circumstances it is not wise to assume that extreme tiredness or weakness is due solely to sleepless nights.

5 Illnesses such as rheumatoid arthritis, to which women are more prone than men, can interfere with the body's ability to use iron. Treatment for the illness should cure the anaemia too.

6 Haemorrhoids are an especial hazard for women during pregnancy and for a while after birth. If a great deal of blood is lost from haemorrhoids, this can increase risk of anaemia. Anaemia can also be a sign of undetected internal bleeding which may be caused by a stomach ulcer, irritation of the stomach lining due to extremely frequent use of aspirin or stomach cancer.

• What to do •

In most cases of anaemia the treatment is to increase your intake of iron. However, if you think you have symptoms it is important to see your doctor for a blood test just to check the degree of anaemia and that there is no underlying cause which does need medical treatment.

Make sure your diet contains plenty of iron-rich foods such as red meat (especially liver, kidneys and heart), fish, eggs, green leafy vegetables, dried fruit, wholemeal bread and breakfast cereals that are fortified with vitamins and minerals. Taking vitamin C at the same time as iron (for example, an orange-juice drink with an iron-rich meal) greatly increases absorption. Using iron cooking pots allows tiny amounts of iron to be added to the food being cooked, further increasing iron in your diet.

Some folic acid-rich foods are liver, wheatgerm, green leafy vegetables, pulses, nuts and yeast extract. Make especially sure you have enough if you use the contraceptive pill or drink quite a bit of alcohol, as your requirements may be more. Drinking too much tea and taking antacids can interfere with iron absorption.

• Arthritis •

See Osteoarthritis, page 477 and Rheumatoid Arthritis, page 484.

• Breast disorders •

See Benign Breast Disorders, page 304, and Breast Cancer, page 322.

• Cancer •

Every year, over 300,000 new cases of cancer are diagnosed in the UK. One in three of us will suffer from cancer in our lives (almost three-quarters of new cases occur in people over the age of 60) and one in four die of it. Currently, about 165,000 British people die of cancer each year.

Although there are very many kinds of cancer, only a few account for more than half of all cancer deaths. Lung cancer by itself accounts for a quarter of all cancer deaths and breast cancer is the biggest cancer killer of women, except in parts of northern England and Scotland where lung cancer deaths are now higher.

The most common cancers in women in the UK are breast (nearly 27,000 cases every year), bowel (nearly 15,000), non-melanoma skin cancer (14,400), lung, (12,600), ovary (5500), stomach (nearly 4900), cervix (4500), uterus (3700), pancreas (3400) and bladder (3250).

Not unsurprisingly, survival from cancer depends to a large extent upon the type suffered and the stage at which it is discovered, with treatment at an early stage leading to a much higher survival rate. Women whose breast cancer is treated at a very early stage have an 80 per cent chance of being alive five years later compared with an 18 per cent chance for women whose breast cancer was treated late. The ten most survivable cancers for women in the UK are non-melanoma skin cancer (97 per cent alive ten years later), placenta (92 per cent), melanoma (75 per cent), uterus (70 per cent), Hodgkin's disease (68 per cent), thyroid (65 per cent), breast (62 per cent), eye (61 per cent), cervix (58 per cent) and bladder (56 per cent).

It is now known that lifestyle and environmental factors play a large part in the development of many cancers and that, with the appropriate changes, a staggering 80 per cent of all cancers could be avoided.

• What is cancer? •

The word cancer covers about 200 different forms of the disease, each of which is different in the way it develops and behaves. All cancers are caused by cells getting out of control and reproducing overly fast, causing a swelling (tumour). As groups of cells are necessary to form all of our organs and tissues, and as cell production in any of these can at some stage go wrong, there is a huge range of potential cancers.

Tumours may be benign or malignant. It is when they are malignant that they are known as cancers. This means that they have the ability to spread to other organs and tissues close by, or that some cells from the tumour may be able to separate and travel via the lymph system (which acts as the body's waste disposal system and helps fight disease), or via the bloodstream, to distant parts of the body where they form new tumours. These are known as secondaries or metastases. A cancer that is not life-threatening in its original site may become so if it spreads to a vital organ such as the liver.

We probably develop potential cancers every day but our immune systems are able to get rid of them. However, if the immune system cannot function at peak for any reason, the cancer will have a greater chance to take hold. It may grow silently for a long time so that even a cancer that is detected 'early' may in fact have been around for years, and there is a chance that there may already be secondaries elsewhere in the body.

Doctors call cancers by different names according to where they develop. For instance, carcinomas occur in the lining of organs while sarcomas arise in fibrous tissue, fat, bone and cartilage. The terms, and there are many, are confusing to anyone not medically trained, and it is important to ask for a simple description of exactly what and where the cancer is.

• Causes •

It is now estimated that diet is the prime cause of 35 per cent of cancers and smoking is the prime cause of 30 per cent. Other contributory causes include infection with certain viruses (such as in stomach cancer and cervical cancer) and occupational hazards. However, pollution, pesticides, radiation and food additives – all variously feared as causes of cancer – do not have much if any part in most cancers, and additives may even help protect against stomach cancer, according to some leading authorities.

In some cases there may be an inherited susceptibility to a particular cancer, which doesn't mean getting cancer is inevitable but that the risks are greater. But nothing is really clear cut with cancer. We all know of many people whose lifestyle might appear to be prime cancer material and yet they are still healthy, while others, who followed all the right rules, may succumb. There are doubtless numerous factors which we have yet to discover or to prove to be linked with cancer, including the role of psychological health.

• Prevention •

There are a number of recommended ways to reduce the overall risk of developing cancer.

1 Don't smoke. Seven out of ten lung cancers in women are caused by smoking. Women develop it at an earlier age than men even though they tend to start smoking later and smoke fewer cigarettes. Smoking is also linked with cancer of the cervix, the bowel and oral cancers.

2 Ensure a healthy diet. Eat foods that are low in fat, particularly saturated fats, and consume plenty of fresh fruit, vegetables and fibre. It is now thought that modifications in diet could reduce risk of cancer by at least one-third and maybe even as much as two-thirds.

The elements in diet deemed most likely to increase risk are meat, total fat, saturated fat, preserved foods (although the amount of smoked, cured, pickled or barbecued foods eaten in the UK is unlikely to be a hazard), alcohol and salt. High fat intake appears to be linked with increased lung and colon cancer and possibly breast cancer, being overweight may be linked with increased endometrial cancer and, in post-menopausal women, with increased breast cancer.

The possible protective factors in food are gained from fruit, vegetables, fibre, antioxidant nutrients (beta carotene and vitamins C and E), fish oils and calcium. Fibre intake is linked with lower incidence of bowel cancer and increased fresh fruit and vegetable intake leads to a drop in lung, breast, cervical, bladder, oral, oesophagal, stomach and colon cancers. Experts usually recommend dietary changes to gain these benefits rather than relying on or adding supplements.

3 Don't get burned by the sun. Most skin cancers are curable but melanoma can be lethal if not diagnosed and treated early.

4 Use a barrier method of contraception if you are not in a steady monogamous relationship. The sexually transmissible genital wart virus is an important risk factor for cervical cancer.

5 Be careful with alcohol. Heavy drinking, particularly if you smoke too, increases risk of the rarer cancers of the mouth, throat and oesophagus.

6 Keep a check on your own body. Take up cervical and breast screening and be alert to any changes in moles on the skin.

7 Try to develop a positive outlook on life, enjoy the moment and cut down on worrying and stress. Feeling good boosts the immune system, whereas feeling oppressed and negative stops it working so well. Express your negative as well as positive feelings instead of keeping painful things bottled up inside. (See Handling Thoughts, Feelings and Needs, page 190.)

8 If you notice a persistent change in bowel or bladder habits, a cough or hoarseness that won't go away, persistent indigestion, difficulty swallowing, unexplained weight loss, any unusual lumps or changes in a mole, any unusual and persistent bleeding or discharge, you should see your doctor. While the causes may well be innocent, if they are signals of a cancer, you will increase your chances of early detection and treatment.

• Treatment •

Orthodox treatment   The mainstay of orthodox treatment is still surgery, radiotherapy (high-energy X-rays or implants designed to kill cancer cells) and chemotherapy (treatment with strong drugs that kill cancer cells but also unfortunately damage healthy cells); in different combinations as appropriate for particular cancers. A course of radiotherapy is usually given over a period of days or weeks, with breaks at the weekends. Chemotherapy may be given as tablets or injections every few weeks for a period of several months.

Radiotherapy and chemotherapy are aggressive treatments and may be extremely unpleasant although the side-effects of both are much fewer nowadays and many women are able to carry on their normal lives and jobs

—————— **Take your time** ——————

If you are told you have cancer, it is important that you are not rushed into treatment. Being given the diagnosis of cancer is inevitably a shock and usually people find it impossible to take in everything a doctor says afterwards about the treatment plans. Take a little time. Cancer is rarely an emergency, as it has already been growing for years. Get whatever information you need in order to understand what is happening, what the treatment offers you and whether you wish to go ahead. You may decide you want a second opinion. Try to find someone you can talk to about it all. Many hospitals have counsellors or, in the case of breast cancer, breast-care nurses. You may also want to contact a self-help or support group through one the the cancer-support charities.

between treatments. The most common side-effect of radiation is tiredness. With chemotherapy there may be nausea, tiredness and loss of hair, but this varies according to the drugs used.

Complementary therapies   Many people nowadays wish to explore complementary methods of treating cancer, either alongside their conventional treatment or instead of it. Complementary therapies put a lot of emphasis on a healthy cancer-fighting diet, on creating a positive and relaxed state of mind and on receiving love, support and encouragement. Some people choose to try methods such as homoeopathy or healing. You can find out more about all of these approaches from the cancer support charities or from the Bristol Cancer Help Centre: see Useful Contacts.

Some people choose to try to boost their immune systems with simple dietary supplements while undergoing orthodox treatments. The Bristol Cancer Help Centre advocates a special programme of vitamin and mineral supplementation to boost the effects of all treatments for cancer but warns that certain vitamins should not be used in certain cancers or alongside certain drugs. Contact them for details of their book called *Cancer and Nutrition: the positive scientific evidence.*

• Coping •

Cancer remains one of the most emotive of illnesses we suffer. We fear it in a way we do not tend to fear heart disease or other chronic diseases. Maybe this is because it is an insidious disease that can take so many forms and can spread unseen and unknown.

For most people there are many emotional issues to sort out when given a diagnosis of cancer. Fears about failing to survive have to be faced, fears about coping with treatment, caring for families while treatment goes on, fears about feeling and looking different after some treatments, fears about cancer coming back. Having cancer can be a time when we re-assess the priorities in our lives and perhaps find that family and friends mean more to us than striving too hard and single-mindedly for success in a career. Fortunately, there is much helpful and sympathetically written information available in the form of books and booklets, and much support to be had from local and national groups. BACUP and CancerLink can advise on both: see Useful Contacts.

• Carpal tunnel syndrome •

This is a numbness and tingling that may develop in the hand, particularly in women over the age of 30. It is caused by swollen tissues trapping the nerve that passes signals from the brain to the hand at the point where it passes through a tiny space – the carpal tunnel – inside the wrist joint. It seems that a change in the balance of sex hormones as women get older can cause fluid to accumulate in the wrist and result in the swelling.

Carpal tunnel syndrome is often a problem during pregnancy. It can also be due, in some cases, to the tissue swelling that occurs with diabetes, thyroid problems or a previous wrist fracture.

Those often especially likely to suffer it are women who have to be dextrous with their hands or who put quite a lot of strain on their wrists, for example in sports such as tennis or in pastimes such as sewing or knitting. The condition may sometimes clear up on its own. This is almost always the case after pregnancy.

• Symptoms •

The first symptoms may be tingling in a few fingers of one or both hands. Tingling and numbness may be intermittent, often accompanied by pain running up the arm from the wrist. Eventually the whole hand may become swollen and heavy and feel extremely painful. Usually the pain is worse at night, when it can be intense enough to wake you up and prevent you getting back to sleep without taking a pain killer.

• What to do •

Sometimes self-help methods, such as sleeping with your arm over the side of the bed, rubbing it or raising it periodically straight into the air so that fluid has a chance to drain downward are sufficient to help you deal with any pain. Occasional pain killers are fine but if you find you need them often you should see your doctor for some help.

First options are a wrist splint, which can be very helpful if worn at night, a small injection of a steroid drug into the wrist to reduce inflammation (instant relief but often temporary) and a diuretic to help reduce fluid retention (which may work or may not, even temporarily).

If these measures do not work, a simple surgical operation can be carried out where, through a tiny incision that leaves minimal scarring, the surgeon can release tough ligaments to create more space for the nerve.

• Fatigue •

According to surveys, feeling tired all the time is a big problem. Population surveys show that at least 30 per cent of women say they always feel tired, compared with 20 per cent of men. But figures based on research into fatigue suggest that three times as many women as men experience extreme exhaustion. There are many possible causes for feeling tired all the time. Those described here should cover most of them.

Overdoing it   Obviously, if you make enormous demands on yourself or have enormous demands made on you, you are extremely likely to become excessively tired. Make sure you build time into your day for proper relaxation (see page 41). Cut down on your activities if you can or try to share out responsibilities at work or home with others.

Sleep problems   Not getting enough sleep happens less than we think (see Sleeping Well, page 36). However, one study of sufferers from chronic fatigue syndrome found a distinct association between fatigue and difficulty sleeping. (Chronic fatigue syndrome is defined as unexplained tiredness which has persisted for more than 50 per cent of the time for more than six months and with mental and physical functioning affected.)

Anaemia   One in ten women suffers from iron-deficiency anaemia. See page 451.

Underactive thyroid   Besides fatigue, other symptoms of this are brittle nails, dry skin, sudden weight gain, and super-sensitivity to cold. Treatment is with a synthetic form of the thyroid hormone.

Hypoglycaemia   This is suffering from low blood sugar, which can make you feel very sluggish. It can be treated by taking glucose.

Magnesium deficiency   A lack of this mineral can cause tiredness, particularly if you are a very active person. Magnesium rich foods are green vegetables, nuts and seeds, wholewheat flour, brown rice and seafood.

Chronic pain   Backache, regular migraines and other kinds of persistent pain can just wear you out and also increase depression, itself a major cause of fatigue. It helps if you can distract yourself from pain as much as possible by trying to do more and stopping negative thoughts (see page 190).

Pollution-induced tiredness   In hot, still weather, traffic congestion and the depleted ozone layer have such an adverse effect on air quality that the young, the elderly, pregnant women and those who suffer respiratory diseases such as asthma may find it difficult to breathe. Avoid outdoor exercise in these conditions; look or listen out for poor air quality readings on weather forecasts.

Viral infections   Illnesses such as flu can leave you debilitated as well as depressed for weeks or months afterwards. Sometimes they may lead to ME (see page 473).

ME   A specific illness with fatigue as a major symptom (see page 473).

Seasonal affective disorder (SAD)   This is a specific form of depression caused by lack of light and occurring in the winter (see page 180).

Food sensitivity   Sometimes fatigue may be a major symptom of a sensitivity to some common food. This kind of sensitivity or intolerance may appear to develop out of the blue, so that a food that you have always enjoyed before with no problem starts to affect you adversely. It is difficult to know which food is the culprit, however, especially as you are likely to be eating it every day. (See Food Allergy and Sensitivity, page 26.)

Under-exercise   Not doing enough exercise stops the body from absorbing essential minerals properly, including iron, lack of which adds to fatigue. Make sure you take at least a brisk ten-minute walk each day.

Boredom   We all need sufficient stimulation to keep us functioning at our best. Boredom at work or at home and lack of responsibility or control in either can have the effect of tiring you out.

Anxiety   If you are anxious about something such as an event you are organising, a holiday you are planning, a difficult situation you have to sort out, you may be using up energy in worry; and are probably lying awake at night worrying as well. Or perhaps there is something in your life that you are frightened to confront – for example, not liking your step-children or not feeling supported by your partner – and feeling tired is a way of avoiding having to do so. (See also Anxiety, page 143.)

Depression   Depression is a major cause of fatigue. Sometimes the cause is easy to identify – the death of someone close, the break-up of a relationship – and you know that, although you feel utterly miserable now, the feelings will lessen in intensity in time. Sometimes the depression is unexplained, its causes unconsciously suppressed since childhood, and you cannot envisage an end to it. Therapy or counselling may help. (See Depression, page 168.)

Unhappiness   If you are unhappy with any important aspect of your life, even if you don't feel overtly depressed or anxious, the most obvious symptom could be a feeling of exhaustion. It takes a lot of effort to suppress negative feelings. Try taking a look at your life, talk with friends or seek professional help to make some re-evaluations, so that you can use your energy in a more constructive and satisfying way.

• Fluid retention •

A number of conditions can lead to fluid retention: an accumulation of fluid in body tissues. It can accompany premenstrual syndrome before a period, particularly if your breasts swell regularly at this time. The contraceptive pill can sometimes cause an increase in weight and breast size.

Some fluid retention is common during pregnancy but any amount signifi-cant enough to make your rings too tight and your face bloated may indicate a potentially dangerous condition called pre-eclampsia which needs urgent attention. It is to spot this in time that women are checked for swelling at each antenatal visit.

Swelling ankles may be a consequence of having varicose veins and stand-ing for too long. Your legs are likely to ache too. Your ankles may also swell if you are sitting down for a long time in an aircraft or on other long jour-neys, because circulation to your legs becomes more sluggish. This passes some hours after you are up and around again.

If your ankles are swollen all the time, however, and you have swellings elsewhere as well as feeling tired and short of breath, you should see your doctor in case this is a symptom of a kidney or heart disease.

There is also a syndrome called fluid retention syndrome which may be poorly recognised by many doctors. Thousands of women are likely to suffer from it. Usual symptoms are bloating, intense thirst, very frequent need to urinate, tiredness, weepiness, irritability and often an irritable bowel, none of which is associated with the menstrual cycle.

Although the causes are unknown, there is a strong genetic predisposition to the condition with three-quarters of women having a family member with the same problem. About 43 per cent have a diabetic relative and a third have a family history of thyroid problems. Putting on weight, entering the menopause or a stressful life event such as marriage, divorce or pregnancy can all trigger it. Many sufferers bloat up almost instantly after a stressful event, such as a row or a distressing telephone call.

Learning what tends to set off symptoms and finding ways to handle stress differently can be extremely helpful for most women with this syndrome. Losing weight, if overweight, can also help dramatically. However, diuretics, often prescribed for fluid retention, do not help at all.

• Gallstones •

These are stones which may form in the gall-bladder. The gall-bladder stores bile, a liquid secreted by the liver to aid in the digestion of fatty foods in the duodenum, the first part of the intestine. The stone is formed from a tiny bit of cholesterol that has solidified and then other solid bits of matter collect around it. No one knows why they occur or why some people keep getting them; nor why women are four times more likely to develop them than men.

Gallstones are more common as we age but up to a half may be symptom-less because they just lie innocuously in the gallbladder, in which case they do not need treatment. The ones which cause trouble are the ones which move with the bile and get trapped in the bile duct which runs from the gall-bladder to the duodenum, causing a severe pain known as biliary colic. If the bile trapped by the stone stagnates there may be inflammation and infection of the gall-bladder, a condition called cholecystitis.

• Symptoms •

The pain of biliary colic is usually intense and gripping. It can be felt in the upper abdomen, the chest or even in the shoulder blades. The pain may increase in severity (while the gall-bladder tries to push bile past the stone that is blocking the way) and then gradually reduce again if the stone eventually flows on into the duodenum or drops back into the gall-bladder. You may have a fever and even vomit while this is going on. Other symptoms that may indicate problem gallstones include excessive wind and heartburn, particularly after a meal rich in cholesterol.

If the gallstone stays blocking the way of the bile, symptoms of jaundice are likely to develop, with yellowing skin and yellowed whites of the eyes.

• Self-help •

Restrict your intake of fatty foods, such as dairy products and fatty meat, and take antacids for indigestion and wind. If you have an attack of biliary colic, take a pain killer and rest. If the pain is still with you after a couple of hours, call your doctor.

• Investigations •

For intense and recurrent biliary pain, you are likely to be referred for investigation for gallstones by ultrasound or X-ray. An attack of cholecystitis can be treated with antibiotics to cure the infection and you may have to avoid all fat in the diet for a while. If you continue to have problems, particularly with evidence of jaundice, you may be advised to have your gall-bladder removed. If an attack is so severe that you need to be admitted to hospital, removal may be recommended on the spot.

• Treatment •

Fortunately, gall-bladder removal (cholecystectomy) is a relatively simple operation nowadays, which can be carried out under general anaesthetic by laparoscopy (see page 218). The gall-bladder is detached and withdrawn through the navel.

This operation can be carried out safely even if a woman is extremely overweight or pregnant. (Only when there are significant complications need a larger incision in the abdomen be necessary.) More than half of all patients leave hospital within 24 hours; the rest within three days.

• Haemorrhoids •

Also known as piles. See Varicose Veins, page 488.

• Headache •

See Migraine, page 475.

• Heart disease •

We are all led to believe that heart disease is mainly a man's problem. Unfortunately this is just not so. While oestrogen levels appear to offer women protection (oestrogen is thought to play a part in relaxing the coronary arteries and other arteries, improving blood flow to the heart), after the menopause women's risk is equal to men's. Indeed more women overall die of heart and circulatory disease than men: over 150,000 in 1992 compared with 140,000 men. Heart disease kills more women under 65 than breast and cervical cancer added together.

Unfortunately, and tragically in many cases, women with heart disease have not received the same attention as men. Pre-menopausal women are six times less likely to have a heart attack than men but more likely to die from it if they do. There may be several reasons for this. Women themselves may not instantly think of heart attack if they have heart symptoms or angina, whereas men are quite likely to think of this at once. When women go to GPs with their symptoms, only the enlightened may suspect heart disease if they are pre-menopausal and refer them for investigation. Cardiologists may be less likely to carry out full investigations on women and more likely to assume symptoms are psychological.

Recent studies carried out around London and in Northern Ireland have found that women are less likely to have surgery than men, even when just as ill, and American studies have shown women are likely to be diagnosed and treated later in their illness than men. After by-pass surgery they are four times as likely to die as men, quite possibly because their condition was by then more serious or because of other complications.

Fortunately this is all beginning to change and the heart-disease statistics for women are starting to be taken seriously. But until recently, few studies were carried out on women and heart disease at all, leaving us forced to assume that risk factors which apply to men apply to women too. One in five women now has three out of the four main risk factors identified for heart disease: smoking, not getting enough exercise, raised cholesterol levels and high blood pressure.

However, although women appear to be able to tolerate higher cholesterol levels than men, one study has found that they might be more vulnerable to high levels of triglycerides, different blood fats which can also clog arteries. Also, high blood pressure appears to be a stronger risk factor for women than for men.

• What exactly is heart disease? •

Heart disease is any kind of disease which affects the heart, including defects a person may be born with. The principal cause of death is from a heart attack, caused by coronary-artery disease.

In coronary-artery disease, the arteries become narrowed and furred up with fatty deposits. Blood fats are transported in the blood by water-soluble particles called lipoproteins. High-density lipoproteins (HDLs or 'good' cholesterol) are responsible for removing excess cholesterol from the blood and high levels of HDLs are associated with lower incidence of coronary heart disease. Low-density lipoproteins (LDLs or 'bad' cholesterol) pick up cholesterol from fat consumed in the diet and from cells that manufacture it in the body, take what is necessary and leave the rest to circulate in the blood. If there is enough of it left circulating, it starts to permeate artery walls and to begin the furring up process.

A heart attack occurs if one or more coronary arteries become totally blocked, preventing it or them from carrying oxygen and vital nutrients to the heart. A blood clot which blocks off the artery is called a coronary thrombosis. When this happens the heart muscle starts to die, causing a heart attack (a myocardial infarction). Chances of full recovery depend upon how much of the heart has been damaged.

• Symptoms of a heart attack •

A heart attack is usually described as a gripping, unrelenting pain over the chest. The pain may spread to the jaw, neck, arms, back and abdomen and you are likely to experience a severe cold sweat.

• Symptoms of angina •

A heart attack can occur out of the blue. More often there are warning pains which occur before the arteries become completely blocked. This is called angina. Its symptoms are:

- tightness or a dull pain in the chest
- breathlessness, even when you are not exerting yourself
- dizziness
- sweating.

• Investigations •

Obviously you or someone with you should call your doctor at once if you have a heart attack. You also need to see your doctor if you start to suffer from angina as you can be given drugs to bring relief from the pain and guidance on how to reduce your risks of further attacks.

Your GP should check your blood pressure and cholesterol levels. You may also need to go to hospital for other tests, including an arteriogram. This involves dye which shows up on X-ray being put into your arteries to see whether they are severely blocked.

• Drug treatments •

For angina, you can be given drugs called nitrates which dissolve under your tongue and end the pain of the attack very quickly by expanding the arteries. Nitrates are also prescribed in sprays or as patches.

• Surgery •

If you need surgery, there are two main methods.

Angioplasty This is a procedure in which a little balloon catheter is inserted into a major artery in the thigh and directed towards the blockage, at which point it is inflated until it can clear the obstruction.

Bypass surgery This involves taking a healthy vein from the leg and sewing it into the affected coronary artery so as to bypass the blockage.

• After effects •

After surgery, there may well be some psychological after effects. Studies have usually looked at men and found that they suffer considerably from anxiety and depression, and have difficulty returning to their normal lifestyle. Recently, a study of women has shown that women may suffer even greater anxiety and depression after a heart attack and are slower to resume interest in sex.

Research in Edinburgh has shown that having help in dealing with stress, anxiety and depression after a heart attack significantly reduces the risk of suffering another one. The British Heart Foundation has published a self-help manual based on the methods used in Edinburgh and these are available to hospital cardiac departments on request. But an increasing number now run their own rehabilitation programmes which have been found to be very valuable indeed.

However, women are less likely to be referred for rehabilitation, or are less likely to attend, and it is now thought that courses specifically tailored to meet women's different needs are also required.

• Prevention •

1 Eat a healthy diet. Cut down on fats, particularly saturated fats, in your diet, as high levels of fat in the blood, including cholesterol and triglycerides, are implicated in heart disease. Have plenty of fresh fruit and vegetables, oily fish twice a week (fish oils are protective) and olive oil (this is a monounsaturated fat which appears to be protective). Garlic is also good for lowering blood-fat levels.
2 Avoid being overweight. It isn't just what you weigh but your weight distribution that is important. Fat that is centred around the abdomen is associated with a higher risk of heart attack.
3 Give up smoking.
4 Take regular exercise, even if it is just a brisk daily ten-minute walk. Exercise raises HDLs or 'good' cholesterol levels.
5 Drink a little alcohol if you like it – this also raises HDLs – but keep your consumption moderate and within the healthy drinking guidelines (see page 57).

6 Have your blood pressure checked every five years. You should be checked more frequently than this if you are on the contraceptive pill.

7 Try to cut down on too much unpleasant stress in your life. Learn to relax and enjoy life a bit more, if you tend to overwork.

8 Make sure you give and receive affection. A little love and support given and received, whether from a partner, close family or close friends, seems to help keep the heart in better health.

9 Consider HRT. If you are going through or approaching the menopause, talk to your doctor about the benefits of hormone replacement therapy (HRT). It appears to reduce the risk of heart disease after the menopause by half and also helps prevent the central distribution of body fat (that is, fat settling around the stomach) which itself increases risk of heart attacks. It also helps prevent osteoporosis and can counter menopausal symptoms. See Menopause and HRT, page 443. However, some cardiologists still have reservations about its being prescribed routinely post-menopause to reduce heart-attack risk.

• High blood pressure •

High blood pressure is not an especial problem for women but is included here because women may not realise that this condition, which affects far more young men than young women, affects the sexes equally after women have passed the menopause and is a greater risk factor for heart disease in women than men. Pregnancy and the combined contraceptive pill also cause high blood pressure in some women and kidney disease can cause it too. Otherwise it is uncommon before the age of 35. There is a considerable genetic element to whether you are likely to suffer from high blood pressure.

• Symptoms •

About 60 per cent of sufferers do not experience any symptoms. Others may experience headaches, shortness of breath, palpitations, chest pain and some-times swelling of the ankles.

Studies show that half of people with high blood pressure don't know they have it, but even just slightly raised levels increase the risk of heart attack while higher levels also increase the risk of kidney failure and stroke.

• What is high blood pressure? •

Blood pressure refers to pressure of blood in the arteries. The beating heart produces a pressure wave, the peak of which is known as the systolic pressure and the lowest point as the diastolic pressure. Doctors measure both and write it as systolic/diastolic. A young woman might, for example, have a blood pressure of 110/70. As we get older blood pressure tends to increase. If it becomes too high, blood vessels narrow and blood clots may form, causing a heart attack or a stroke.

There isn't one systolic and diastolic figure that signifies normal blood pressure for everyone. Our blood pressure will rise when we are feeling angry, excited, scared or worried. It usually goes down when we are feeling calm and relaxed.

A high blood pressure is one that doesn't go down when we are resting or asleep but remains permanently raised.

Experts believe that 40 per cent of us ought to do something about our blood pressure. Ten to 15 per cent of people may need treatment with drugs as well as making the following lifestyle changes, which an additional 25 per cent of us should also make.

• Self-help •

1 Avoid being overweight. High blood pressure and body weight are directly related.
2 Don't drink too heavily and try to give up smoking as this is a very strong risk factor for a heart attack, although it doesn't in itself raise blood pressure.
3 Take exercise. Exercise of the rhythmic kind, such as walking, jogging, cycling and swimming is good. If you already have high blood pressure, avoid weight-lifting exercises.
4 Take care with every sort of medication. Always be aware that certain cold cures, nasal drops and drugs, such as antidepressants, may increase blood pressure.
5 Try to cut down on stress. Sustained high-stress levels are likely to make blood pressure rise. Relaxation methods, meditation and yoga are worth the general benefits they bring, although their actual effect on blood pressure is uncertain, according to research for the American National Institutes of Health.
6 Reduce your salt intake if you have high blood pressure, but eating less salt does not affect normal blood pressure.
7 Have blood-pressure checks. Ask your GP to check your blood pressure every five years. (You have a right to do this.) If you have been hurrying or are under stress, the reading may come out higher than normal. It is never safe to rely on one blood pressure reading for this reason. If your blood pressure, after a few readings, is found to be at a level just below where treatment might have to be considered, you should be re-checked six months later and at six-monthly intervals.

• Drug treatments •

Drugs, if you need to take them, usually have to be taken for life (along with making the above changes to your lifestyle). The main drugs used to treat high blood pressure are diuretics, beta blockers, calcium antagonists and ACE-inhibitors. Experts claim they are all very safe but they may all have some minor side-effects.

• Incontinence •

There are various causes of incontinence but the two which most often affect women are stress incontinence and urge incontinence.

Stress incontinence   This is a leakage of urine which may occur during sudden physical activities such as coughing, laughing, sneezing or lifting something heavy, all of which put pressure on the bladder. It occurs because support of the bladder neck has become weakened, making the bladder unable to hold on to all its contents in such circumstances. This condition affects an enormous number of women of all ages. The main cause is child-birth which weakens the pelvic floor unless you take steps to prevent it. Stress incontinence is very common after a prolapse (see page 251) which occurs when the pelvic floor relaxes.

You are even more likely to suffer stress incontinence if you are over-weight, have a chronic cough, suffer from constipation, suffer repeatedly from urinary tract infections or have to do a lot of heavy lifting.

Urge incontinence   This is the sudden urgent need to pass urine which is caused by an irritable muscle in the bladder (the detrusor muscle) going into spasm. It is the second most common form of incontinence in women after stress incontinence, although elderly men may also suffer it.

• Self-help •

1 Lose weight if you need to. Excess weight puts extra pressure on the bladder.
2 Practise pelvic-floor exercises. These can cure or considerably improve both conditions for very many women. If you can contract your pelvic

GETTING HELP

If you cannot contract your pelvic-floor muscles without help (up to 30 per cent of women cannot do this at will), or if you have been doing the exercis-es for a couple of months with no success you should see your GP who may refer you to a specialist physiotherapist or put you in touch with a specialist nurse called a continence advisor.

After assessment, you may be given a vaginal cone of the appropriate weight to place in the vagina like a tampon. The sensation of the cone start-ing to fall out makes the pelvic floor muscles contract to hold on to it. The aim is to be able to go about normal daily living, including laughing and coughing, without losing the cone.

If the pelvic floor needs strengthening, specialist physiotherapists may apply vaginal/anal electrodes to stimulate the muscles (creating a prickly sensation), or you can do this at home using a battery-operated muscle stimulation unit. It is necessary to keep going at this for three to six months, so regular visits to the physiotherapist for encouragement and support may be necessary to keep enthusiasm up.

floor without help, try doing ten sets of ten pelvic-floor contractions every day for at least eight weeks. (Physiotherapists recommend doing them every day for life, whether you have stress incontinence or not). Find a position in which you can do the exercise most easily. Some women like to lie on their backs with their knees raised, others may prefer to sit. Squeeze the muscles you would use to stop a flow of urine. Squeeze in slowly for about five seconds, then relax for five seconds before doing the exercise again.

3 Eat lots of fibre Eating plenty of cereals, fresh fruit and vegetables will help prevent any need to strain when you pass stools.

4 Try to give up smoking You are likely to cough less, along with all the other benefits.

5 Bladder training for urge incontinence can be very helpful. Here the aim is to build up the amount of urine you can hold on to and how long you can hold on to it. The problem may not be a full bladder but having got into the habit of going to empty the bladder too frequently, when it is only half full, so that the bladder becomes accustomed to holding only a little at a time and you receive the signal to empty more frequently than you should.

Try increasing the amount of fluid you drink (preferably water) and wait a little longer than you are comfortable before going to pass urine. When you have the urge before time, do pelvic floor exercises or, if these aren't strong enough yet, apply pressure to the perineum (the groin area) by sitting on a rolled up bath towel. Also do something to distract yourself from the desire to pass urine.

6 Resist the urge to wear pads in your pants (you need to learn to rely on yourself) or to cut down on your fluid intake. But drink less tea, coffee, cola and alcohol. The first three contain caffeine which can increase urgency, and alcohol is a diuretic (a drug that increases urine flow).

7 For further information, see Useful Contacts.

• Treatment •

If self-help measures for stress incontinence fail to work and you are really bothered by it you might want to consider an operation to strengthen the pelvic-floor muscles and tighten the neck of the bladder. Many women are horrified by the thought of an operation and would rather soldier on; others are very happy to have had it. For urge incontinence, treatment with a drug called oxybutynin can try to stabilise the irritable bladder. An expected side-effect with oxybutynin is a dry mouth. If you don't get a dry mouth, the treatment is unlikely to work and the dosage may need to be manipulated, within the drug guidelines, until you do get one.

• Irritable bowel syndrome •

Irritable bowel syndrome is the name given to a group of symptoms, a number of which may occur when the bowel muscle stops working properly.

Doctors may refer to it as a functional bowel disorder because the problem is with the way the bowel works but, unlike in inflammatory bowel disorders such as Crohn's and ulcerative colitis, there is no disease or any abnormality that is causing the difficulty.

It is estimated that up to a third of the population may suffer symptoms which would be diagnosed as irritable bowel syndrome if they went to a doctor. Most don't go. However women are more likely to go to their doctor, which is why it is commonly thought that women suffer much more often than men. In reality they only suffer slightly more often and, due to the proximity of the pelvic organs and the bowel, symptoms may worsen during a period or during sex. One in ten people has symptoms severe enough to warrant some kind of medical attention.

• Symptoms •

There are a vast variety of these, which most commonly start between the ages of 15 and 40, although they can occur for the first time at any age. Most sufferers have some of the following:

- Abdominal pain or gripes in the abdomen (caused by the bowel muscle going into spasm).
- Diarrhoea (caused by the muscle moving the contents of the bowel along too quickly).
- Constipation with pain (caused by the muscle working too slowly).
- Alternating diarrhoea and constipation.
- Small pellety stools which may be covered in mucus.
- Wind.
- Bloated feeling in the abdomen.

These main symptoms may be accompanied by others such as an urgent need to empty the bowels occasionally leading to accidents, a feeling that the bowels have not been emptied completely, a need to pass urine very frequently (caused by an irritable bladder), nausea, belching, indigestion, an unpleasant taste in the mouth, rumblings in the stomach, tiredness, irritability and mild depression. Women particularly may suffer backache, headache and painful periods and may find sex painful as well.

• Causes •

Exact reasons for why the bowel muscle should develop problems are unknown. Some doctors think the cause may be lack of fibre in the diet, although this wouldn't explain all symptoms and many sufferers find taking more fibre worsens symptoms. Some believe stress and anxiety may cause it. Certainly, stress and anxiety can have an effect on the bowel and worsen symptoms but it is probably not true that stress causes the problem in the first place.

There is some evidence that in irritable bowel sufferers normal sensation in the bowel becomes heightened and there is currently research interest in a drug that blocks the action of the hormone serotonin which appears to increase sensitivity of the bowel.

• Investigations •

If your symptoms are severe enough to cause you concern, you should see your GP. Very importantly, do tell your GP about your bowel symptoms as well as about any general abdominal pain, or else he may assume the problem is gynaecological and send you off to a gynaecologist instead.

You may need to be referred to a gastroenterologist for investigations to ensure that no bowel disease is present. These may include blood tests, examination of stools for blood, a sigmoidoscopy (where a special telescope is inserted in the anus so that the bowel can be examined) and a barium X-ray. If no problem is found, you may want to consider some of the approaches described below.

• Approaches that may help •

1 Eating more fibre may benefit about a third of sufferers. Try it in the form of cereals, wholewheat bread, fresh fruits and vegetables.
2 Learning to relax can be enormously helpful (see page 41) as stress and anxiety exacerbate the problem.
3 Peppermint oil can relieve many of the symptoms of irritable bowel, including pain from wind. Capsules to swallow are available from pharmacies and health-food stores.
4 Hypnosis may help sufferers learn to control their own gut and therefore vastly reduce symptoms (but hypnosis in which the aim is purely to reduce anxiety and stress is not so effective). A particular technique has been pioneered by a Manchester consultant gastroenterologist, Dr Peter Whorwell. He uses hypnosis to put patients into a relaxed state and encourages them to visualise a scene appropriate to their own need: for example, seeing their gut as a river flowing slowly if they suffer from diarrhoea, or flowing faster if they suffer from constipation. In addition, or if this is difficult, he suggests they put a hand on their stomach and think of the warmth from their hand soothing the gut, taking away spasms and helping to control pain. The prime aim is to teach the brain to control the gut. His laboratory research has shown that these methods really do influence the activity of the gut.

Although his method is not widely available, a number of gastroenterologists in hospitals in the UK have now taken courses with him to learn how to use it.
5 An operation, pioneered by consultant surgeon, Mr Bernard Palmer, at the Lister Hospital in Stevenage, may help sufferers who experience a sense of incomplete emptying of the bowels and who, on rectal examination, are revealed to have prolapsing rectal tissue or asymptomatic piles (piles which don't cause any symptoms). These can irritate the anal sphincter and send it into spasm, affecting the messages it sends to the muscle of the large bowel

which in turn starts behaving oddly. If bands (known as Baron's bands) are put around the excess rectal mucosa to tighten them up, the cycle may cease. In a number of patients, this operation has been sufficient to eliminate symptoms of irritable bowel.

6 Sufferers from irritable bowel syndrome are particularly likely to try complementary medicine, such as homoeopathy, acupuncture, medical herbalism and reflexology. Some may find relief through particular methods, others not.

7 See Further Reading for details of several useful books.

• Lupus •

Correctly called systemic *Lupus erythematosus*, this illness is generally known as lupus. It is an auto-immune disease, meaning a disease in which the body attacks itself in some way. In lupus, the body produces excess antibodies which may accumulate and cause problems in various organs such as the skin, blood vessels, joints, kidneys, brain and lungs.

It first affects mainly young women, particularly in their teens and twenties, and it is relatively rare for lupus to be diagnosed after the age of 45, although many mild cases go undiagnosed altogether and a woman who is diagnosed in her fifties may have had unrecognised symptoms for decades. Women suffer from lupus nine times as often as men and there are an estimated 26 sufferers per 100,000 population in the UK. It is not known what causes the disease.

• Symptoms •

Lupus is a disease which takes varying forms. It can cause acute flare-ups with very noticeable and often unpleasant symptoms or, as mentioned, it may be so mild that it isn't even recognised. It can also come and go altogether. Although lupus can affect very many parts of the body, individual sufferers usually find that most of the problems lupus causes for them are in one area of their body only.

Lupus can affect the skin, causing pink spotty rashes. (It is from this that the name is derived, because the word 'lupus', Latin for wolf, was originally used by physicians to describe certain rashes on the cheek and nose that resembled wolf bites). Lupus sufferers very commonly suffer allergic skin reactions to things, particularly drugs such as penicillin. Many sufferers also have Raynaud's, where the fingers and toes are severely affected by cold (see page 481).

One form of lupus which affects the skin only is known as discoid lupus. Unlike the systemic type, where skin rashes are relatively mild, discoid lupus may cause a severe and scarring rash on the face and scalp and some hair loss. Rarely are other organs affected in any way.

Hair loss also commonly occurs, when there is an active flare-up of the disease. It does, however, grow back although not until some months after the attack is over, as it takes many months for hair to grow.

Most women with lupus have aches and pains in muscles and joints. However, although this can be very painful, the joints are not actually damaged or deformed as in arthritis (although this symptom may lead initially to a misdiagnosis of rheumatoid arthritis). Tendons in the fingers may periodically become inflamed, preventing the fingers from extending fully.

Many sufferers find they are very sensitive to sunlight, coming out in rashes after even minimal exposure, or experiencing more joint pains.

Sharp pains may be experienced in the chest or shortness of breath if the heart and lungs are affected. If the brain is affected, the sufferer may experience depression or possibly have a history of epilepsy. Anaemia is common and kidney disease can occur if antibodies accumulate in the kidneys. When lupus is diagnosed early this can usually be prevented. If not, kidney failure can occur but this is now rather rare.

• Diagnosis and treatment •

Lupus can be diagnosed from blood tests. Kidney function is tested at the same time by urine analysis.

There are various drugs which may be used in the treatment of lupus. Aspirin and non-steroidal anti-inflammatory drugs (NSAIDs) may often be all that is needed if the main symptom is joint pain. Anti-malarial drugs work well when there is both skin and joint disease and also for discoid lupus, but doses have to be carefully calculated because otherwise there is a risk of affecting vision.

Steroids are the mainstay of treatment as these can deal with all lupus symptoms. However these do cause side-effects, such as weight gain, indigestion and mood disturbance and, in long-term treatment, softening of bone and thinning of skin, although to some extent this can be reversed when treatment is gradually brought to a stop.

Some people with lupus develop high blood pressure and this has to be treated with drugs too, otherwise there is a higher risk of kidney damage.

For further information on lupus see Useful Contacts.

• Pregnancy •

In the past, lupus sufferers were advised against pregnancy. This is not the case now. There is no increased risk of suffering a flare-up during pregnancy and the pregnancy itself is usually without extra complications, although there is a slightly higher miscarriage risk. If a woman is having to take steroids for her symptoms, these can safely be continued during pregnancy. However, in the first few months after the baby is born, there is a high likelihood that she will experience a flare-up of her lupus symptoms, the reasons for which are unknown.

• Lymphoedema •

See All About Breasts, page 340.

• Myalgic Encephalomyelitis (ME) •

Myalgic encephalomyelitis means muscle pain affecting the brain, spinal cord and nerves. It can strike at any age although most sufferers are aged 20 to 40 when they first fall ill and a slight majority are women.

It is estimated that there are over 150,000 sufferers in the UK although ME's existence is still a matter of some controversy. Some doctors do not accept it, preferring to diagnose chronic fatigue syndrome, defined as fatigue which has a definite onset, is unexplained, is experienced more than half of the time with adverse effects on both mental and physical functioning and has lasted more than six months. But this may cover a number of conditions whereas the main symptoms of ME are very specific. ME is now recognised as a severely disabling disease by the Department of Health and the Department of Social Security.

• Symptoms •

The major symptoms are:

- a crippling fatigue often brought on by the tiniest exertion
- impaired short-term memory
- severe muscle pain.

These symptoms are essential for a diagnosis of ME. Other possible accompanying symptoms include poor concentration, aching back or neck, shaking legs, blurred vision, hypersensitivity to sound and light, sleep disturbance, smelling strange odours, racing heart, profuse sweating, poor circulation, an irritable bowel and difficulty passing urine. Some people suffer untypical mood changes or develop allergies to chemicals or foods.

• Causes •

Viruses are thought to be responsible in at least 80 per cent of cases and those which so far seem most suspect are enteroviruses (which cause gastric flu, hepatitis and some respiratory infections among other things) and the herpes virus (the strains responsible for chicken pox and glandular fever). Both of these types of viruses are able either to persist in the body or be reactivated a long time after the initial illness is over.

Of course, only a minority who catch the common illnesses they cause ever develop ME.

Most of those who do develop it tend to be very active people or those who drive themselves very hard, and say they were fit and well until they caught one of these illnesses. Too much physical activity while incubating a virus can reduce the body's chances of getting rid of it. It is said that ME also sometimes occurs when someone incubating a virus undergoes an extreme stress or has an immunisation at this time.

The immune system appears to be affected in ME but quite how and with what effects remains uncertain. One study has found the immune system to be over-stimulated, so that it is in effect in a permanent state of fighting foreign bodies: not only the virus but any foreign substances, which could help explain the incidence of allergies. Others have found parts of the immune system to be depressed.

Brain scans clearly show structural abnormalities and abnormalities in blood flow to the brain stem and in the hypothalamus, the part of the brain concerned with temperature control and sleep patterns. There is also evidence of low blood cortisol which could also help explain allergies because cortisol normally suppresses allergic responses.

• Self-help •

1 The single most important self-help remedy is to get plenty of rest, particularly when the illness is in its initial stages. Unfortunately, this is usually the time when normally active people are keen to get back to their usual daily lives and try to do too much. Being overactive at this stage can cause ME to become chronic whereas, given rest and gradual exercise, it could disappear in a few months.

2 Take careful exercise. Exercise should be very gradually built up. It is not a good idea to start a programme of activity prescribed by a well-meaning GP and stick to it, however you are feeling. Graded exercise is often helpful in chronic fatigue syndrome but not in ME. Individuals need to experiment for themselves with only as much physical and mental exercise as they can manage. Initially, even reading or watching television may be too exhausting.

• Treatments •

There are, unfortunately, no treatments which routinely work for everyone, although many approaches have been tried. Only three treatments have been demonstrated in trials to be of benefit:

• magnesium injections (six at weekly intervals, often requiring boosters)
• high doses of evening primrose oil
• high doses of intravenous immunoglobulin (not usually given in the UK).

Although ME is definitely not caused by magnesium deficiency nor does magnesium therapy cure it, treatment with magnesium may help because the symptoms of deficiency do include many common symptoms of ME, such as changes in heart rhythm, palpitations, poor blood circulation and gut disorders. Evening primrose oil may help because it contains an essential fatty acid which has a direct anti-viral approach. Anti-depressants may help some, but only if the symptom of depression is present, and antiviral drugs and calcium antagonists may also be prescribed by doctors to try to reduce muscle pain.

As none of these treatments necessarily helps, many people with ME try alternative therapies. The most popular include homoeopathy, allergy testing and desensitisation, and dietary measures. These include vitamin and mineral supplements; cutting out certain foods thought to adversely affect the immune system (such as sugar, alcohol, wheat, dairy products and processed foods); and going on special diets designed to eliminate candida, a yeast claimed to get out of control and invade various organs if the immune system isn't working.

ME experts believe that if something works for an individual, then it is right for them. But there is no point putting the body through the stress of any method which makes you feel miserable and doesn't seem to achieve anything. Certain elimination diets need to be treated cautiously, as a diet plentiful in all necessary nutrients is essential in any chronic illness.

The charity, Action for ME (see Useful Contacts), can provide information about all the types of treatments described above.

• Outlook •

Estimates on the chances of full recovery from ME range from 20 to 35 per cent within two years. Unfortunately, 20 per cent of sufferers find their condition deteriorates and may become permanently disabled, in wheelchairs or bedbound. The majority, however, is able to learn to manage their illness by resting sufficiently and cutting down on activities.

• Migraine •

Migraine can be a miserable condition. It is suffered by 15 per cent of the population and 65 per cent of sufferers are women. The pain and degree of disability which can be caused by it is horribly underestimated by the unafflicted. One survey of attitudes about migraine found that four out of ten people thought it was often just an excuse given by others to get time off work, and about the same number thought that having a migraine didn't warrant being absent from work.

• Symptoms •

Migraine attacks usually start during childhood or in the teens. A migraine is a severe headache which can last from two hours up to three days and which may be suffered frequently or infrequently. Migraines vary from individual to individual and even from migraine to migraine.

Commonly, there is a warning or prodomal phase which occurs some hours before the headache actually comes on. You may find yourself in a suddenly inexplicable buoyant mood, feel full of energy, have a craving for sweets or sweet foods or feel tired and yawn a lot.

A minority experiences an 'aura' before the headache starts. You may notice a small blind area in the centre of your field of vision which then extends to blur half your vision. You may see flashing sparks or zigzags.

When the headache comes on, the pain may be throbbing or piercing and is usually on one side of the head only. Many migraine sufferers cannot bear light or sound at this time and cannot stand certain smells. You may feel hot or cold and shivery, feel or be sick and suffer from diarrhoea or, occasionally, an increased need to pass urine. Often there is a fleeting sensation of pins and needles, usually on one side of the body, and speech may slur. It can also become hard even to string a sentence together. Most people don't want to eat during a migraine but some sufferers actually have an increased desire for food.

When the headache has gone away, you may feel very weak and drained, often for a day or more.

Headaches which are not migraines are muscle tension headaches, caused by stress, and which are usually experienced across the forehead or at the back or top of the head or on both sides of the head simultaneously. Non-migraine headaches may also occur for other reasons, for instance if you suddenly stop drinking caffeine (caffeine-withdrawal headache) or if you are sensitive to monosodium glutamate in Chinese food. Very rarely is headache the sign of a brain tumour, although most new migraine sufferers fear at first that it is.

• Causes •

These are not fully understand but it is believed that changing levels of the brain chemical serotonin is involved in the mechanism of migraine. Serotonin acts on blood vessels in the brain, narrowing and expanding them, and is also involved in pain-control pathways.

Some complementary health practitioners believe that migraine is a symptom of a masked food allergy: that is, a response to some common food that is eaten almost every day (perhaps bread or potatoes) and not realised to be causing problems.

• Triggers •

Some people cannot explain their migraine at all; others have fairly clear triggers. These include eating certain foods such as, commonly, cheese, chocolate, fried foods or citrus fruits; drinking coffee, tea or red wine; missing meals; exercise; sleep disturbance; taking the contraceptive pill; relaxing (particularly if having a lie-in at weekends); stress. Some women have menstrually related migraines, suffering them only in the week prior to a period or at ovulation.

• Drug treatments •

For many sufferers, taking a pain killer at the start of an attack is sufficient to make it go quickly. If non-prescription pain killers do not work for you, your doctor can prescribe a stronger drug and, if necessary, a drug to stop you being sick (anti-emetic). Some tablets combine the two.

A very powerful migraine treatment which used to be very popular and is still quite widely used is ergotamine. It can be very effective taken early in an attack but can be addictive and should not be used as a main treatment by anyone who has one or more migraine attack a month. If you become dependent on ergotamine, you develop withdrawal symptoms similar to your migraine when you do not take it, leading to more and more ergotamine being taken.

A new treatment which has had a dramatic effect on severe migraine is sumatriptan (Imigran). Unfortunately it is expensive and so likely only to be prescribed by GPs in dire cases. However, migraine experts and members of the support group the British Migraine Association have found that taking half a tablet (50mg instead of 100mg) is just as effective in most cases, and reduces side-effects, such as transient tingling, sensations of warmth and tightness in the chest.

For those who suffer very frequent migraine – severe attacks more than twice a month – preventive therapy may be recommended. Preventive treatments used are beta blockers (drugs which act on blood vessels and lower blood pressure), pizotifen and methysergide (which belong to a group of drugs called 5-HT blockers), calcium channel blockers, which dilate blood vessels in a similar way to beta blockers, clonidine (another high blood pressure drug) and amitriptyline, an antidepressant which can be effective even when no depression is suffered and at lower doses. It is usually a case of trial and error with these drugs, especially as it may take a couple of months before any beneficial effect is seen.

• Self-help •

Many people try acupuncture for migraine, with varying degrees of success. Also possibly helpful are leaves from the feverfew plant. You can take tablets or chew the slightly bitter-tasting leaves (two or three chopped up in a sandwich every day). Tablets or capsules are available from health-food shops and many pharmacies. If you wish to grow the plant, ask your local garden or herb centre where you can get it or contact the British Migraine Association for information.

Most migraine sufferers find it very useful to learn relaxation techniques, as attacks are commonly triggered or worsened by stress.

An aid which many sufferers have found helpful is the Headaid Migraine Reliever, a portable battery-operated machine which stimulates the skull, triggering production of the body's own natural pain-killing chemicals and reducing stress hormones. A trial at the City of London Migraine Clinic found it could reduce the number and duration of migraine attacks. It costs £185 (1994 prices) but if it doesn't work for you you can return it within 30 days for a full refund. See Useful Contacts.

• Osteoarthritis •

Osteoarthritis affects half of all adults, usually later in their lives. Women and men suffer equally but a crucial difference is that for women the usual pattern of the disease is for several joints to become damaged by arthritis whereas only one joint is usually affected in men.

In osteoarthritis the cartilage of the joint affected starts to disintegrate. The process can result from natural wear and tear over the years or it can be precipitated by an injury or by too much strain on a particular joint. Usually it doesn't start occurring till at least the fifties. However an injury, even a forgotten childhood one, could cause arthritis in a single joint, such as the big toe joint, at an early adult age.

• Symptoms •

There is pain and inflammation in the affected joints, but the inflammation is not destructive as in rheumatoid arthritis. Fingers, knees and hips are particularly likely to be affected. (One type of arthritis suffered almost always only by women causes swellings on the finger joints which start as soft raised areas and then become bony.)

At first there may be only slight stiffness in affected joints but gradually pain develops. Depending upon the site of the arthritis, there may be pressure on nerves causing pain to radiate down the arms or through the buttocks and down the legs. The pain can sometimes be enormously disabling and mentally all-consuming, unless a sufferer learns techniques for coping.

• What to do •

X-rays can confirm whether you are suffering from osteoarthritis. Aspirin or paracetamol may deal with the pain if it is not too severe. If it is, the non-steroidal anti-inflammatory drugs can usually help. These should not be taken long-term unless a drug to prevent the damage they may do to the lining of the stomach is prescribed as well. However, it may be preferable to try non-drug methods of reducing pain and to keep these drugs for short-term use in particularly painful flare-ups.

There is a self-help tape for beating chronic pain, based on the psychological approach taught to chronic pain sufferers at the world-famous Walton Centre in Liverpool devoted to treating and researching pain.

TENS MACHINES

TENS (transcutaneous electrical nerve stimulation) machines are portable devices smaller than a personal stereo, and run on a low-voltage battery. You put two or four self-adhesive electrodes over the parts of the body you want to treat and then press a button on the machine to receive a pulsed current which is like a tingling sensation. The current stimulates the body to produce endorphins, the body's natural pain killers.

Machines can be bought (most cost a little under or somewhat over £100) or may be borrowed from some pain clinics. Some people experience a beneficial effect when the machine is used just for half an hour a day, others safely use them for up to eight hours a day. For more information phone the TENS Careline or write: see Useful Contacts.

The tape includes relaxation instructions and techniques for changing thoughts and feelings about pain and pain behaviours. See Useful Contacts.

Exercise should be avoided when joints are acutely swollen or inflamed but it is a good idea at other times to keep the joint as mobile as possible. Gentle exercise that does not strain or jolt the joints is best. Other simple means of pain relief, such as ice packs, heat pads or hot water bottles wrapped in towels can be comforting when pain is acute.

Massage, osteopathy, chiropractic and the Alexander Technique may all be helpful. Some sufferers swear by the TENS machine (see above).

If hips are affected by osteoarthritis and the disintegration of the joint is severe, hip replacement (with joints of metal or metal and plastic) can be simply performed with very beneficial effects. However, the NHS waiting lists for this operation may be dauntingly long.

• Osteoporosis •

Osteoporosis is thinning of the bone to a degree that causes fragility and easy fracture. It is estimated that one in three women who has passed the menopause suffers from it. But it isn't just a disease that may come with increasing age. Women in their twenties, thirties and forties may also sometimes suffer from it. Men can suffer it too, although far less frequently than women.

Bone mass increases through childhood until it reaches its peak strength between the ages of 25 and 35. Sufficient calcium intake is important for creating strong bone. After the age of 35 bone density starts to decline and becomes particularly rapid after the menopause because of loss of oestrogen with its beneficial effects on bone.

• Women at especial risk •

Women most at risk of osteoporosis are those who:

- Had their menopause before the age of 45.
- Had a hysterectomy before they reached the menopause.
- Have had no periods for prolonged lengths of time because of hormonal irregularities; for example, as caused by polycystic ovarian syndrome.
- Have suffered in the past from anorexia or bulimia, particularly if severe enough to have caused their periods to stop.
- Had periods that stopped as a result of over-exercise.
- Have been on steroids for a long time. (They appear to weaken bone.)
- Smoke or drink a lot (alcohol prevents calcium absorption while tobacco may lower oestrogen levels).

• Symptoms •

Usually the first symptom is a broken wrist, hip or vertebra which occurs in a minor injury or fall. A fracture in these circumstances after the age 50 is highly likely to mean osteoporosis because a little bump or trip does not break bones if they are healthy.

Another sign is loss of height. One survey of 500 women over 50 found that nearly a third had lost height in recent years but only a fifth had thought to mention the fact to their doctor. If the bones in the spine weaken, they may squash together, making you look shorter and also curving the spine so that you have a slight stoop. When this happens, you may sometimes, but by no means always, experience backache. If the curve is pronounced, however, you may develop difficulties in breathing because the ribs get squashed.

• Prevention •

1 Hormone replacement therapy (HRT). The National Osteoporosis Society believes very firmly that all women should consider HRT at the menopause (whether naturally or artificially induced), regardless of whether they have menopausal symptoms or not. (See page 446.) Women who start taking HRT soon after the menopause and continue for at least five years more than halve their risk of suffering a fracture. It is effective even if not started until 11 or 15 years after the menopause.

   Most women should be able to take HRT if they want to but for some it may not be suitable. You should discuss it with your GP. However, as not all GPs are up on the research or are not in favour of it as a routine prescription at the menopause, you may need to arm yourself with further information. The National Osteoporosis Society will be very helpful: see Useful Contacts. If you cannot take HRT, following the advice below is particularly important.

2 Have plenty of calcium in your diet. Research now shows that not only is sufficient calcium important when we are young and bone is growing but sufficient calcium later in life can also prevent loss of bone. The National Osteoporosis Society recommends 1000mg a day up until the age of 45, then 1500mg daily if you are not on HRT. Pregnant and breast-feeding women need at least 1200mg a day. Taking calcium through diet is better than taking a supplement, but you may wish to add a supplement as well. See under Calcium, page 18, for details of calcium-rich foods.

3 Take regular exercise to help keep your bones strong. Weight-bearing exercise such as walking, dancing and playing tennis is what you want for this purpose. Exercise also helps the body absorb calcium better.

4 Try to give up smoking if you are a smoker and cut down on alcohol. Women who smoke 20 cigarettes a day throughout adulthood have a 5 to 10 per cent deficit in bone density by the time they reach the menopause. However the picture for alcohol is not so entirely bleak. One study has shown that a moderate amount of alcohol can actually be beneficial for bone density.

5 Ask your GP to arrange a bone scan if you are at high risk of osteoporosis (for example if you had a premature menopause or have had to take steroids for a long time). A bone scan shows bone density. Unfortunately

there aren't that many machines available in the UK as yet but it is now government policy that access to DEXA (dual-energy X-ray absorptiometry) should be improved. At present most machines are in the private sector and a scan may cost between £30 and £250. However, there is still some controversy over how effective these machines are in detecting fracture risk.

• Treatment •

Spinal osteoporosis may be treated with a drug called etidronate. It is given in a 14-day cycle followed by 76 days of calcium supplementation. This three-month cycle has to be carried on for at least three years. Studies show that it can increase bone mass in the spine and reduce the likelihood of further spinal fractures in women with osteoporosis. It also appears to be able to prevent bone loss at the hip, although not to increase bone there, but it doesn't seem to have any role in preventing wrist fractures. The major downside of taking it is that the tablets must be taken two hours before or after food (that is, in the middle of four hours without food), otherwise it will not be absorbed properly.

Another drug which can also increase bone mass slightly is calcitonin, a natural hormone derived from salmon or eels. It also requires supplementation with calcium. Unfortunately it has to be administered daily by injection, although a nasal spray version is currently being developed.

Two other treatments which have not been highly successful and which need extremely careful usage are anabolic steroids, which can increase bone density but cause rather a lot of undesirable side-effects, and sodium fluoride, which is supposed to increase bone density (and needs calcium supplementation) but at too high doses may increase risk of fractures.

Physiotherapy can be important to to improve mobility and relieve pain. Some sufferers find acupuncture helpful.

For up-to-date advice on self-help and on what treatments are on offer, write to the National Osteoporosis Society for details of their booklets on osteoporosis, HRT and the menopause, hysterectomy and HRT, exercise, physiotherapy and osteoporosis in men. See Useful Contacts.

• Piles •

See Varicose Veins: Haemorrhoids, page 488.

• Raynaud's •

This is a disorder of the circulation (variously known as Raynaud's phenomenon, Raynaud's Disease and Raynaud's syndrome but most usually nowadays just as Raynaud's) in which the blood supply to the fingers and toes and sometimes to the ears and nose is badly affected. A spasm of the small arteries serving the extremities causes restriction of the blood flow, with a resultant lack of oxygen.

Nine out of ten Raynaud's sufferers are women and are usually in their teens or early twenties when they first notice symptoms, although Raynaud's can occur for the first time at any age. One in ten women will suffer it at some point in their lives. There is probably some hormonal connection, as puberty is often the time when symptoms first develop and symptoms tend to be worse around the time of ovulation, while during pregnancy and after the menopause they tend to improve. Raynaud's isn't necessarily a life sentence. Most teenagers grow out of it.

• Symptoms •

The affected extremities first become numb and turn white, then blue once all the available oxygen is used up, then red when the spasm is over and more blood reaches the tissues. The whole process can be very painful, lasting from a few minutes to a few hours and with an unpleasant or painful tingling and burning sensation as circulation returns.

• Triggers for attacks •

Exposure to cold is particularly often the trigger for attacks but experiencing any dip downward in temperature can do it, for instance when moving from a warm room to a cooler one. Putting a hand in the fridge or under a cold tap can easily trigger an attack.

Emotional stress or anxiety can exacerbate the problem. Certain other physical conditions such as hardening of the arteries (arteriosclerosis), clots in the blood vessels (thrombosis) and rheumatoid arthritis can also trigger Raynaud's. Taking certain drugs such as beta blockers for high blood pressure or angina, or ergotamine, present in some migraine treatments, may set Raynaud's off or worsen it.

• Scleroderma •

A small number of sufferers from Raynaud's may be at especial risk of the condition progressing further and developing into scleroderma (literally meaning hardening of the skin), a disease of the connective tissue which can affect both the skin and the internal organs.

Scleroderma can be suffered mildly or severely. In the mild form, which affects 60 per cent of sufferers, the skin on the hands and feet becomes stiff, tight and shiny and there may be some problems with swallowing and eating. In the severe form, known as diffuse scleroderma, much of the skin and the whole of the digestive system may be affected. In some cases there is a degree of calcinosis (calcium deposits which may stick up from under the skin), ulceration and extremely poor blood circulation.

Although scleroderma cannot be cured, there are many treatments which can alleviate specific symptoms effectively, especially if the disease is detected early. There are two tests which can show whether someone with Raynaud's is at risk of developing scleroderma: a blood test to check for circulating anti-nuclear antibodies and an examination of the small blood vessels at the base of a nail. These tests can be organised through your GP.

• Self-help •

If symptoms of Raynaud's are mild, keeping warm may be all the treatment you need. In general, keeping warm is extremely important indeed. As far as possible you should try to avoid sudden changes in temperature and keep hands and feet warm all the time, for example with the aid of small portable hand and foot-warmers, heated car seats, thermal underwear and socks, and glove liners as necessary. The rest of the body needs to be kept warm too because the warmth of the extremities depends upon how warm the main organs are.

Trials have shown that extracts from the ancient *Ginkgo biloba* tree appear to increase blood flow to the extremities in some people with Raynaud's. *Ginkgo biloba*-leaf extract is available from health food shops. Oil of evening primrose oil has also been found helpful by many.

If you are a smoker, do try your hardest to stop. Smoking further impedes blood circulation.

• Treatments •

In more severe cases of Raynaud's it is especially important to do all you can to reduce the number of attacks suffered, as repeated episodes of oxygen star-vation can eventually damage the tissues and in the worst cases can lead to gangrene. There are now a lot of new drugs available which can dilate the blood vessels without all the adverse side-effects that used to accompany older drugs used before. These drugs, called vasodilators, include calcium-channel blockers, ACE inhibitors and prostaglandins. If you are prescribed one of these and it doesn't work, it is worth trying another one, as different types of drugs appear to suit different people.

For anyone who suffers very numerous attacks and is at high risk of gan-grene, or where gangrene has already started to set in, intravenous treatment with vasodilators can help enormously. Some doctors still think, erroneously, that amputation is the only option if gangrene has set in, so it is very impor-tant to ensure that intravenous vasodilators are tried before any such drastic step is taken.

Sometimes an operation called a sympathectomy may improve circulation to the feet. A sympathectomy is the surgical division of sympathetic nerve fibres, part of the nervous system which controls unconscious bodily func-tions. The sympathetic nerves to the feet lie in the back and if these are cut the arteries may relax and blood circulation improve. A similar operation on the neck, where the sympathetic nerves serving the hands and face lie, unfortunately doesn't seem to improve circulation and is usually not to be recommended.

• Rheumatoid arthritis •

Rheumatoid arthritis is a chronic disease in which the body becomes allergic to the lining of the joints, called the synovial membrane, which becomes inflamed and swollen. It is one of the auto-immune diseases, where the body attacks itself.

Rheumatoid arthritis affects about five women for every two men. It tends to develop after the age of 30 (although there is a form which affects children, known as Still's Disease). Three quarters of sufferers are likely to be aged between 25 and 65.

Incidence of rheumatoid arthritis may be decreasing. One large GP study of 45- to 64-year-old women found almost half as many currently affected by rheumatoid arthritis as in the years between 1955 and 1960 when a similar study was carried out. Symptoms were also found to be less severe.

• Symptoms •

The symptoms of rheumatoid arthritis can be extremely unpredictable, flaring up and then disappearing for weeks, months or years. Usually the finger joints are affected first and you may notice pain, tenderness and stiffness. This may then spread to the knees, elbows, ankles, shoulders and hips. However, it is equally possible for the other joints to be affected first and the fingers last. Hips are the least often affected.

Sometimes the stiffness which is worst in the morning may wear off quite quickly; at other times it may not be quick to disappear. Whenever the condition is acute, there is likely to be fever, loss of appetite, tiredness, risk of anaemia and a general feeling of not being well. The swollen inflamed joints all become extremely painful to touch.

Deterioration occurs most quickly in the first two years of having the disease (which makes it important to try and diagnose it early). All of the joints may become deformed, as the inflammation attacks tissue, cartilage, bone and muscle and eventually may destroy the joint. Deformity is most obvious in the fingers. Where muscle wastage or destruction occurs, there may be complete loss of control of movement and, if the disease hasn't been arrested by any means, a sufferer may become severely crippled.

• Diagnosis and drug treatments •

Rheumatoid arthritis should be diagnosed as early as possible because drugs commonly used in treatment have little effect on the course of the disease if given too late. As most deterioration occurs in the first two years and only slowly thereafter, the aim is to start treatment before two years have elapsed, when it might be possible to reverse decline. There are a number of early referral clinics in the UK for this reason.

It is important that the diagnosis of rheumatoid arthritis is made by a rheumatologist. One UK study found that 40 per cent of people referred early did not definitely have rheumatoid arthritis and therefore risked unnecessary treatment. Blood tests, X-rays and urine analysis are amongst the initial investigation methods.

The main treatment in orthodox medicine is with the slow-acting anti-rheumatic drugs (SAARDs) which include methotrexate, sulphasalazine, gold, penacillamine and azathioprine. These all carry risks of various side-effects, such as auto-immune complications or effects on the eyes or liver, and patients prescribed them have to be monitored carefully and have regular blood tests. Methotrexate seems to have fewer adverse effects and to be more effective. However, this drug and azathioprine increase the risk of infertility and so must be used with care in younger women.

Unfortunately, if treatment with these drugs is started late (after the first two years of symptoms), they are unlikely to be able to halt the march of the disease much at all, with the result that up to 80 per cent of patients with symptoms severe enough to warrant treatment from hospital specialists are suffering moderate or severe disability after 20 years.

It would seem that, to be effective as a means of long-term suppression, SAARDs need not only to be started early but may need to be given continuously throughout the course of the disease (although, for unknown reasons, in some patients they cease to have any beneficial effect after a couple of years).

However, within two years there is a high discontinuation rate with these drugs (except methotrexate) because of apparent lack of efficacy or adverse side-effects. With methotrexate, 65 per cent of those prescribed it are still likely to be taking it two years later, and 50 per cent after five years. Even so, there is no certainly that the SAARDs can achieve the improvements that were once hoped for them.

Other drugs commonly prescribed to help relieve pain are aspirin, which reduces inflammation as well as pain, and non-steroidal anti-inflammatory drugs. However, these can all irritate the stomach so, if used very frequently, should be balanced with a drug to protect the gastrointestinal tract (such as misoprostol or an H2 antagonist). Low-dose long-term tricyclic antidepressants may also help relieve pain. Some doctors may still prescribe systemic steroids in the short term. However, these can have nasty side-effects and, in the view of many, shouldn't be prescribed to young women. However researchers in Bristol have found that low-dose steroids can prevent, slow or halt bone damage in half of all sufferers, so steroids may come back into more general favour again.

One treatment possibility being explored is therapy with the monoclonal anti-TNF antibody. (TNF is a cytokine, part of the body's defence system which turns on inflammation. Monoclonal antibodies are synthetic forms of antibodies.) However, despite the raised hopes when some success with this treatment was first announced in 1994, most researchers are cautious because TNF is unlikely to be the cause of rheumatoid arthritis; and suppressing it, while having the effect of reducing inflammation, may not actually prevent joint destruction. Several different molecules in the joints are being targeted for monoclonal antibody therapy by researchers world-wide, and it may turn out that some are involved in rheumatoid arthritis.

Another possibility is that photosensitising drugs, compounds which can be concentrated in target tissues where they remain inactive until exposed to (laser) light, may be of use to treat auto-immune diseases. To date, these have been used mainly in advanced cancers but it is now suggested that overactive inflammatory processes in arthritic joints could possibly be targeted by this means.

Also exciting interest is a treatment with oral collagen (an important body protein) in the form of an orange drink. American researchers found, in a small study, that the condition reversed completely after three months of daily drinks. They are now running larger trials.

• Non-drug treatments •

Physiotherapy can be very helpful for sufferers and enable them to retain some movement and use of affected joints. Exercises devised to suit each individual, ice packs, heat pads and hydrotherapy (exercise in heated pools) may all be used to help achieve this. Also extremely important is rest, especially whenever there is an acute flare-up of a joint. Splints to be worn round the affected joint at night and maybe through the day may be recommended at these times.

Many sufferers may discover drugs don't suit them and find regular physiotherapy gruelling. They prefer to find their own ways for achieving relief, with a third of chronic sufferers trying complementary therapies. In one study of patients by rheumatologists at a London teaching hospital, over half who had tried acupuncture, osteopathy, homoeopathy or herbal medicine said they had benefited.

Manipulating diet is an approach tried by many sufferers. Eating a diet low in saturated fat, refined sugars and refined starches, and high in whole-grains, vegetables and fibre is claimed by many to help reduce symptoms. Taking fish oils or evening primrose oils daily for at least six months may reduce pain and swelling. Some sufferers may find improvement in symptoms from taking tablets containing the antioxidant nutrients selenium and vitamins A, C and E.

For pain relief the use of TENS (transcutaneous electrical nerve stimulation) machines may be helpful (see page 478). For details, and other further information, see Useful Contacts.

• Rosacea •

See page 108.

• Thyroid disorders •

These problems are quite common and are usually caused by disturbances in the immune system. An underactive or an overactive thyroid gland each affect about two in every 100 people, but women are ten times more likely to have an underactive thyroid than men. The thyroid gland produces hormones that are needed for numerous bodily processes.

Symptoms of an underactive thyroid   These usually include weakness, dry skin, coarseness of the skin, fatigue, slowed-down speech, swollen eyelids, feeling cold, failure to sweat much and cold skin. Other common or possible symptoms include thick tongue, coarsened hair, weight gain, hair loss, bloodless lips, shortness of breath, loss of appetite and a hoarse voice.

Symptoms of an overactive thyroid   Most common symptoms are nervousness and edginess, sudden mood changes, swollen neck, a tendency to sweat, feeling hot, palpitations, tiredness, weight loss, fast beating heart, shortness of breath and increased appetite. Eye problems (such as blurring of vision, double vision), swollen legs, diarrhoea and weight gain may also occur. Women often find they start blushing extensively. When eyes protrude or become staring, along with other symptoms above, this is known as Graves disease.

• Diagnosis •

Your doctor will refer you for tests. These are likely to include blood tests to check thyroid function, a radioactive iodine scan which identifies thyroid overactivity, and probably an electrocardiogram, to check heart activity. For an overactive thyroid, liver function may also be tested.

• Treatment •

For underactive thyroid   Treatment involves the replacement of the thyroid hormone thyroxine. It is usually for life but as it is a natural hormone which is being replaced there should be no side-effects. Symptoms will return if the dose is too low.

For overactive thyroid   Treatment involves drugs, surgery or radioactive iodine. One of these methods may be more suitable than another for particular individuals, but often doctors have their own preferences too.

There are a number of drugs which can help stabilise an overactive thyroid, some with more side-effects than others. They may need to be taken for just weeks or maybe years, according to the degree of the problem.

If the thyroid swelling is very large, part of the gland may be removed surgically but this has to have been preceded by drug treatment.

Radioactive-iodine treatment is radioactive iodine given as a drink. The iodine is taken up by a number of the thyroid cells (iodine is necessary for the production of thyroxine; see above) and these are then destroyed by the radioactivity, reducing the output of thyroxine. Some doctors calculate how much to give so that there is the greatest chance of thyroid function returning to normal while others prefer to knock out the thyroid function completely and give thyroxine therapy for life.

• Further information •

Learning you have a thyroid disorder is likely to be alarming and treatment options and possible side-effects may initially seem daunting. See Further Reading for a very helpful book.

• Toxic shock syndrome •

Toxic shock syndrome is a very rare illness but it is potentially fatal very quickly. It is caused by a common type of bacteria called *Staphylococcus aureus* which lives without causing problems on the skin, in the nose, armpit or vagina in a large minority of the population. Rarely, however, certain strains may produce a particular toxin which triggers a massive attack on the immune system. Only about 18 people a year in the UK suffer toxic shock syndrome however, because most people are able to produce antibodies against the toxin.

Although toxic shock syndrome can affect women, men and children, often as a result of infection following burns, stings or surgery, half of all cases are in women using tampons. However tampons do not cause toxic shock and your risks are tinier than minute if they are used correctly.

• Symptoms •

Symptoms are sudden high fever (over 102 °F or 39 °C), vomiting, diarrhoea, sore throat, aching muscles, dizziness, feeling faint and a rash that looks like sunburn. If left untreated for 24 hours, heart and kidney failure can occur.

• What to do •

Toxic shock syndrome is a medical emergency and you must contact a doctor immediately. If you are using a tampon, remove it at once. If treated early enough, antibiotics can cure the infection. Other drugs may be prescribed if any complications have occurred. If you have been using tampons, do not use them again unless your doctor approves this.

It is thought that the increased risk with tampon use is linked with the absorbency of the tampon. You should never use a tampon that is more absorbent than you need (to avoid having to change it too often) and you should never leave it in place for more than six hours, unless instructions by the manufacturers supplied with the packet allow use overnight.

• Varicose veins •

A varicose vein arises because of some defect in one of the valves that help blood flow from the legs back to the heart. If a valve doesn't work properly, there is a back-flow of blood, causing the affected vein to dilate to cope and gradually its elasticity is lost. As it expands, it puts pressure on other valves, stopping them from working properly and increasing the problem. The vein eventually becomes varicosed, with a bluish-black, knotted appearance.

Valves are often damaged by thrombosis (blood clots) in the vein that may occur after childbirth, operations or accidents, but damage may also occur for no known reason. Women are much more likely to suffer from them than men and a susceptibility to them can be inherited. They often first appear or may worsen during pregnancy, when the veins around the vulva are quite likely to swell too. Varicose veins of the anus are called haemorrhoids or piles. They usually occur if you have to strain to pass stools, putting pressure on the veins. They are very common towards the end of pregnancy and after birth, when the size of the uterus impedes blood flow from the rectum.

• Symptoms •

Varicose veins   Twisted, swollen blue veins are visible under the skin, usually on the calves and inner side of the thigh. If you lie down and put your leg in the air, they probably disappear because all the blood flows out of them. You may find your ankles swell and your legs ache if you have been standing for a long time.

Haemorrhoids   Symptoms include soreness around the anus and often a little bleeding when you pass stools. If the haemorrhoids prolapse, they can be felt or seen outside the anus. They feel a bit like a little bunch of grapes. If they get twisted outside the anus (strangulated haemorrhoids) they cause extremely severe pain.

• Self-help for varicose veins •

1 Don't stand for longer than necessary, but take plenty of exercise so that the muscles in your legs keep pumping the blood back to your lungs.
2 Whenever you have a chance to relax, put your feet up. If your feet are higher or at the same height as your heart, blood will be able to return along the veins from your legs to your heart without having to defy gravity and therefore putting pressure on the dilated veins.
3 In bed, rest your heels on pillows or cushions or raise the foot of the bed about 30cm (12in) above the head by putting blocks or some other firm support underneath it.
4 Lose weight, if you need to. Being overweight doesn't cause varicose veins but it makes surgical treatment more difficult should you need it.
5 Ask your GP whether support stockings would be appropriate for you. If so, these can be prescribed. Support stockings can help relieve discomfort because by compressing the swollen veins on the surface of the leg, they help return the blood to where it can be carried back to the heart. You should walk a lot while wearing them, as this helps the stockings do their work, and keep your feet up when you aren't moving around. Take the stockings off at night but still sleep with your feet raised, to prevent blood pooling again.

• Help for haemorrhoids •

1 Try to push any prolapsed haemorrhoids back up into position. If you cannot do this or there is pain, your doctor should do it. See your doctor if there is any bleeding, as there can be other more serious causes which need eliminating.

2 Take more fibre in your diet to prevent constipation. Increase your intake of cereals, wholemeal bread, fruits and vegetables, and drink plenty of fluids.

3 Ask your doctor to prescribe a cream or suppository to make the area around the anus less painful, if necessary.

• Treatments •

Varicose veins   There are two main types of treatment used if treatment is necessary. One involves injecting a chemical solution into the vein to produce a controlled amount of inflammation which in turn will lead to the formation of scar tissue that should block the back-flow of blood through the vein. This can be done on an out-patient basis.

Surgery is the other method used, usually when varicose veins are more extensive. Either the vein is stripped out or it is separated and tied off. The procedure can be carried out under local or general anaesthetic and many hospitals allow you to go home the same day.

You will need to wear bandages for a while and it will be some weeks before all the discomfort disappears when you walk, although it is important to get moving as soon as possible after the operation.

Unfortunately, treatment doesn't stop more varicose veins developing. This happens to about one in five sufferers after treatment.

Haemorrhoids   Injections can be given to shrink haemorrhoids. In very severe cases, surgery can be carried out, as described above.

USEFUL CONTACTS

Subjects are listed in A–Z order within the sections where they are mentioned in the book.

Please send a large SAE if writing, as many organisations are charities with only modest funding.

Part I: Staying Healthy

Acupuncture

British Medical Acupuncture Society
Newton House, Newton Lane,
Lower Whitley, Warrington,
Cheshire WA4 4JA
Tel 01925 730727
Can provide names of medical doctors who have trained in acupuncture.

The Council for Acupuncture
179 Gloucester Place,
London NW1 6DX
Tel 0171 724 5756
Register of traditional acupuncturists.

Alcohol

Alcohol Concern
275 Gray's Inn Road,
London WC1X 8QF
Tel 0171 833 3471
Ground Floor, 4 Dock Chambers,
Bute Street, Cardiff CF1 6AG
Tel 01222 488000

Alcoholics Anonymous
Local groups are listed under Alcohol in phone directories, or you can contact the head office in York on 01904 644026.

Alexander Technique

Society of Teachers of the Alexander Technique (STAT)
20 London House, 266 Fulhan Road,
London SW10 9EL

Aromatherapy

Aromatherapy Organisations Council
3 Latymer Close, Braybrooke,
Market Harborough,
Leicester LE16 8LN
Tel 01858 434242

Chiropractic

British Chiropractic Association
29 Whitley Street,
Reading, Berks RG2 OEG
Tel 01734 757557
Enclose a £1 cheque for a register copy or ask for information over the phone.

Complementary Medicine

Institute for Complementary Medicine
PO Box 194, London SE16 1QZ
Ask for a list of local approved practitioners of the therapy you are seeking.

Eyes

Bates Association of Great Britain
Friars Court, 11 Tarmount Lane,
Shoreham by Sea,
West Sussex BN43 6RQ

Corneal Laser Centre
St James Infirmary, Leeds, and
Clatterbridge Hospital, Wirral
Tel 01484 688118

Royal College of Ophthalmologists
17 Cornwall Terrace,
London NW1 4QW

Feet

The Society of Chiropodists
53 Welbeck Street,
London W1X 7HE
Tel 0171 486 3381

Podiatry Association
Swaynes Cottage, Fore Street,
Weston, Hertfordshire SG4 7AS

Hair

Hairline International
Lyons Court, 166a High Street,
Knowle, West Midlands B93 OLY

Homeopathy

British Homoepathic Association
27a Devonshire Street,
London W1N 1RJ
Tel 0171 935 2163
Can provide a list of medically qualified homoeopaths.

Society of Homoeopaths
2 Artizan Road,
Northampton NN1 4HU
Tel 01604 21400

Osteopathy

General Council and Register of
Osteopaths
56 London Street, Reading,
Berks RG1 4SQ
Tel 01734 576585/566260

Plastic Surgery

British Association of Aesthetic Plastic
Surgeons (BAAPS)
Royal College of Surgeons,
35-43 Lincoln's Inn Fields,
London WC2A 3PN
Tel 0171 636 4864

National Hospital for Aesthetic Plastic
Surgery
Bromsgrove, Worcester,
Tel 01527 575123
Telephone information service in the form of a recorded message on all the cosmetic procedures they offer. Phone switchboard on number above for the number of the procedure you are interested in.

Self-help Associations

Patients Association
8 Guilford Street, London WC1N 1DT
Tel 0171 242 3460
Organisation that puts the patient's point of view. Holds details of organisations and support groups for different disabilities and illnesses.

Shiatsu

Shiatsu Society
5 Foxcote, Wokingham,
Berks RG11 3PG
Tel 01734 730836

Skin

The National Eczema Society
163 Eversholt Street,
London NW1 1BU
Tel 0171 388 4097

The Psoriasis Association
7 Milton Street,
Northampton NN2 7JG

Sleep

Medical Advisory Service
Insomnia Helpline 0181 884 9874
(5–10pm, Mon–Fri)

Teeth

British Society for Mercury-free
Dentistry
Flat 1, Welbeck House
62 Welbeck Street,
London W1M 7HB
Tel 0171 486 3127

Missing Teeth Clinic
Eastman Dental Hospital,
Grays Inn Road, London WC1

British Dental Health Foundation
Eastlands Court, St Peter's Road,
Rugby, Warwickshire CV2l 3QP

Tranquillisers

Council for Involuntary Tranquilliser
Addiction
Cavendish House, Brighton Road,
Waterloo, Liverpool L22 5NG
Tel helpline: 0151 949 0102

Working Conditions

London Hazards Centre
3rd Floor, 308 Grays Inn Road,
London WC1X
Tel 0171 837 5605

PART II: Emotional and Mental Health

Bereavement

The Compassionate Friends
6 Denmark Street, Bristol BS1 5DQ
Tel 0117 929 2778
*Bereaved parents can offer support to others.
Local branches.*

Cruse
126 Sheen Road, Richmond,
Surrey TW9 1UR
Tel 0181 940 4818
*Branches throughout Britain offering advice,
information, social support and counselling
to bereaved people.*

National Association of Widows
Neville House, 14 Waterloo Street,
Birmingham B2 5TX
Tel 0121 643 8348
*Information, advice and practical and emo-
tional support for widows. Local branches.*

Carers' Support

Carers National Association
20 Glasshouse Yard,
London EC1A 4JN
Tel 0171 490 8818
Carers' helpline 0171 490 8898
*Offers practical advice and emotional sup-
port to anyone looking after a person who
needs full-time care: child or adult.*

Complementary Medicine

See Institute for Complementary
Medicine, page 491

Counselling (see also Marriage Guidance and Counselling)

British Association for Counselling
(BAC)
37a Sheep Street, Rugby,
Warwickshire CV21 3BX
Tel 01788 78328

Depression

Association for Postnatal Illness
25 Jerdan Place, London SW6 IEA
Tel 0171 386 0868

Depression Alliance
PO Box 1022, London SE1 7QB
Tel 0171 721 7672
*Charity offering support and information,
run by sufferers and carers.*

Depressives Anonymous
36 Chestnut Avenue, Beverley,
Humberside HU17 9QU
Tel 01482 860619
*Telephone number is for information, in
office hours, not a helpline.*

The Manic-Depressive Fellowship
13 Rosslyn Road, Twickenham,
Middlesex TW1 2AR
Tel 0181 892 2811
A self-help network for sufferers and families.

Meet-a-Mum Association (MAMA)
14 Willis Road, Croydon,
Surrey CRO 2XX
Tel 0181 655 0357

Seasonal Affective Disorder Association (SADA)
PO Box 989, London SW7 2PZ

The Samaritans
17 Uxbridge Road, Slough,
Berks SL1 1SN
The Samaritans have listening services available all around the country 24 hours a day every day of the year. Anyone who feels despairing or suicidal and needs to talk can ring at any time. Local numbers can be found in phone directories.

Eating Disorders

Eating Disorders Association
Sackville place, 44 Magdalen Street,
Norwich, Norfolk NR3 1JE
Helpline 01603 62 1414
Can offer advice to sufferers and families about the condition and how to find help, and recommend reading materials. Also runs a network of self-help groups.

Humanistic Psychotherapies

Association for Humanistic Psychology Practitioners (AHPP)
l4 Mornington Grove,
London E3 4NS
Tel 0181 983 1492
Supply a membership directory. The association advises contacting several practitioners to discuss your needs and to find out what is offered. This may be done by phone or by an initial meeting which many offer free.

Gestalt Centre London
c/o 64 Warwick Road.
St Albans, Herts AL1 4DL

Institute of Psychosynthesis
The Barn, Nan Clark's Lane,
London NW7 4HH

Institute of Transactional Analysis
BM Box 4104, London WC1N 3XX

Marriage Guidance and Counselling

Catholic Marriage Advisory Council
Clitherow House, 1 Blythe Mews,
Blythe Road, London W14 ONW
Tel 0181 371 1341

Jewish Marriage Council
23 Ravenhurst Avenue,
London NW4 4EL
Tel 0181 203 6311

Relate (Marriage Guidance)
Herbert Gray College,
Little Church Street,
Rugby CV21 3AP
Tel 01788 73241
Phone for details of local branches or look in local phone directory.

Parents and Families

Contact a Family
16 Strutton Ground,
London SW1P 2HP
Tel 0171 222 2695
Head office for organisation which puts families with children with disabilities or special needs in touch with each other. Lots of local groups

Gingerbread
33 Wellington Street,
London WC2E 78N
Tel 0171 240 0953
Provides practical and emotional support for single parents. Self-help groups around the country.

National Council for the Divorced
and Separated
c/o 13 High Street, Little Shelford,
Cambridge CB2 5ES
Tel 01533 708880
*Has local branches where people can meet
supportive others and make new friends.*

National Council for One Parent
Families
255 Kentish Town Road,
London NW5 2LX
Tel 0171 267 1361
*Offers advice for legal and practical prob-
lems.*

National Family Mediation
9 Tavistock Place,
London WC1H 9SN
Tel 0171 383 5993
*Local services provide mediators to help
couples who are separating or divorcing
settle disputes and come to agreements,
particularly over children.*

Organisations for Parents under Stress
(OPUS)
106 Godstone Road, Whyteleaf,
Surrey CR3 OEB
Tel 0181 645 0469
*Can refer parents to a local group or group
nearest to them.*

The Parent Network
44 Caversham Road,
London NW5 2DS
Tel 0171 485 8535
*Organisation dedicated to supporting
parents with children at any age through
groups in which new and more effective
means of family communication are
explored.*

Parents Anonymous
9 Manor Gardens,
London N7 6LA
0171 263 8918
*Sympathetic phone helpline and a listening
ear for parents who feel they may abuse
their children.*

Stepfamily
Chapel House, 18 Hatton Place,
London EC1N 8RU
Tel 0171 209 2460
Helpline 0171 209 2464, Mon–Fri
2–5pm and 7–10pm.
*Provides practical information and emotion-
al support for those in stepfamilies.*

Phobias

The Institute for Neurophysiological
Psychology
Warwick House, 4 Stanley Place,
Chester CH1 2LU
Tel 01244 311414

MIND
Granta House, 15-19 Broadway,
London E15 4BQ
Tel 0181 519 2122
*A charity that can provide information,
advice and which publishes a number of
helpful books and booklets. It also has local
associations around the country.*

The Open Door Association
447 Pensby Road, Heswall,
Wirral, Merseyside L61 9PQ.

The Phobics Society
4 Cheltenham Road,
Chorlton-cum-Hardy,
Manchester M21 1QN
Tel 0161 881 1937 or 626 509

Post-traumatic Stress Disorder

MIND: see Phobias, above.

Psychotherapy

British Psychoanalytic Society
63 New Cavendish Street,
London W1M 7RD
Tel 0171 580 4952

Society of Analytic Psychology
1 Daleham Gardens,
London NW3 5BY
Tel 0171 435 7696

The United Kingdom Council of Psychotherapy
Regent's College, Inner Circle,
Regents Park, London NW1 4NS
Tel 0171 487 7554

Self-help Associations

See Patients Association, page 492.

Single People

The National Federation of Solo Clubs
Room 8, Ruskin Chambers,
191 Corporation Street,
Birmingham B4 6RY
Tel 0121 236 2879
Clubs throughout the country run social events so that people can meet each other.

Part III: Our Sexual Selves

Abortion & Unplanned Pregnancy

British Pregnancy Advisory Service
Austy Manor, Wootton Wawen,
Solihull, West Midlands B95 6DA
Tel 01564 793225
Non-profit-making (but fee-charging) charity. Provides pre- and post-abortion counselling. Can arrange abortions as appropriate at their nursing homes around the country.

Pregnancy Advisory Service
13 Charlotte Street, London W1P 1HD
Tel 0171 637 8962
Non-profit-making (but fee-charging) charity which offers pre- and post-abortion counselling and can arrange abortion as appropriate at their clinic in Greater London.

Support Around Termination for Abnormality (SAFTA)
29-30 Soho Square, London W1V 6JB
Helpline 0171 439 6124

Women's Health
52 Featherstone Street,
London EC1Y 8RT
Tel 0171 251 6580
Can provide information about abortion services and post-abortion groups, as well as women's health, especially gynaecological health.

The Women's Therapy Centre
6 Manor Gardens, London N7
Tel 0181 263 6200
Services include post-abortion counselling and groups. Fee-charging.

British Agencies for Adoption and Fostering
11 Southwark Street, London SE1 1RG
Tel 0171 409 8800

Health Information Service
Tel 0800 665544

Cancer

BACUP
3 Bath Place, Rivington Street,
London EC2A 3JR
Tel 0800 181199 (Mon–Thurs 10–7pm, Fri 10–5.30) and 0171 613 2121
Cancer nurses can provide information and support about all aspects of cancer to those with cancer, their families and friends. Publishes many booklets, including several on specific aspects of breast cancer.

Breast Cancer Care
15-19 Britten Street,
London SW3 3TZ
Nationwide Freeline 0500 245345
London Helpline 0171 867 1103
Glasgow Helpline 0141 353 1050
Edinburgh Helpline 0131 221 0407
Provides help, information and support, information on obtaining prostheses and a service of trained volunteers who have had breast cancer and who visit or support by phone.

Bristol Cancer Help Centre
Grove House, Cornwallis Grove,
Clifton, Bristol BS8 4PG
Tel 0117 9743216

Can offer guidance for playing an active part in one's own recovery through a variety of complementary therapies. Can offer help with physical, psychological and emotional problems experienced by those with cancer.

CancerLink
17 Britannia Street,
London WC1X 9JN
Tel 0171 833 2818
Edinburgh: 0131 228 5557
Provides information and support on all aspects of cancer. Publishes a number of booklets on coping with cancer and can give details of support groups in your area.

Penguin Cold Cap System
Medical Specialties of California,
274 Hither Green Lane,
London SE13 6TT
Tel 0181 244 4040/697 5424

Radiotherapy Injured Patients Support
Tel 01206 395610

Contraception

See British Pregnancy Advisory
Service, page 496
Offers, amongst other services, contraception advice and services, including sterilisation.

The Family Planning Association
27–35 Mortimer Street,
London W1N 7RJ
Tel 0171 636 7866
Can provide information about contraception and availability of local family-planning services.

National Association of Natural Family
Planning Teachers
Natural Family Planning Centre,
Birmingham Maternity Hospital,
Queen Elizabeth Medical Centre,
Birmingham B15 2TG
Tel 0121 472 1377 ext 4219
Can provide a list of local NFP teachers.

NHS Helpline
Tel 0800 224488

Natural Family Planning Service
Catholic Marriage Advisory Council,
Clitherow House, 1 Blythe Mews,
Blythe Road, London W14 ONW
Tel 0171 371 1341
Can provide a list of NFP teachers. You don't have to be Catholic to use this service; nor do you need to be married.

See Pregnancy Advisory Service, page 496.
Offers, amongst other services, emergency contraception and sterilisation.

Endometriosis

The Endometriosis Society
65 Holmdene Avenue, Herne Hill,
London SE24 9LD
The Society produces a range of leaflets on all sorts of treatments, including complementary ones, publishes regular newsletters and can put women in touch with others who have or have had endometriosis.

Herpes

Herpes Association
41 North Road, London N7 9DP
Tel 0171 609 9061
Provides information sheets.

HIV & AIDS

Body Positive
51b Philbeach Gardens,
London SW5 9EB
Tel 0171 835 1045
Details of Body Positive self-help groups around the country for people who are HIV positive.

National AIDS Helpline
Tel 0800 567123
A 24-hour service with calls free from anywhere in the UK. A list of needle exchanges is also available from this number.

Positively Women
Tel helpline 0171 490 2327 (12–2pm, Mon–Fri)
Tel 0171 490 5515 (10am-5pm, Mon-Fri)
A woman can ring either of these numbers for advice or support for HIV. The helpline is operated only by women who are HIV positive themselves.

The Terrence Higgins Trust
52–54 Grays Inn Road,
London WC1X 8JU
Tel helpline 0171 242 1010
(12 noon–10pm daily)
Administration and advice 0171 831 0330 (10am–5pm, Mon–Fri)
Legal line 0171 405 2381(7–10pm, Weds only)
Provides an enormous range of services and booklets. They can offer advice on testing, treatment, legal matters, welfare matters and information about other relevant organisations or groups.

Infertility

CHILD
Suite 219, Caledonian House,
98 The Centre, Feltham,
Middx TW13 4BH
Tel 0181 893 7110 (24 hours)
Self-help charity that offers advice, information and support, produces a quarterly newsletter and co-ordinates regional groups.

Childlessness Overcome Through Surrogacy (COTS)
Loandhu Cottage, Gruids,
Lairg, Sutherland IV27 4EF
Tel 01549 402401
Offers support and advice about surrogacy.

Diagnostic Andrology Service
112 Harley Street, London W1N IAF
Tel 0171 224 2849
Testing service for men which carries out tests on sperm, for a fee. Men can refer themselves for diagnosis, but GPs must refer for treatment.

Human Fertilisation Embryology Authority
Paxton House, 30 Artillery Lane,
London E1 7LS
Tel: 0171 377 5077
Provides list of all licensed infertility clinics and the services offered, both NHS and private, although it isn't specificed which is which.

ISSUE
509 Aldridge Road, Great Barr,
Birmingham B44 8NA
Tel 0121 344 4414
Self-help advice and support group that produces fact sheets, a quarterly magazine and co-ordinates a network of self-help and support groups.

IUD Problems (Missing Threads)

Margaret Pyke Centre,
15 Bateman Buildings, Soho Square,
London W1V 5TW
NHS free helpline 0800 22448
Tel 0171 734 9351
NHS family-planning service and research centre which runs a missing threads clinic and takes referrals from all over the country.

Lymphoedema

Clare Maxwell School of Massage
PO Box 457, London NW2 4BR
Tel 0181 450 6494

The British Lymphology Interest Group
Sir Michael Sobell House,
Churchill House, Oxford OX3 7LJ
Can supply directory of treatment centres. Send an SAE for details of cost ($£5$ plus p&p at time of writing)

Lymphoedema Support Network
Appeal Office,
The Royal Marsden Hospital,
191 Fulham Road, London SW3 6JJ
Tel 0171 433 3410/727 6973/ 748 2403

MLD UK
8 Wittenham Lane,
Dorchester on Thames,
Oxfordshire, OX10 7JW

Menopause

Amarant Trust
Grant House, 50–60 St John Street,
London EC1M 4DT
Tel 0171 490 1644
HRT helpline 01338 400190
Charity that is very strongly in favour of HRT and of increasing its general availability.

See Women's Health, page 496
Can provide all the information, pros and cons about HRT, but won't advise.

Women's Health Concern
PO Box 1629, Earls Court,
London W8 6AU
Tel 0171 938 3932
Provides information on many aspects of women's health and in principle supports HRT

Miscarriage

Miscarriage Association
c/o Clayton Hospital, Northgate,
Wakefield, West Yorkshire WF1 3JS
Tel 01924 200799
For information, advice or the chance to talk to someone else who has had a miscarriage.

Premenstrual Syndrome

National Association for Premenstrual Syndrome
PO Box 72, Sevenoaks,
Kent TN13 3PS

The Premenstrual Society
PO Box 102, London SE1 7ES

Women's Nutritional Advisory Service
PO Box 268, Lewes,
East Sussex BN7 2QN
Tel 01273 487366

Psychosexual Counselling

Association of Sexual and Marital Therapists
PO Box 62, Sheffield S10 3TS.
Send sae for list of NHS clinics in your area with qualified sex therapists.

See Family Planning Association, page 497.
The FPA can advise on clinics or other services which offer psychosexual counselling in your area.

Institute of Psychosexual Medicine
11 Chandos Street, Cavendish Square,
London W1M 9DE.
Can provide list of NHS and private doctors in your area approved by the Institute to treat psychosexual problems.

See Relate, page 494
There are trained sex-therapy counsellors at many of the local branches of Relate. Look in the telephone directory for your nearest branch.

Rape

Rape Crisis Centre
PO Box 69, London WC1X 9NJ
Tel 0171 837 1600 (24 hours)
Afrisian Black Women's Line
Tel 0171 916 5656

Self-help Associations

See Patients Association, page 492

Women's Health – General

See Women's Health, page 496

PART IV: A–Z of Women's Health Problems

Cancer

See BACUP, page 496 and
CancerLink, page 497
Both of these charities can provide details of other groups set up specifically to serve people with a particular form of cancer or to offer help with after care, etc.

Cancer Relief Macmillan Fund
15–19 Britten Street,
London SW3 3TZ
Tel 0171 352 7811
A national charity that aims to improve life for people with cancer and their families. It is responsible for the establishment within the NHS of Macmillan nurses, who help and advise on all aspects of coping with cancer. Also publishes a leaflet lists of cancer-help charities and a directory of specialist breast-cancer services.

Incontinence

The Incontinence Foundation
2 Doughty Street,
London WC1N 2PM
Free leaflet on incontinence.

Incontinence Information
Tel helpline 0191 213 0050
(9am–6pm, Mon–Fri)

Lupus

The following organisations provide support and information, publish booklets and help raise money for research.

The British SLE Aid Group
25 Lynden Crescent,
Woodford Green, Essex

Lupus Group
Arthritis Care,
8 Grosvenor Crescent,
London SW1X 7ER
Tel 0171 235 0902

ME

Action for ME
PO Box 1302, Wells,
Somerset BA5 2WE
Tel 01749 670799
Can provide extensive information on all aspects of ME including alternative approaches. Send a large SAE for an information pack.

Information tel 01891 122976
Taped information about ME, its symptoms, causes, how to diagnose it, how to cope, details of recommended consultants and latest information on treatment and therapies. Calls charged at 39p per minute cheap rate and 49p per minute at other times, with 30 per cent of revenue donated to Action for ME.

ME Association
Stanhope House, High Street,
Stanford le Hope, Essex SS17 OHA
Tel 01375 642466
More orthodox in its approach than Action for ME.

Migraine

Headaid Migraine Reliever
Natural Medical Ltd,
PO Box 15, Rye,
East Sussex TN31 6TZ
Costs £185 (1994 prices) but if it doesn't work for you you can return it within 30 days for a full refund.

The City of London Migraine Clinic
22 Charterhouse Square,
London EC1M 6DX
Tel 0171 251 3322
A medical charity that can see patients from throughout the UK if referred by their GP.

British Migraine Association
178a High Road, Byfleet,
Weybridge, Surrey
Tel 01932 352468
Run by migraine sufferers to provide information about migraine and support.

Osteoarthritis

WLAP Ltd,
Pain Tape, PO Box 1,
Wirral L47 7DD.
Self-help tape on beating pain; write for current details and prices.

TENS Machines
Spembly Medical Ltd,
Newbury Road, Andover,
Hants SP10 4DR
TENS Careline 0800 515413

Osteoporosis

National Osteoporosis Society
PO Box 10, Radstock,
Bath BA3 3YB
Tel 01761 432472
Tel helpline 01761 431594.
Booklets on osteoporosis, HRT and the menopause, hysterectomy and HRT, exercise, physiotherapy and osteoporosis in men.

Raynaud's

Raynaud's and Scleroderma
Association
112 Crewe Road, Alsager,
Cheshire ST7 2JA
Tel 01270 872776
Information and advice about all aspects of Raynaud's, including conventional and alternative treatments.

Rheumatoid Arthritis

Arthritis Care
18 Stephenson Way,
London NW1 2HD
Tel 0171 916 1500
A voluntary organisation providing information and advice on arthritis, particularly self-help.

FURTHER READING

Part I: Everyday Health

Hair

Hair Loss: Coping with Hair Loss and What to do About it, Elizabeth Steel (Thorsons, 1995)

Hair Today, Gone Tomorrow?: Dealing with Unwanted Body Hair, Dr Antonia Bradbury.

Healthy Eating

Understanding Additives, Which? Books (Consumers Association and Hodder and Stoughton, 1988)

The New E for Additives, Maurice Hanssen (Thorsons, 1987)

The Food Trap: a Self-help Plan to Control your Eating Habits, Paulette Maisner with Rosemary Turner (Allen and Unwin, 1985)

Professional Help for Health

HEA Guide to Complementary Medicine and Therapies, Anne Woodham (Health Education Authority, 1994)

Relaxation

The Complete Book of Massage, Clare Maxwell-Hudson (Simon & Schuster, 1988)

Simple Relaxation, Laura Mitchell (John Murray, 1987)

Part II: Emotional and Mental Health

Depression

SAD: Seasonal Affective Disorder, Angela Smyth (Thorsons, 1990)

Handling Thoughts, Feelings and Needs

A Woman in Your Own Right, Anne Dickson (Quartet Books, 1982)

Obsessive-compulsive Disorder

Understanding Obsessions and Compulsions: a Self-help Manual, Dr Frank Tallis (Sheldon Press, 1992)

Panic Attacks

Don't Panic: a Guide to Overcoming Panic Attacks, Sue Breton (Macdonald Optima, 1986)

Self Help for your Nerves, Claire Weekes (Thorsons, 1995)

Post-traumatic Stress

Post-traumatic Stress Disorder: a Practical Guide to Recovery, David Kinchin (Thorsons, 1994)

Understanding Post-traumatic Stress Syndrome, MIND,
(Available from MIND Mail Order Service, Granta House, 15-19 Broadway,
   London E15 4BQ: 45p inc p&p)

Where to Go for Help
What is psychotherapy?, Sidney Bloch (OUP, 1982)
Introduction to the Psychotherapies, Sidney Bloch (OUP, 1986)
Innovative Therapy in Britain, edited by John Rowan and Windy Dryden (OUP,
   1988)

Part III: Our Sexual Selves

Breast Cancer
Always a Woman: a Practical Guide to Living with Breast Surgery, Carolyn Faulder
   (Thorsons, 1992)
Lymphoedema: Advice on Treatment by Claud Regnard, Caroline Badger and Peter
   Mortimer (Beaconsfield Publishers Ltd, 20 Chiltern Hills Road, Beaconsfield,
   Bucks HP9 1PL or from the Lymphoedema Support Network – see Useful
   Contacts. Send SAE for details of price.)

Cancers of the Reproductive System
Cervical Smear Test: What Every Woman Should Know, Albert Singer FRCOG and
   Anne Szarewski (Macdonald Optima, 1988)
Positive Smear, Susan Quilliam (C Letts, 1992)

Contraception
The FPA Guide to Contraception, Suzie Hayman (Thorsons, 1993)

Endometriosis
Understanding Endometriosis, Caroline Hawkridge (Macdonald Optima, 1989)

Hysterectomy
Hysterectomy: the Woman's View, Anne Dickson and Nikki Henriques (Quartet
   Books, 1994)

Infertility
Infertility: a Sympathetic Approach, Professor Robert Winston (Macdonald Optima,
   1994)
Coping with Childlessness, Diane and Peter Houghton (Unwin Paperback, 1987)
Adopting a Child: a Guide for People Interested in Adoption, Prue Chennells (British
   Agencies for Adoption and Fostering, 1990)

Sex and Sex-related Problems
When a Woman's Body Says No to Sex: Understanding and Overcoming Vaginismus,
   Linda Valins (Penguin, 1992).
   (As well as being ordered from bookshops this can be bought by mail order from
   Healthwise, the bookshop of the Family Planning Association, 27–35 Mortimer
   Street, London W1N 7RJ. Price approx £6.99 plus £1.50 for p&p.)

Urinary-tract Infections
Understanding Cystitis: a Complete Self-help Guide, Angela Kilmartin (Arrow, 1985)

Cystitis: How to Prevent Infection and Inflammation, Angela Kilmartin (Thorsons, 1994)

Vaginal and Sexually Transmitted Diseases
Herpes: What it is and How to Cope, Dr Adrian Mindel and Orla Carney (Optima Positive Health Guide, 1991).

Part IV: A–Z of Women's Health Problems

Women's Health Problems
Coping Successfully with your Irritable Bowel, Rosemary Nicol (Sheldon Press, 1989).
Irritable Bowel Syndrome, Geoff Watts (Mandarin, 1991)
ME: How to Live With It, Dr Anne Macintyre (Thorsons, 1992)
Living with ME: a Self-help Guide, Dr Charles Shepherd (Mandarin, 1992)
Thyroid Disorders, Dr Rowan Hillson (Macdonald Optima, 1991).
Women's Waterworks: Curing Incontinence, Pauline Chiarelli (available from Incontinence Foundation, price £4.95 plus £1 for p&p.)

INDEX